Psychophysiological Aspects

of SPACE FLIGHT

Psychophysiological Aspects of SPACE FLIGHT

Edited by BERNARD E. FLAHERTY, LT.COL.,USAF(MC)

Columbia University Press, New York, 1961

SYMPOSIUM ON PSYCHOPHYSIOLOGICAL ASPECTS OF SPACE FLIGHT
May 26 *and* 27, 1960

Otis O. Benson, Jr., Maj. Gen., USAF (MC), Co-chairman

Bernard E. Flaherty, Lt. Col., USAF (MC), Co-chairman

Jack Harmon, Symposium Coordinator, Southwest Research Institute

David L. Black, Southwest Research Institute

Douglas H. Hagen, Lt., USAF

This research was supported in whole or in part by the United States Air Force under Contract AF41(657)–319, monitored by the School of Aviation Medicine, USAF, Brooks Air Force Base, Texas.

Published in Great Britain, India, and Pakistan
by the Oxford University Press
London, Bombay, and Karachi

Library of Congress Catalog Card Number: 60–15809

Manufactured in the United States of America

Preface

OTIS O. BENSON, JR.

One can say with confidence that we now possess all the basic knowledge required to keep man alive in space for a limited, yet significant, period of time. Although there is room for refinement and simplification, and although the development of equipment continues to pose difficult problems, all the essential knowledge is at hand.

By contrast, our position with respect to man's behavioral capabilities in space is not nearly so well established. Human history provides no example of what would seem to be such an unfavorable combination of psychic stressors. Isolation, confinement, weightlessness, unusual and distasteful methods of coping with personal problems, anxiety over the reliability of equipment—all these factors, individually as well as collectively, would seem to jeopardize human capability in ways which we have only begun to assess.

The foregoing circumstances clearly called for a conference of informed physicians and scientists for the purpose of surveying our present knowledge and recommending the directions which future research must take in order to provide the required technology within desirable time periods. Such a conference, believed to be the first of its kind, was sponsored at Brooks Air Force Base on May 26 and 27, 1960, by the School of Aviation Medicine, in keeping with its long tradition of leadership in the solution of aeromedical problems. We are pleased to acknowledge here the administrative assistance provided by Southwest Research Institute, and the editorial efforts of the Columbia University Press in making the proceedings available to an interested public.

The reader will note that the conference agenda embraced an unusual variety of topics ranging from the psychosocial problems of

General Benson is Commander, Headquarters USAF Aerospace Medical Center (ATC), Brooks Air Force Base, Texas.

small groups, through the medical and psychological problems of selection, training, and maintenance, to the bedrock problems of neurophysiology and endocrinology. Correspondingly, the reader will note that the speakers represented a variety of professional and scientific persuasions—a variety that was no less evident among those who were invited to attend. It was no accident that we took this approach to the central theme of the symposium. Rather, it was a deliberate approach, calculated to lend substance to our perspective that man's behavior is a joint function of many kinds of influences arising both inside and outside the body, and that the understanding and control of this behavior can be achieved only through the joint efforts of all the life sciences. This is the frame of reference within which we pursue behavioral research at the School of Aviation Medicine, and it is typical of much of the research throughout the remainder of the United States Air Force.

It will be evident to even the most casual reader that the symposium has not provided an exhaustive treatment of the central theme, either in breadth or depth. Nevertheless, he will find provoking discussions of those topics which have the most critical relevance for manned space flight, and it is sincerely hoped that these will generate further thought, imagination, and active research planning for our future needs. If we can but realize this consequence alone, the symposium will have served a vital purpose.

Contents

PART 3
PROBLEMS OF HUMAN RELIABILITY

PART 4
SPECIAL TECHNIQUES OF CONTROL

Psychophysiological Aspects

of SPACE FLIGHT

Introduction

BERNARD E. FLAHERTY

In the man-machine system essential to space flight, man's limitations are the baseline which determine the degree of efficiency of the total system (1). Man's psychophysiological limitations are less well-defined than the limitations of any other part of the man-machine system; his total behavior is most meaningful only when we are able to integrate the psychosocial facets of his performance into a framework of genetics, anatomy, physiology, and chemistry.

It is possible to predict some of the stresses which will be encountered by the astronaut in space travel; we know that they will arise from forces outside the capsule, within the capsule, and within man himself (2). Stresses may be exclusively external—e.g., engineering failure, radiation, forces of gravity; or, they may be entirely internal—in the sense of psychophysiological malfunction. It will be virtually impossible to isolate a single stress and the immediately resulting psychophysiologic response, because man, as a complex, constantly interacting psychophysiologic unit, is demonstrated most classically in the man-machine system. Furthermore, man is an integral part of the total machine; the contributions of the machine to the final system output cannot be differentiated from the contributions of man. A stress of any type or quantity will initiate a series of interlocked physical and psychophysiological reactions in the total system. Within a matter of seconds (or fractions of a second) it will be necessary for the human operator to isolate from this series of interactions a basic *gestalt* problem and the major components intrinsic in this problem. He must immediately select the best available finite solution; the accuracy of this solution

Colonel Flaherty has been Chief, Neuropsychiatric Branch, School of Aviation Medicine, USAF Aerospace Medical Center (ATC), Brooks Air Force Base, Texas. He is presently Head, Department of Neuropsychiatry, USAF Hospital, Tachi Kawa AFB, Japan.

will depend on appropriate past experience in a framework of his potential, current psychophysiologic efficiency, and the availability of reliable data from the machine.

The over-all purpose of this symposium is the definition and suggested resolution of the psychophysiological problems implicit in space flight. To achieve this goal it is necessary to answer these questions:

1. *Where are we now?* It is imperative that we assess realistically our current basic achievements in science as they apply to these problems. Our urgent need for resolution of these problems may force us to apply our knowledge prematurely. On the other hand, unnecessary repetition and reduplication of basic science effort, a pleasant but expensive academic luxury, frequently delays immediately available "application."

2. *Where do we go from here?* An appraisal of our current status must force us to determine how psychophysiologic research and application in the problems of space flight can proceed most expeditiously. We must utilize the appropriate efforts of physiologists, anatomists, and chemists—as well as those of researchers engaged in the various "pure" behavioral disciplines.

If these interdisciplinary efforts are to succeed, we must establish a common language. There is increasing evidence that psychologists and psychiatrists must become more substantially grounded in anatomy, chemistry, and physiology; "organicists," in turn, must learn functional psychological principles.

Compartmentalized thinking, occasionally noted in scientific thought, is probably seen most frequently in the various behavioral disciplines. Two problems of this type are most evident: First, there is understandable loyalty on the part of adherents to a particular discipline toward the codes, hypotheses, and systems of interpretation peculiar to that discipline; occasionally this loyalty assumes an emotionally burdened, cult-like fervor that can lead to rejection of all clinical and basic science evidence which would contradict its beliefs.

It is evident the several behavioral groups (including the biochemist and neurophysiologist with a primary interest in behavior) need each other if they are to make a meaningful whole of many separate parts. Both semantics and working concepts must reflect an emotional insight that behavior occurs in an *organism*, the fabric of which limits behavior and is changed by behavior. This is a truism, accepted intellectually, but denied too often in emotionally charged interpretations.

A second problem area, related to the first, is common to all behavioral disciplines. I refer here to the principle of causality, as it relates to psychic determinism. With few exceptions up to the present time, all behavioral phenomena have been evaluated and interpreted essentially in terms of simple "cause and effect." There is increasing evidence that behavior may be based, in part at least, on random, variable factors. Eccles (3) considers the manner in which the brain achieves liaison with the "mind" as the essence of this problem. Livingston's recent work (9) suggests one possible neurophysiological mechanism of hallucination is associated with space and time distortion, emphasizing central control of peripheral sensory receptors. This is of immediate interest to workers attempting to explain hallucinatory phenomena seen frequently in isolation and sensory deprivation experiments.

Increasing experimental evidence, and the fact that causality has long ago been discarded as a fundamental axiom of the advanced physical sciences (4, 5), suggests that we may wish to revise basic tenets in the interpretation of behavior (6). In attempting to establish "mind" into these current concepts of the physical sciences, we might consider seriously the edict of Philip Morrison (7):

> In the end, . . . no view of the world can remain unchallenged by the physicists' findings; the future of every philosophy can be measured by the degree to which it can admit to the world of the mind the physical map of the atomic universe.

A sense of urgency pervades our study of the psychophysiological aspects of space flight. Already the United States and Allied Nations have sent over three hundred mammalian creatures into flight within, or approaching, the boundaries of space. Data obtained from these flights and from simulated flights have helped us to anticipate the reactions of space flight on the various body systems in the human being. The void that remains, the human element, cannot be determined until a significant number of astronauts have returned from flight through space. However, we can anticipate, from what we know already of space flight and its environment, many of the problem areas; and we can predict with some degree of accuracy the psychophysiological reactions of man to this environment.

Realization that the critical problem areas which threaten man's effective conquest of space are largely psychophysiological in nature results in an appreciation of the urgent responsibilities of this symposium. The definition of neurophysiologic effects of stress, with particular emphasis on endocrine and endogenous rhythm factors, is essential. The requirement that physiologic data from the human operator be constantly available to earthbound observers must be resolved. We must establish allowable quantitative and qualitative deviations in sensory input—and the manner in which these deviations effect psychophysiologic response. We must evaluate all possible techniques—such as chemotherapy, hypnosis, conditioning, or thermal variations—by which the pioneer human operator might be assisted in withstanding his many stresses.

These are but a few of the critical problems we discussed during this symposium. The product of our work must establish our current achievements and blatant deficiencies; it must serve as a stimulus for rapid resolution of the psychophysiologic impasse which delays man's entry into space. "Man is a sea-level, low-speed, one-g, 12-hour animal" (8), representing the weakest link in our aerospace development to date.

This symposium was organized to strengthen this "weakest link," and to force an exchange of ideas between disciplines which communicate rarely and poorly—despite a mutual, urgent need to share research efforts in approaching a common goal. One facet of this common goal is an evaluation of the psychophysiological aspects of space flight.

REFERENCES

1. Gantz, K. F., ed., Man in Space. New York, Duell, Sloan & Pearce, 1959.
2. Flaherty, B. E., Psychiatry in space flight, in *Proceedings*, Detroit Regional Meeting of APA, October, 1959.
3. Eccles, J. C., Neurophysiological Basis of Mind. Oxford, The Clarendon Press, 1953.
4. Russell, B., On the notion of cause, in *Mysticism and Logic and Other Essays*, pp. 180, 194, 199. London, Allen and Unwin, 1951.
5. Tarski, A., Introduction of Logic and Methodology of Deductive Sciences, p. 98. New York, Oxford University Press, 1941.
6. Angel, Ronald W., The concept of determinism, Am. J. Psychiat., 116:405, 1959.

7. Morrison, Philip, Cause, chance, and creation ("Adventures of the Mind, 51"), Saturday Evening Post, 232:No. 44:32, 110, 111, 112, 114, April 30, 1960.
8. White, General Thomas D. (Chief of Staff, USAF), The inevitable climb to space, Air Univ. Quart. Rev., X:No. 4, Winter, 1958–59.
9. Livingston, R., Reticular Formation of the Brain, An International Symposium. Detroit, Mich., Henry Ford Hospital, 1958.

PART 1

Technical Background and Experience

Operator Requirements

ERNST STUHLINGER

Among the thousands and thousands of questions which are raised and discussed every day by the members of our space vehicle development teams, there is one question which is distinguished by its persistent absence: the question whether man himself, as a living astronaut, should go into space. He should, of course, and this fact is well understood today by everyone who takes an active part in our space projects. Man will be guided and driven into space by the same motives that drove him to the poles of the earth some sixty years ago.

A question of a very different nature is what should the astronaut be required to do on his flight through space. There is no clear-cut consensus of opinion on this question. The answer which I will try to give reflects the thinking of many of those who contributed, and will contribute, to the development of space-going vehicles and their guidance and communication systems, but who would feel on uncertain grounds if they were called to make a meaningful, psychophysiological analysis of a human operator.

We will divide the great number of possible manned space missions into two categories: the first comprises flights through satellite orbits, flights around the moon and around planets, and flights through deep space. The second consists of flights which include lunar landings and planetary landings. All flights in both categories, of course, hopefully end with the safe return of the astronauts to Earth.

Flights in the first category are distinguished by the relative simplicity of their flight-mechanical requirements. While the required accuracies of trajectory parameters are high, the motion of

Dr. Stuhlinger has been Director, Research Projects Office, Army Ballistic Missile Agency, Huntsville, Alabama. He is presently Director, Research Projects Division, National Aeronautics and Space Administration, George C. Marshall Space Flight Center, Huntsville, Alabama.

the spacecraft is a function of well-known laws of celestial mechanics. The elements of this motion will be precalculated with the necessary accuracy; guidance functions will be programmed into automatic devices, and the entire flight will be supervised by telemeter and radar observations from the ground. If necessary, radio commands will overrule the programmed guidance devices in order to improve the accuracy. The various guidance phases of a circumlunar flight are illustrated in Figure 1. The reentry phase will be by far the most

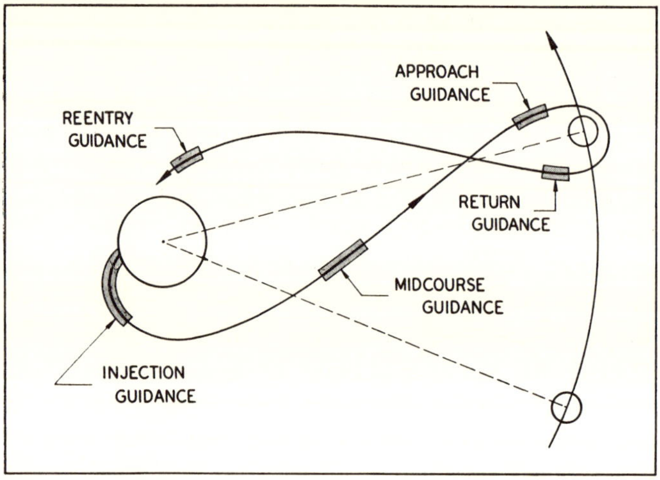

Figure 1. Guidance Phases of Manned Lunar Circumnavigation

critical part of the flight, not only because of the stringent accuracy requirements with respect to angle and time of arrival at the outer fringes of the atmosphere, but because the density of the atmosphere at high altitudes seems to be subject to severe fluctuations. Figure 2 shows how sensitively a circumlunar trajectory depends upon the angle of injection, provided that there is no midcourse and no approach guidance, and Figure 3 depicts a similar situation at reentry. The guidance requirements imposed by these sensitive interrelations, however, can be fully met by a combination of onboard and earthbound devices. In fact, all space projects in this category will be flown a number of times without a human passenger aboard. When the astronaut finally mans the capsule, he will not

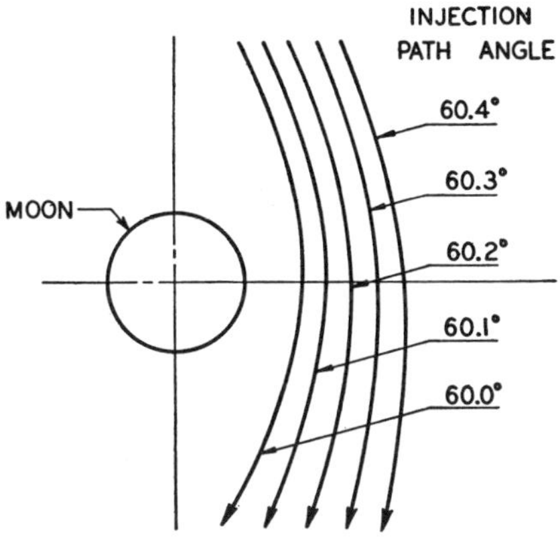

Figure 2. Variation of Circumlunar Trajectory as a Function of Injection Angle

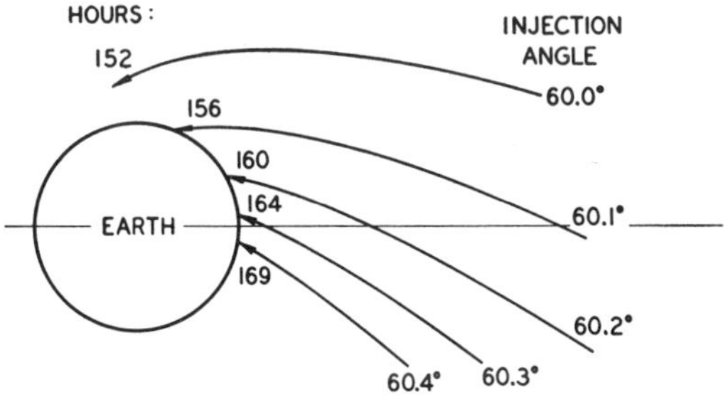

Figure 3. Variation of Reentry Trajectory as a Function of Injection Angle

represent an integral part of the guidance or control system. He will be required, though, to oversee continuously the proper functioning of at least some of the devices. If a component needs adjustment, repair, or substitution, he will perform the necessary operation. If a parameter should vary beyond the range for which the instrument is prepared, the astronaut will correct the situation. Beyond these functions, the human operator will not be required to make any decisions which are essential for the flight. By supervising the proper functioning of the instruments he will, of course, increase very substantially the over-all chance for a successful flight. On the other hand, a manned flight will not be considered successful unless the mission is accomplished and the astronaut reaches his home base safely, while an unmanned space project may be satisfactory even if only 60 or 70 percent of the flights complete their missions.

The purpose of the man in this first category of space flights is twofold: first, he should provide information about himself, his reaction to prolonged weightlessness, his ability to cope with the eating and breathing conditions aboard a spacecraft, his usefulness as an observer, his capability of making technical decisions which influence flight parameters, his proficiency in case he would take an active part in guidance and control functions, his psychological stability in the strange environment of outer space—in short, he should try out his spaceworthiness under real space flight conditions.

Second, the astronaut should make observations of those unexpected events for which the programmed instruments are not prepared. In spite of the marvelous progress of our computer technology, the human mind is still far superior to any electromechanical device when it comes to reasoning and judgment, to decisions among a large number of possibilities, or to a distinction between the usual and the unusual. For example, when traveling close to the lunar surface, the astronaut will decide to which particular objects the cameras should be directed, and which part of a certain area deserves closer scrutiny.

Besides these two functions, the supervision and adjustment of the automatic instruments will occupy the astronaut's attention during the entire flight. Although this latter function will definitely increase the success probability of the flight, it will not in itself represent a justification of human flight. If other purposes for the man in space did not exist, this latter function would lead to the meaningless cycle where the vehicle serves only to carry the man, and the man serves only to keep the vehicle flying.

At the time when flights of the second category are initiated, the human astronauts will be well prepared for their roles through the experience gained in orbital, circumlunar, and circumplanetary missions. As a first operation in space in which man will probably participate as an integrating part we may select orbital refueling. Figure 4 shows an artist's conception of three Saturn vehicles in an earth orbit; two of them gas up the third, which then will be capable of taking two or three men to the surface of the moon, and back to Earth again. Everyone who has ever participated in a missile fueling operation on a launching pad will agree that it would be a very cumbersome and frustrating experience, to say the least, to align the vehicles, to connect the fueling hose, to check and operate

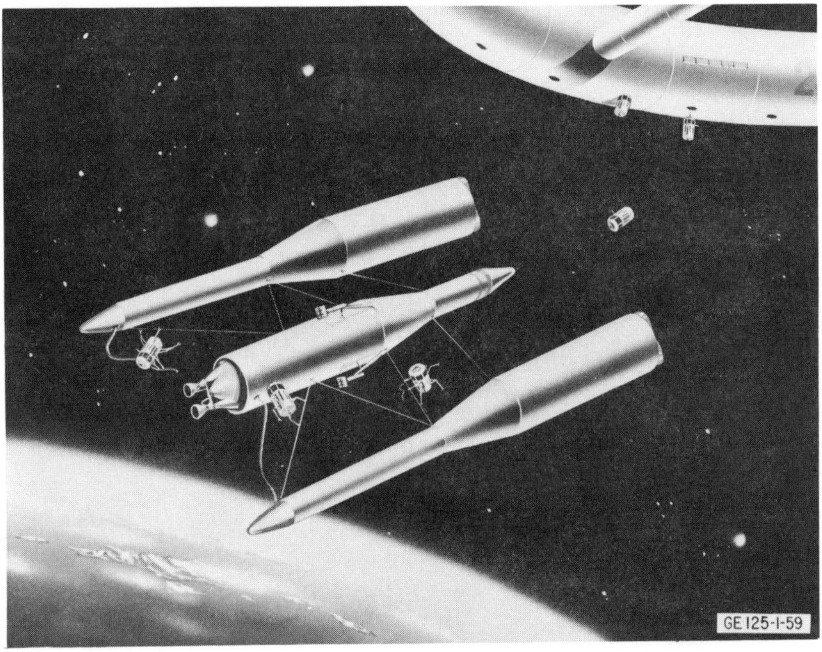

Figure 4. Refueling Maneuver in Orbit

all the components, and finally to prepare the spacecraft for take-off —all this under conditions where the vehicle assembly sweeps around the earth once every ninety minutes. Even though a fully automatic or a remote-controlled operation of this kind may be possible, the immediate presence of a few human operators will be invaluable.

As the next operation which will definitely profit from the active participation of a man we will consider a lunar landing maneuver. A counterrocket decelerates the spacecraft during its approach to the moon. At the end of the landing operation, the spacecraft must touch down with a velocity that approaches zero in the moment of lunar contact. However, for fuel economy, the hovering period must not be too long. Besides, the spacecraft must be controlled in its lateral motions in such a way that it settles down on a suitable spot which was selected by inspection during the approach maneuver. Again, a procedure which is partly programmed, and partly remote-controlled through television and radio-command links from Earth,

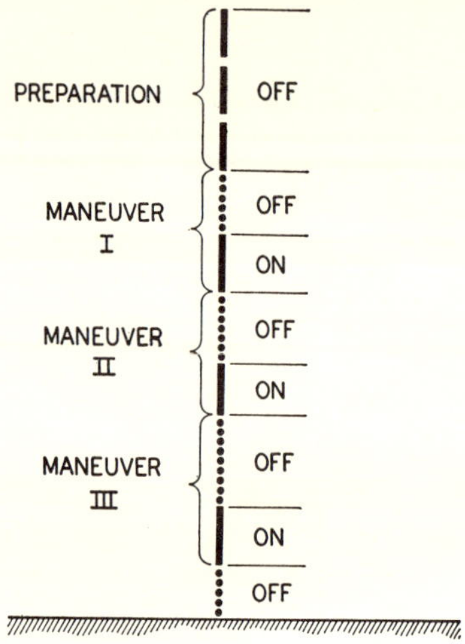

Figure 5. Lunar Approach Scheme

might be capable of achieving such a landing, but a human operator would decisively increase the chance of success.

Man's main purpose on the moon, however, will be to search the lunar surface with the discerning mind of the scientist, with his ability to distinguish between the common and the unusual, with his keen eye for the unexpected, and with his most remarkable capacity for observational data. He will drive across the lunar surface, avoiding boulders and crevices, but studying unusual formations, taking measurements at well selected points, drilling holes at promising sites, and observing simultaneously as many lunar features as he possibly can. It is very likely that unmanned vehicles such as the one shown in Figure 6 will roam across the lunar surface long before man sets foot there, but the wealth of observations and carefully selected samples that a live man can retrieve from the moon

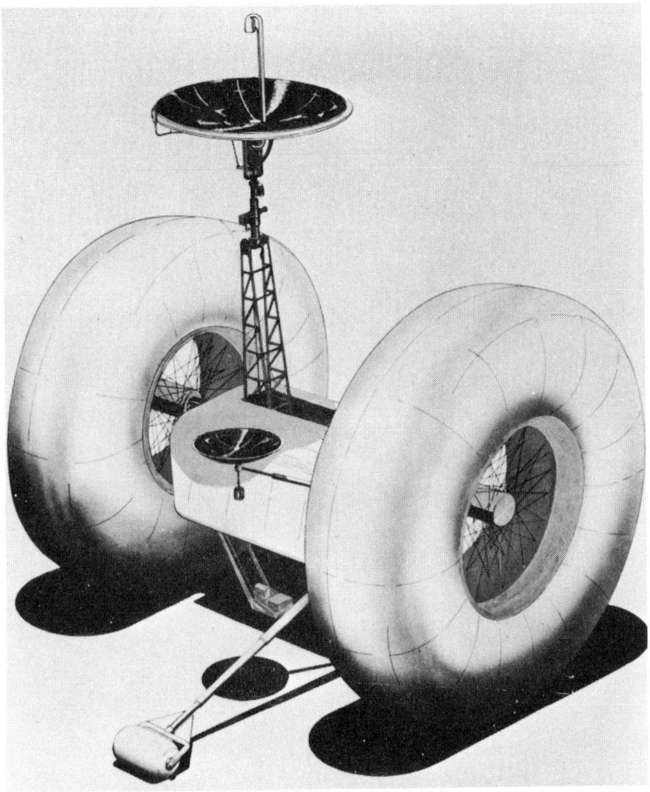

Figure 6. Unmanned Lunar Roving Vehicle

will always be immeasurably greater than what a preprogrammed, remote-controlled robot can achieve.

Man's abilities will be called upon heavily when the return flight is initiated. He will check and adjust the launching position, make sure that all the instruments work properly, stow the samples safely in the hold of the spacecraft, and prepare the take-off procedure. Take-off, return flight, reentry into the earth's atmosphere, and terrestrial landing, however, will again be programmed and controlled from Earth. The human operator will only supervise the correct functioning of all devices.

Many of the phases of manned lunar landing will be repeated when a planetary landing is to be made, with the difference,

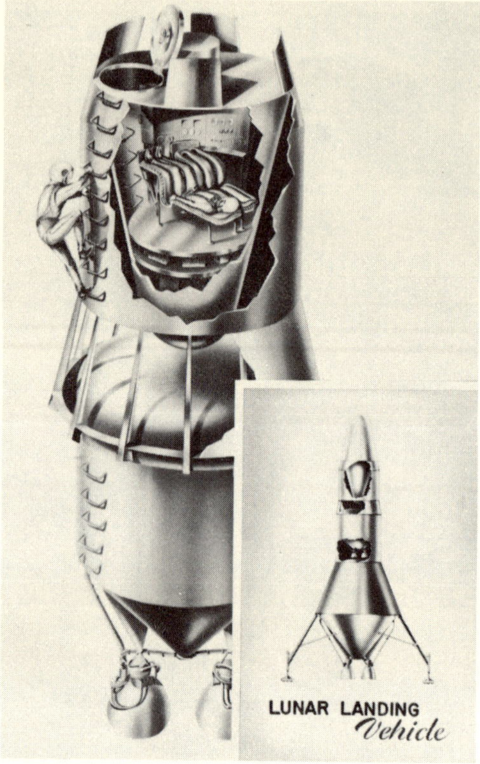

Figure 7. Manned Lunar Landing Vehicle and Lunar-Earth Return Vehicle

however, that a landing on a planet will be much more challenging, much more intriguing, and much more demanding for the human operator than a lunar landing. Mars, for example, has an atmosphere which allows the use of wings or parachutes. We know very little about its surface structure, and even less about its possible forms of life, either extinct or presently existent. The value of human exploration on the Martian surface cannot be substituted by any amount of automatic devices. Just let us imagine how much we can observe when we walk across the Texas prairie, how many plants and animals we discover, how well we can become acquainted with their life habits, with their development history, with their adaption to their environment—and how little we would ever know of them if we were to look at the prairie only through the medium of a television camera sweeping quickly across the surface!

The role of the human operator during a Martian landing maneuver will be more decisive than his role during a lunar landing, simply because of the much greater distance between Mars and Earth. Fewer details concerning the landing procedures can be transmitted by radio and television, and, most important, the one-way trip of a radio signal from Mars to Earth lasts between 2.5 and 18 minutes. Remote control of the landing maneuver will not be feasible. In fact, an astronaut landing on Mars will probably "fly" or "parachute" his spacecraft to a selected landing site very much as he would do it over terrestrial terrain which he knows from photographs, but which does not have an Instrument Landing System that takes him safely to the landing strip while he keeps his eyes on the instruments.

While unmanned landings on a planet with instrumented capsules are certainly possible, and very probably will be made before the first manned landing, it is most likely that manned descent to a planet will always be made under immediate control by the astronaut. The same will be true for the manned ascent from the planetary surface. On the long trajectory between planet and Earth, however, the spacecraft will be guided by programmed automatic devices, and man's role will be reduced to that of an overseer.

Man's role in space is undoubtedly focused most strongly on the surfaces of the moon and the planets. Even though he can, and will, perform valuable functions during flight, a flight scheme should always be arranged so that the spacecraft can continue its flight by automatic or remote control back to Earth in case the astronauts should be stricken by unconsciousness. Once the spacecraft has landed on foreign terrain, the further success of the mission, and the safe return of the astronaut, will depend decisively on the man. But before he goes there, his ability to brave the many hostile attributes of extraterrestrial space will be extensively probed and tested on space flights in the Mercury capsule, in the X-15, in the Dynasoar, in Saturn space vehicles, and in larger spacecraft. It is very reassuring to see that our National Aeronautics and Space Administration and the Air Force place very strong emphasis on these projects.

During our last annual ARS meeting, Professor Sedov, the well-known Russian space scientist, was asked about Russian long-range space planning. He had this to answer: "The goal of Russian space plans—and I have no doubt that you here have the same plans—is man in space, not as a strapped-down, half-conscious bundle, crammed in a narrow capsule and whirling through an orbit, but as an active, discerning scientist who explores the moon and the planets. The reward which will come out of this scientific exploration will be so great that it easily justifies any effort which we can possibly take."

ACKNOWLEDGMENT

The figures in this paper are based on reports by the Aeroballistics Laboratory, the Structures and Mechanics Laboratory, the Systems Support and Equipment Laboratory, and the Guidance and Control Laboratory of the Army Ballistic Missile Agency, Huntsville, Alabama, which were used in a comprehensive report, "Lunar Exploration Based on Saturn-Boosted Vehicles" (February, 1960). Permission to use these figures is gratefully acknowledged.

Project Mercury: The Program and Its Objectives

CHARLES J. DONLAN *and* JACK C. HEBERLIG

Project Mercury is this nation's initial program for manned orbital flight. It received official status on October 5, 1958, when it became an active NASA program, although a good deal of the preliminary planning in research activity began twelve to eighteen months before this date. At that time the following guidelines were adopted by NASA for the implementation of this project. These original guidelines still constitute the basic program for Project Mercury.

PROGRAM CONCEPTS

Objectives
1. Orbital flight and recovery
2. Man's capabilities in space environment

Basic principles
1. Simplest and most reliable approach
2. Minimum of new developments
3. Progressive build-up of tests

Method
1. Drag vehicle
2. ICBM booster
3. Retrorocket
4. Parachute descent
5. Escape system

Objectives. The main objectives of Project Mercury are (1) to insure safe orbital flight and recovery of a man in the space capsule and (2) to study man's capabilities in a space environment. In the

Mr. Donlan is Associate Director of Project Mercury, National Aeronautics and Space Administration Space Task Group, Langley Field, Va. Mr. Heberlig is Technical Assistant, Office of Project Director.

initial manned orbital flight of Project Mercury, the first objective will undoubtedly receive much popular emphasis. However, the more far-reaching and scientific objective of the program is to study man in a space environment. This study may well influence the next generation of spacecraft. This objective will be discussed more fully subsequently.

Basic Principles. In regard to the basic principles, the approach taken was to use the simplest and most reliable methods known and to minimize new developments. Also, systems reliability was to be demonstrated by a progressive buildup of tests. In this way, the primary objectives could be attained in the most reliable manner in the least amount of time.

Method. The method used to carry out the program has been outlined above. A high-drag ballistic reentry shape was selected for the basic design. In the present state of technology, this decision still appears to be a sound one. By modifying the adapter section of the Atlas ICBM booster to receive the capsule, this booster can be used to put the capsule in orbit. A cluster of solid-propellant retrorockets were adapted for positive reentry. After the high reentry velocity is reduced because of aerodynamic drag on the blunt shape, a parachute recovery system will lower the capsule to Earth. In order to provide the astronaut with a positive means of escape from a malfunctioning rocket, an escape system was provided. Recent tests of this system, simulating an off-the-pad abort, an abort at maximum dynamic pressure on exit, and an abort at a very high altitude and velocity, have all been successful. The parachute recovery system is also being extensively tested to assure high reliability. Nevertheless, the astronaut is provided with a backup reserve parachute in case malfunction of the primary parachute occurs.

CAPSULE AND ESCAPE SYSTEM CONFIGURATION

Figure 1 shows the capsule with and without its escape system. The retrorocket package and heat shield can be seen on the bottom of the capsule. The heat shield is of the ablative type and is made of a phenolic resin. Three retrorockets are used to initiate the descent from orbit. The metal shingles on the afterbody are made of cobalt alloy, which dissipates the reentry heat by radiation. This type of construction allows full expansion in all directions. The parachute recovery system is contained in the upper cylinder. The maximum diameter of the capsule is about 74 inches. The launch configuration (shown at left of Figure 1) is approximately 25 feet in height.

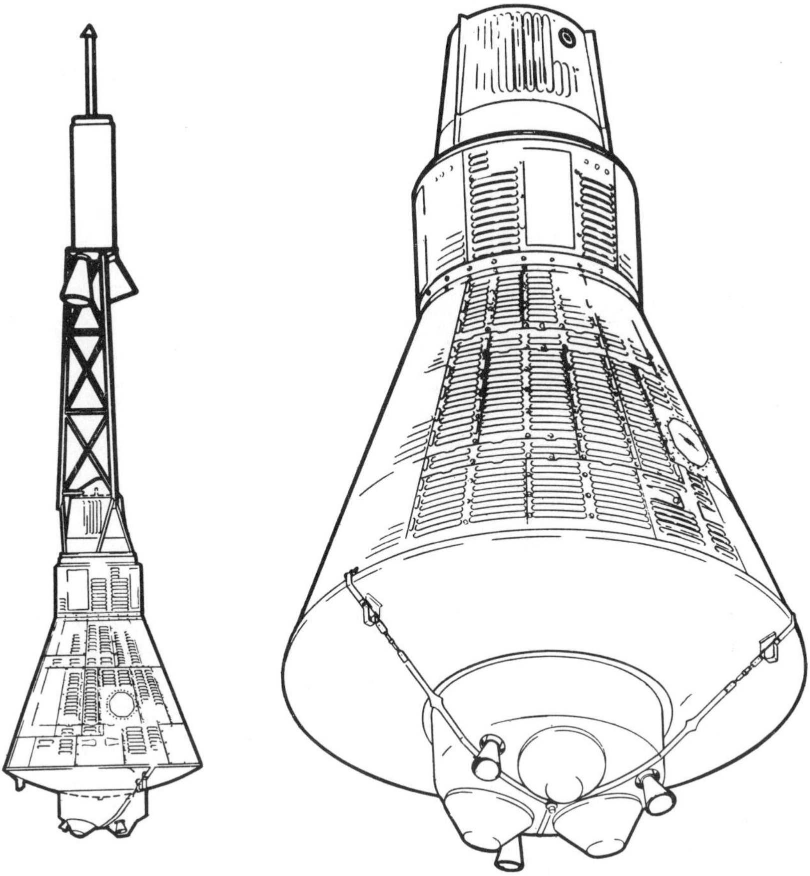

Figure 1. Capsule and Escape System Configuration

The tower escape system allows the capsule to be pulled away from the immediate vicinity of the booster at any time. To date, there have been no booster malfunctions that would have prevented a safe escape of the capsule from the scene of immediate danger.

Figure 2 has been prepared to show the relative position of the astronaut, the window, and the emergency egress hatch. The astronaut is shown in a semisupine position, with his back toward the heat shield. The window and egress hatch are two modifications that have been made in the design of the capsule since its initial stages. The window, directly above the astronaut's head, has been added to allow him to make observations independent of the periscope. The hatch, on the astronaut's right, has been developed so the astronaut could, in case of some unforeseen emergency

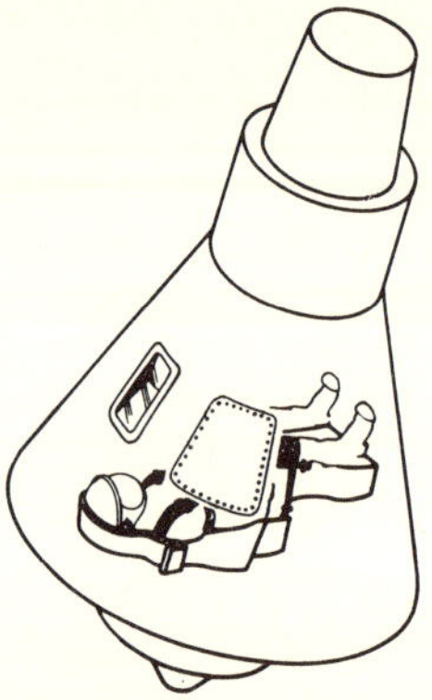

Figure 2. Diagram Showing Relationship of Pilot, Window, and Emergency Egress

after landing, exit from the capsule quickly. As the astronaut turns the hatch handle, primacord is exploded in such a manner as to cause the hatch structure to fail and thus fall free.

When all the many systems and subsystems are consolidated and integrated within the capsule structure, the Mercury capsule interior arrangement will be similar to the sketch in Figure 3. The capsule is complicated by the redundant systems which have been added for increased safety. Starting from the small end of this sketch (from right to left), one can distinguish the antenna can, the two horizon scanners, the parachute package, the pitch and yaw jets and associated plumbing, the periscope housing, the astronaut's instrument panel, the side-arm controller, and sundry electronic and power packages. The environmental control system is mainly below the astronaut's couch. The capsule is completely automatic, but provisions have also been made for piloted operation. Each system has a backup; in the communications systems there are several

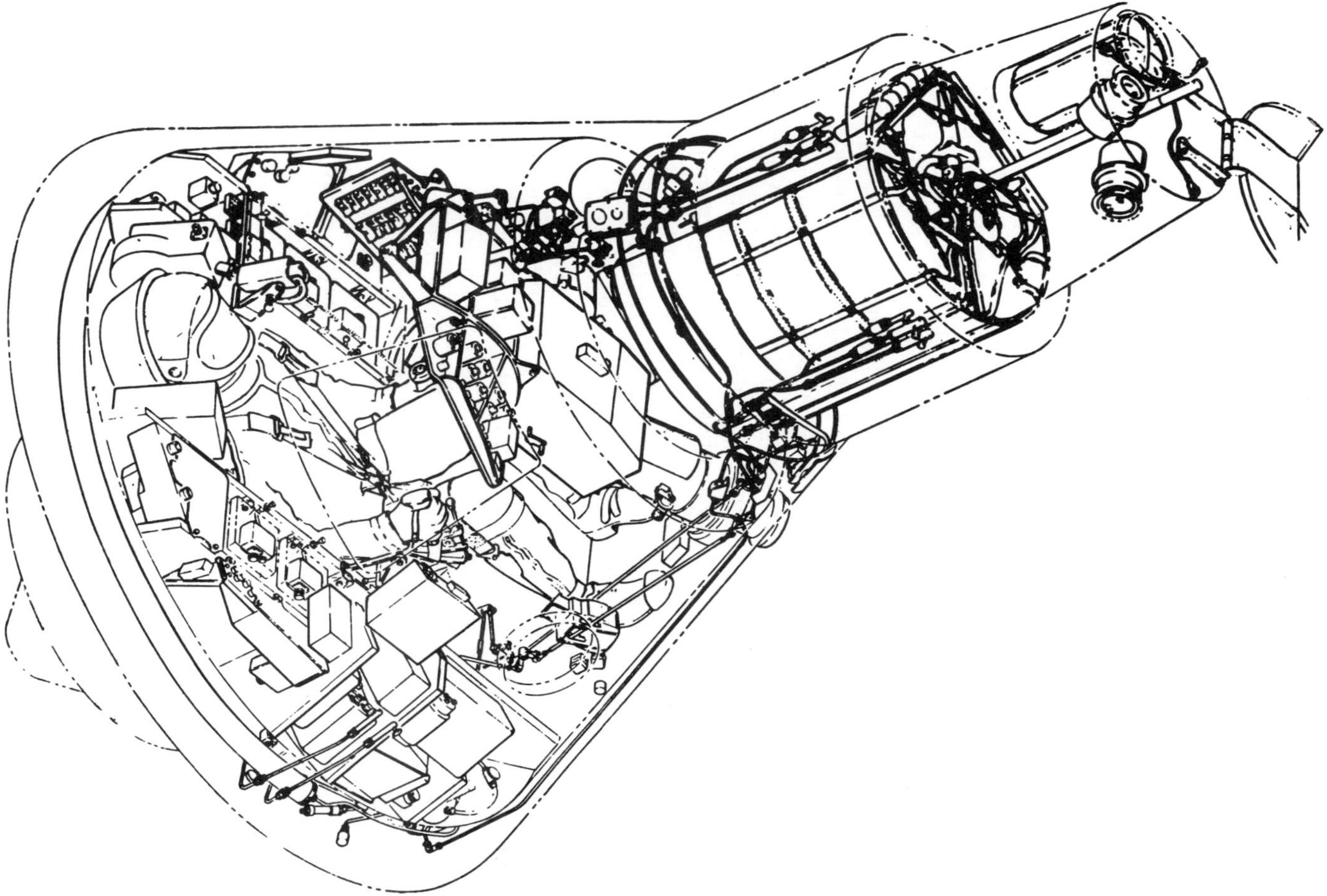

Figure 3. Internal Arrangement of Capsule

backups. There are two telemetry systems for sending back capsule data and pilot data. Also, there are onboard recorders which collect the same information sent by telemetry.

The astronaut may take over completely and perform all the functions of the automatic control system. Because of the parallel manual system, he will also be able to fly any mode that might fail on the automatic system.

MAJOR CAPSULE SYSTEMS

All the major Mercury capsule systems have been described (1). Some facts on a few of the systems of special interest are discussed briefly in the following sections.

Instrument Panel. The instrument panel is shown in Figure 4. The controls and displays on this panel are grouped as to function. The group on the left side has various pilot controls, such as those concerned with the attitude control system and the retrorockets. The two large handles are for decompression and repressurization. Decompression would be the method used for extinguishing a fire.

The next group is a sequencing display. This consists of a series of lights arranged in sequence and designed so as to indicate whether the various functions occurred, or did not occur, at the proper time. A green light comes on when the function does indeed occur, and a red light comes on when there is some failure in the automatic functioning. The handle just to the left of each light is the pilot's control to override and correct the failure of any particular function. The light at the very top of this group is the abort light which comes on in the event an abort is initiated. If the abort does not occur, the pilot can abort by using his left-hand grip. The switch immediately under the abort light is the pilot's "ready" switch. This switch is used prior to launch to light up a "ready" light on the test conductor's panel in the blockhouse.

The next series of dials are flight instrumentation. The dials indicate acceleration, rate of descent, altitude, and the fuel supply in the hydrogen peroxide tanks. The top center of the panel is the attitude display. This combination display shows rate and attitude in pitch, roll, and yaw. The rate display is in the center, surrounded by the attitude displays consisting of three dials. This particular display for attitude control was arrived at after a number of simulation

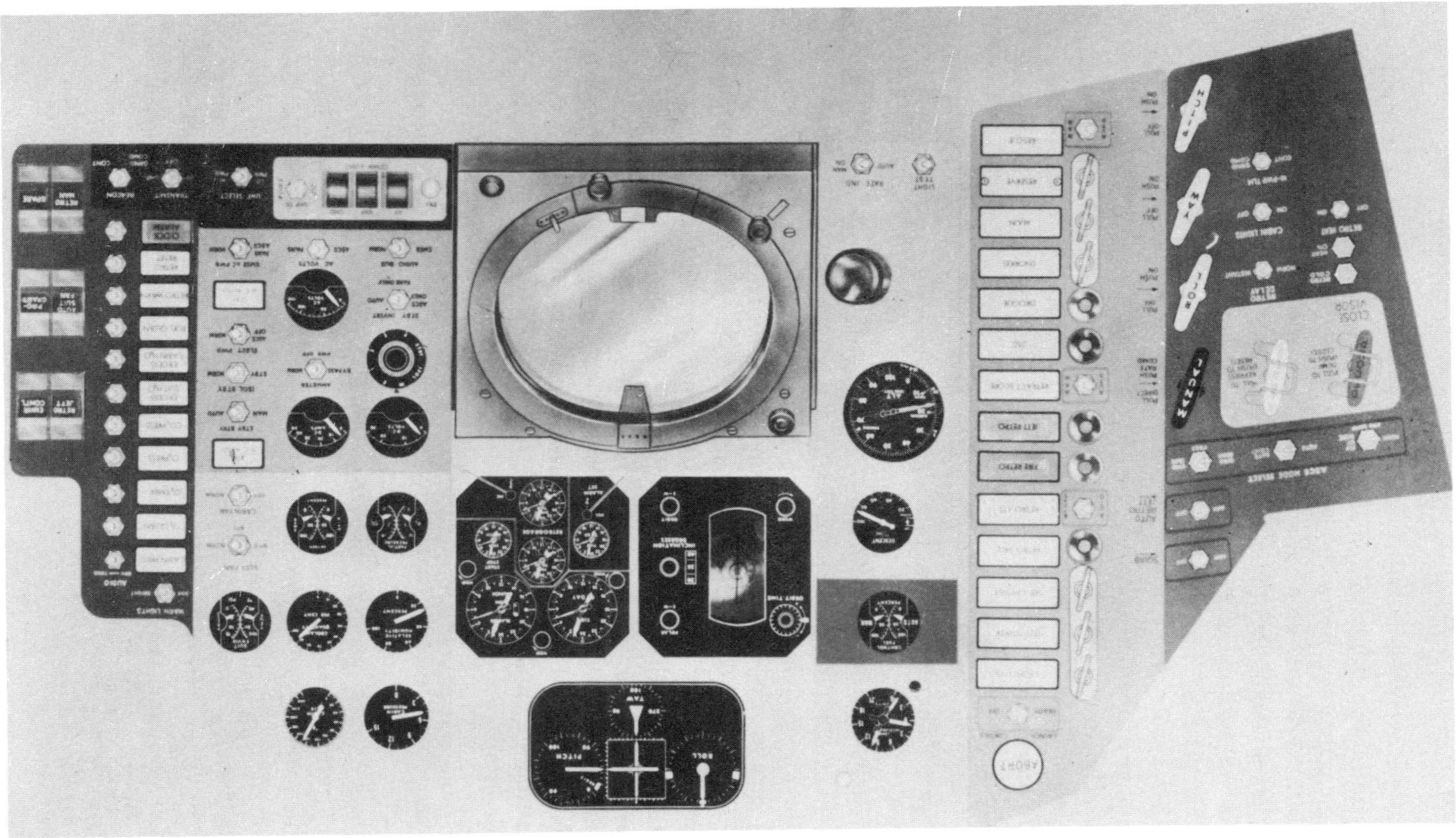

Figure 4. Pilot's Instrument Panel

flights were made with various types of displays. The astronaut control of attitude will be aided by the periscope, which is located in the center and below the instrument panel, and a window, which is located directly above the panel. The astronaut will be able to see the horizon in back of the capsule through this window in the normal orbital attitude of $14\frac{1}{2}°$ as well as in the retrofiring attitude of 34°. The periscope provides the astronaut with a view of the earth beneath the capsule. He can control the attitude by location of the earth's image in the periscope.

The instrument in the left center is a dead-reckoning type of device which consists of a small model of the earth, clock-driven to rotate in time with the orbit. In the right center is the satellite clock, which, in addition to firing the retrorockets, indicates time of day, the lapsed time since launch, and time-to-go for retrorocket firing. The astronaut is provided with an additional time-to-go dial which he may set for any desired event and also a separate stop watch.

The environmental control system instrumentation is grouped in the upper right-hand corner of the instrument panel. This group indicates the following: cabin pressure, temperature, relative humidity, and oxygen partial pressure; primary and emergency oxygen supply pressure; and carbon dioxide partial pressure downstream of the lithium hydroxide canister in the pressure suit control system. Controls for the cabin pressure system fans are provided on this panel. A warning-light panel is installed adjacent to the environmental control system instrumentation. This panel gives the astronaut visual warning of major systems failures. At the same time, an auditory warning system is actuated when failure occurs. The astronaut would turn off the auditory warning signal by actuating a switch located by the light and then take corrective action. Warning lights are provided for loss in cabin pressurization, depletion of primary oxygen supply, emergency-rate mode of operation, decrease in cabin oxygen partial pressure below 3 psi, increase of carbon dioxide partial pressure to 3 percent in the pressure suit circuit, and excessive cooling water to the suit and cabin heat exchangers. A telelight panel is located on the left console to give the astronaut indication of flight-event sequential operation. On this panel the launch oxygen supply and snorkel operation are presented. Manual backup controls are installed adjacent to the lights. A green light indicates that the event has occurred; a red light indicates the event has not occurred. Heat-exchanger water-flow controls and the emergency-rate valve control are located on the right console, which is not shown in this figure.

The instrument panel and astronaut will be photographed in flight. In addition, the data from the system instrumentation will be telemetered and recorded by onboard recorders. Continuous physiological data on the astronaut's condition in flight will be made with electrocardiogram, body temperature, and respiration rate and depth measurements. These data will be recorded by onboard recorders and will be telemetered.

Environmental Control System. The Mercury environmental control system (Figure 5) maintains the environment for the astronaut at a temperature between 50° and 90° F. (2). The astronaut may manually select the temperature in this range that makes him most comfortable. During reentry, when the cabin air temperature may approach 180° F., the suit environmental control systems will still maintain the air in the pressure suit within the desired temperature range. The system is capable of operating for about 32 hours. Body odor is removed by use of activated charcoal, and carbon dioxide is removed by the use of lithium hydroxide. Fresh oxygen enters the suit at the torso and exits at the helmet. As the oxygen leaves the helmet, it enters a debris trap where small particles are removed and then it moves through the odor absorber and carbon dioxide absorber. A filter is provided downstream of the carbon dioxide absorber in order to prevent lithium hydroxide dust from contaminating the suit oxygen. The temperature of the gas is lowered in the heat exchanger and water is removed in the water absorber. The resulting drop in pressure is counteracted by an increased supply of gas from the oxygen bottle. Ten cubic feet per minute is the flow rate through the suit at approximately 5 psi. Considering the fact that this system only weighs about 130 pounds, it represents indeed a noteworthy engineering accomplishment.

Automatic Stabilization and Control System. One of the more complex systems in the capsule is the automatic stabilization and control system. Figure 6 shows the normal operation of this system. The Atlas and capsule configuration at lift-off is shown at the left of this

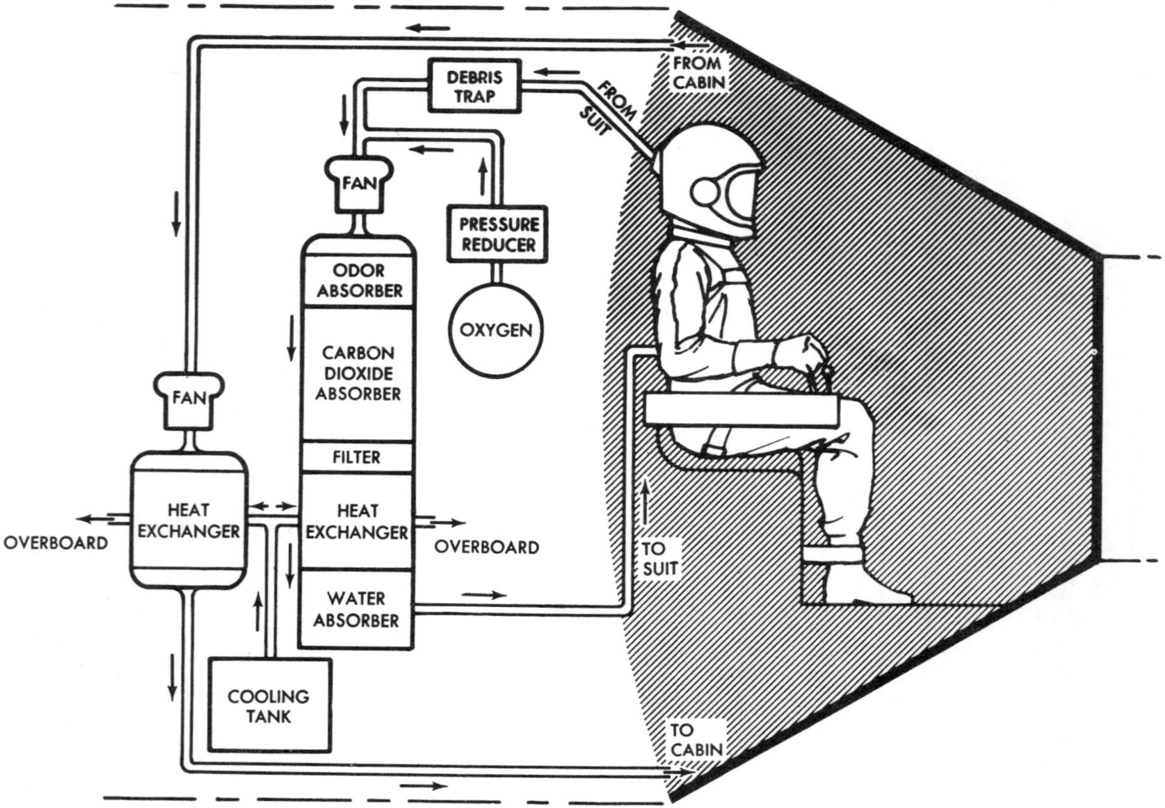

Figure 5. The Mercury Environmental Control System

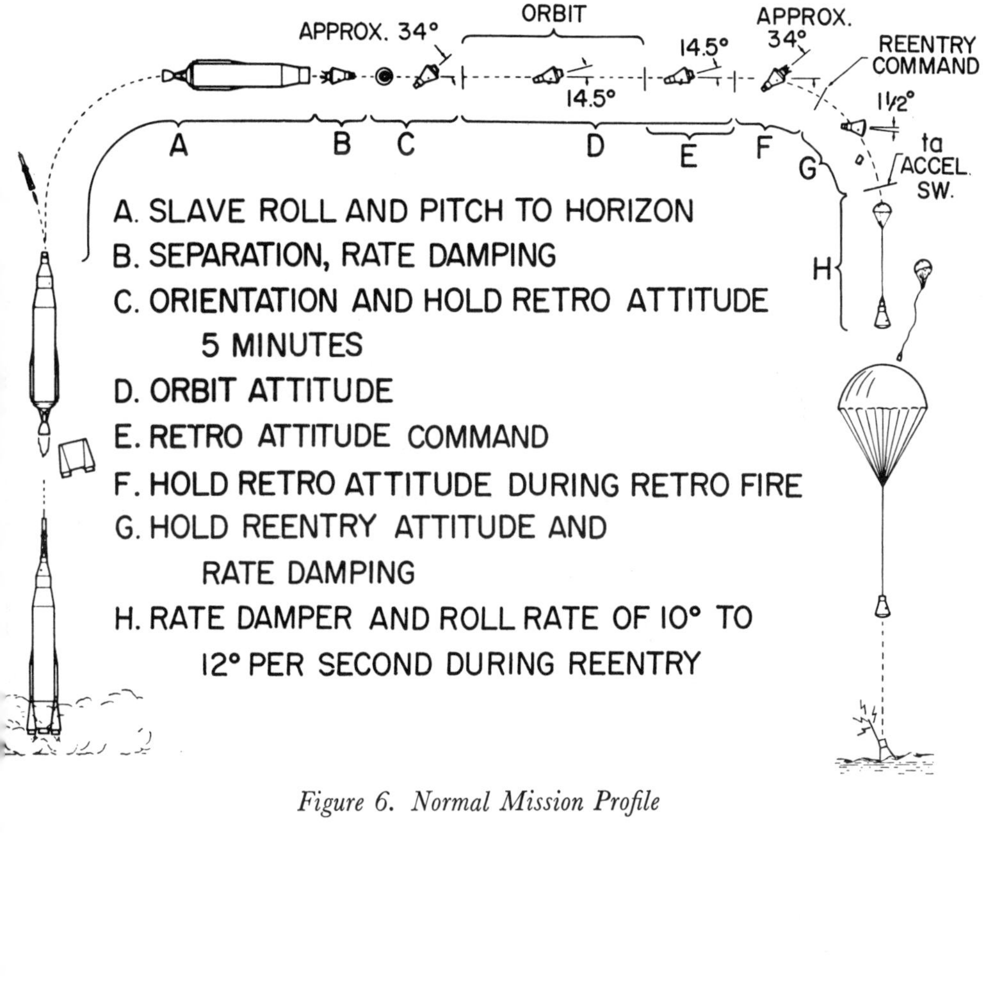

Figure 6. Normal Mission Profile

figure. When the Atlas drops its booster engines, an event known as staging, the capsule removes the escape rocket by firing a special jettison rocket. The Atlas booster then follows a tilt program which yields an orbital altitude of approximately 105 nautical miles at the time of insertion. At booster cutoff the capsule's posigrade rockets fire, separating the capsule from the booster, as shown in position B in Figure 6. The stabilization system maintains capsule rate damping for 5 seconds, until all oscillations of the capsule have been stopped. The capsule then is oriented to the retrorocket firing attitude, as shown in position C. The capsule is maintained in this attitude for 5 minutes. In this time period, ground tracking stations can determine if capsule orbital velocities and insertion angles are correct enough to allow the capsule to maintain itself in orbit. The capsule is then oriented into the normal orbital attitude, as shown in position D. The capsule is maintained in a 14½° blunt-end-up position. This permits the astronaut, with the aid of the periscope, to see past the larger heat shield end. Also, the retrorockets are in the right position for reentering immediately in case of emergency. The automatic stabilization and control system next orients the capsule into the retrofiring attitude, as shown in position F. After retrofiring, the capsule is oriented to the reentry attitude, as shown in position G, and the retropackage is jettisoned. As the capsule enters the atmosphere, the control system introduces a roll rate of 10° to 12° per second and also maintains rate damping, which prevents large capsule oscillations from building up. At about 42,000 feet the drogue parachute is deployed, and its action gives stability to the capsule prior to deploying the main parachute at 10,000 feet. Upon landing, capsule recovery is aided by the use of UHF and HF transmitters and receivers, a Sofar bomb, dye marker, and flashing light.

ACCELERATION AND IMPACT ATTENUATION

One of the major concerns in the design of the Mercury capsule is to protect the pilot from excessive accelerations during flight and in landing. The escape rocket, if fired in an off-the-pad abort or at high altitude where the drag forces are low, would place upon the astronaut an acceleration level of 20g for a period of almost 1 second. Impact on the water would give acceleration levels as high as 40g for a few milliseconds. A contoured couch which evenly distributes a man's weight was developed and tested. Normal exit g profiles were run, and the subjects demonstrated ability to control and do tasks which are necessary for normal capsule functions. Tests in which accelerations reached values as high as 25g were also conducted, and they demonstrated the validity of this support system in case of the escape-rocket firing. However, a major problem still

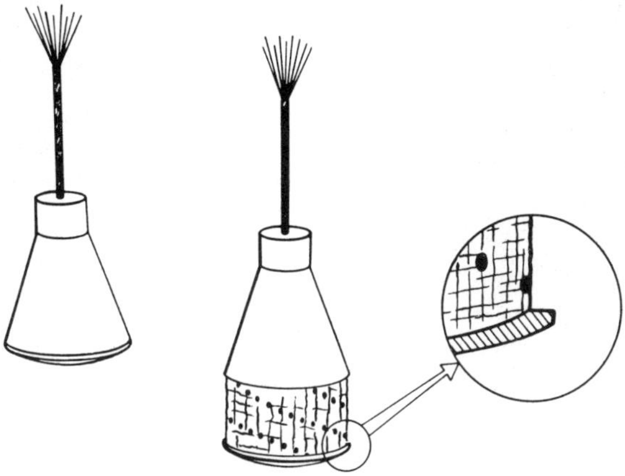

Figure 7. Air Cushion for Impact Attenuation

existed for the case of land impact or impact on the water with a high horizontal wind profile. It is believed that a satisfactory solution to this problem has been accomplished by the accordion-like air cushion design shown in Figure 7. The air cushion consists of a 4-foot skirt made of rubberized Fiberglas that connects the heat shield to the rest of the capsule. After the main parachute is deployed, the heat shield is released from the capsule and the bag fills with air. Upon impact, the airtrap between the heat shield in the capsule is vented through holes in the skirt as well as through portions of the capsule which are not completely airtight. Thus the desired cushioning effect is provided.

MERCURY FLIGHT TEST VEHICLES

Figure 8 shows the three rocket flight test vehicles used in Project Mercury. The Little Joe system shown at the left is a cluster of solid-propellant rocket motors used in the research and development

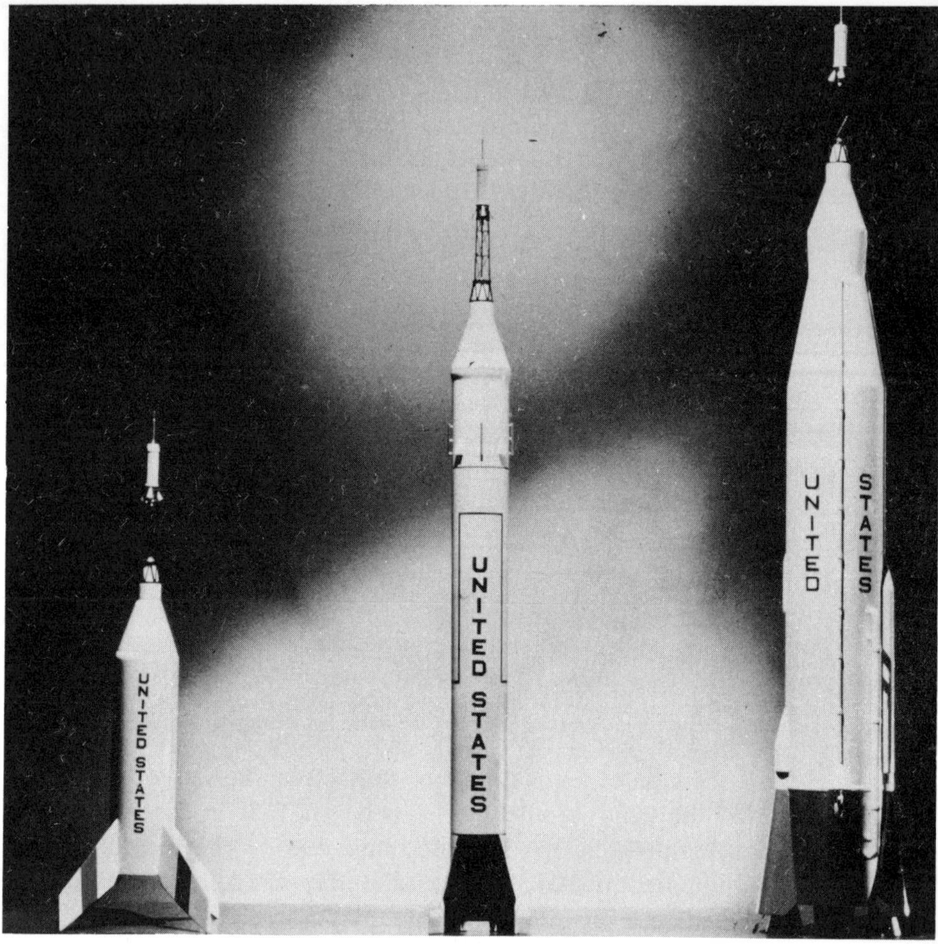

Figure 8. Project Mercury Flight Test Vehicles
Left, Little Joe. Center, Redstone. Right, Atlas

program. No manned flights are contemplated with this booster, although successful flights have been made with small primates aboard the capsule. The Redstone Booster, shown in the center, will be used for training flights for astronauts. Before the astronauts' training program begins, an animal will be sent aloft to demonstrate the system. The Mercury-Atlas combination is shown at the right. In the Atlas program, animals will also be sent aloft before a man is put in orbit.

The reliability of each of these systems is of obvious importance in this program. The booster quality assurance program includes the following:

Standard booster hardware
Selection of individual components and subsystems
  Nominal performance
Marking of parts
100-Percent inspection of parts
Comprehensive roll-out inspection
Flight safety review

Standard booster hardware is being used to take advantage of all the experience gained in conducting the weapons system program of which the basic boosters are a part. The reliability of each system will be based upon the nominal performance of each individual component and subsystem. Also, as these systems are assembled in the various industrial plants, each part is being marked or tagged with a Project Mercury label. Although the assembly-line technique has been established for these boosters, 100-percent inspection of all parts will take place to assure the highest quality control possible. Upon assembly of a booster system, a comprehensive roll-out inspection will be made. The history of all parts going into a particular booster will be carefully documented and reviewed. In this manner, the operational proficiency of all systems and their individual components is made known. After the capsule has been mated to the booster and the mechanical and electrical integration is completed, a flight safety review board will be held. This review board reports on the over-all expected reliability of the two systems—that of the capsule and booster together. Only after the capsule-booster combination meets the requirements of the flight safety review board will approval for flight be given.

MERCURY ORBIT, TRACKING, AND RECOVERY

Orbit Selection Criteria. Selection of the firing azimuth is very important in the over-all Mercury operation. The orbit selection criteria are as follows:

1. Use of existing tracking stations
2. Use of Atlantic Missile Range for normal landing
3. Remain over continental U.S. for considerable time for tracking during orbit and reentry
4. Orbit over friendly territory and in temperate zone

It was most advantageous to use the existing tracking stations established for other national programs (3). Thus, only a minimum of additional stations had to be implemented. A total of 17 stations, including the control center at Cape Canaveral, will be active while the Mercury capsule is in orbit. Of these 17, two of the stations will be located onboard ship in the mid-Atlantic and Indian Oceans. At each tracking station there will be telemetry read-out giving the personnel real-time indication of the pilot's condition and the capsule systems. Prior to each flight aeromedical and capsule systems specialists will be sent to each of the monitoring stations facilities. After each flight these specialists will aid in evaluating the pilot and capsule systems' performance. The down-range tracking facilities of the Atlantic Missile Range will be used for the normal reentry tracking. In this way the capsule may be followed on radar from the time it begins its reentry until impact. Constant communication by voice will be possible during this time. In order to determine the exact altitude and velocity of the capsule, the tracking facilities in the continental United States will be used extensively for determining the correct time of retrofiring so that the capsule will land in the predicted impact area. In the United States, there are six such tracking installations. Another requirement for the orbit selection is that the capsule should pass over friendly territory and maintain itself in a temperate zone. It is of interest to review the philosophy used in establishing the ground-station requirements.

Ground Stations. The ground-station selection criteria are as follows:

1. Continuous tracking from Hawaii to Bermuda
2. Retrotimer reset and ground command capabilities during each orbit

3. Continuous contact during launch and through insertion
4. Maintain frequent voice and telemetry contact
5. Continuous impact prediction

Continuous tracking is required from Hawaii to Bermuda. During each orbit, the retrotiming device must be capable of being reset along with other ground command capabilities. Continuous

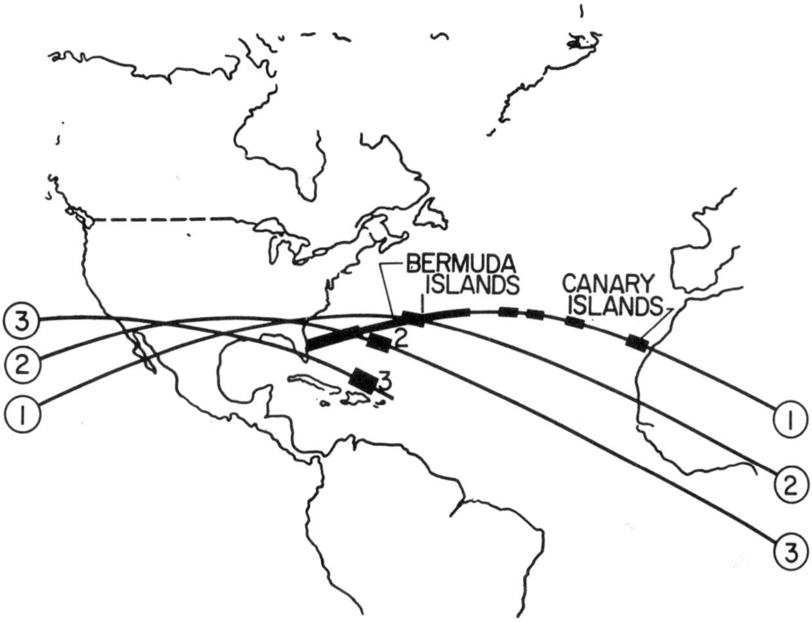

Figure 9. Project Mercury Anticipated Recovery Areas

contact during launch and through insertion is required to determine the orbit characteristics and pilot's well-being. Frequent voice and telemetry contact must be maintained throughout the orbit. There must exist sufficient tracking information to provide continuous impact prediction; that is, at any time during the flight, the recovery forces should know exactly where the capsule would impact if the retrorockets were fired at that time.

Recovery. It is not feasible to provide world-wide recovery forces; therefore, certain areas have been designated as primary recovery areas (Figure 9). A long recovery area is provided (from Cape

Canaveral toward the Bermuda Islands) to include all impact points which might occur due to an early abort. Between the Bermuda Islands and the Canary Islands are other primary recovery areas. These areas are so located that if orbital velocity or insertion angle is not correct, firing of the retrorockets would cause the capsule to impact in these designated areas. If the initial orbit is not correct, and conditions were to prevent the capsule from making three orbits, a second impact area is established at the end of the second orbit, as shown. The impact area from a nominal flight, however, occurs at the end of the third orbit down the Atlantic Missile Range, designated here as area 3. As mentioned previously, this would mean continuous tracking of the capsule during entry from Hawaii until impact.

THE ASTRONAUT AND HIS TASK

The flight of a Mercury capsule into orbit and return, fundamentally, is an extension of the flight envelope of aircraft. The majority of sensations and demands on the astronaut are similar to those imposed on the pilot of any highly maneuverable, high-performance aircraft. For this reason, the prime technical qualification for the Mercury astronaut was that he should be an experienced pilot, trained in objective flying; i.e., test flying. His presence in the Mercury capsule can be expected to increase the chances of a completely successful mission, because he has the capability and ability to take control of the capsule in the event of a malfunction of many of the automatic systems.

The astronaut in Project Mercury will furnish other important milestones in man's conquest of space. Some examples of the kind of scientific information that this first venture of man-into-space makes possible are listed in the accompanying table.

Some Examples of Research Observations of the Biological Effects of Prolonged Weightlessness Which Project Mercury Makes Possible

Physiological	*Psychological*	*Task Performance*
Function of the circulatory system	Orientation	Attitude control
Eating and drinking	Time estimation	Capsule systems monitoring
Pre- and post-flight tests of stress reactions	Autokinesis and oculogyric illusions	Navigation

The Mercury orbital missions will permit the study of the effects of prolonged weightlessness on the physiological reactions, the subjective psychological reactions, and the performance of the astronaut. Of particular interest will be the effects of weightlessness on the function of the respiratory and circulatory systems. Telemetered electrocardiogram and breathing rates will make it possible to determine not only the effects of prolonged weightlessness itself, but the effects of transition from high accelerations to zero-g and back to the high accelerations associated with launch and reentry. Problems associated with eating and drinking in prolonged weightless flight can also be studied. Stress hormone studies, together with pre- and post-physical examinations, will allow assessment of the body's physiological reaction to the total envelope of flight stresses.

Subjective psychological phenomena likely to be effected by the weightless environment can be studied through voice reports and capsule instrumentation. The ability of the astronaut to orient himself in space can be determined. The effects of the reduction in proprioceptive cues in time estimation can also be determined. The extent of the autokinesis and oculogyric illusions in a weightless environment should also be of interest.

Of utmost practical importance to future manned space flight efforts will be the quality of the astronaut's performance in space. Accuracy of manual attitude control should provide a good test of psychomotor performance capability. Monitoring of the capsule orbital systems should provide an indication of the vigilance and perceptual accuracy. Navigation will test reasoning and visual discrimination of earth terrain features and heavenly bodies outside the capsule.

The following statement has been made (4) in regard to the importance of Project Mercury:

> It has become increasingly evident that the full utilization of space flight for scientific and exploration purposes will depend on man's ability to participate in the flight mission. While, in principle, it is possible to devise increasingly complex instruments and automatic systems, in practice, the availability in the vehicle of human intelligence and decision-making capacity will prove to be essential for successful accomplishment of many advanced space missions.

It is believed that Project Mercury will provide the baselines by which the future space vehicles will be built, around the most valuable and useful machine—man himself.

REFERENCES

1. Faget, M. A., and R. O. Piland, Mercury Capsule and Its Flight Systems. Paper No. 60-34, Inst. Aero. Sci., January, 1960.
2. Johnston, R. S., Mercury Life Support Systems. S. M. F. Fund Paper No. FF-25, Inst. Aero. Sci., New York, N.Y., January, 1960.
3. Mathews, C. W., Review of Operational Plans for Mercury Orbital Mission. IAS Preprint No. 60-36, Inst. Aero. Sci., January, 1960.
4. Gilruth, R. R., and H. K. Strass, Present and Future Steps in Manned Space Flight. Manned Space Station Symposium, April, 1960.

Personal Experiences in Space Equivalent Flight

DAVID G. SIMONS, B. W. HENDERSON, *and*
JEAN-LOUIS RIEHL

This paper considers from a psychophysiological point of view three experiences related to space flight. Many of the similarities and differences among them are identified, and the neurophysiological implications of several of the most impressive phenomena are discussed. The three experiences include the MANHIGH II flight and the MANHIGH III flight, in which the senior author participated as pilot and as flight surgeon, respectively, and a 30-hour chamber run in which the same author participated purely as a subject.

MANHIGH II FLIGHT

Complete descriptions of the equipment used on this flight and the facts associated with it have been published (1, 6). The 32-hour flight, reaching an altitude of 101,000 feet, involved a total of 42 hours continuous "on-duty" time. This was broken only by occasional naps of 10 to 20 minutes' duration. Additional reports of flight experiences, observations, and comments are available (1, 2, 3, 5).

In a review of the psychophysiological aspects of the MANHIGH flights (4), the concepts and techniques for monitoring both the psychological and physiological status of the pilot have been described. On the MANHIGH II flight the pilot was required to submit hourly subjective ratings on three items. They included thermo-comfort (scored on a 6-point scale), personal condition (scored 0–100 percent), and confidential subjective comments and objective observations recorded on tape. On the MANHIGH II flight a special effort was made to report functional efficiency in a realistic and

Colonel Simons, Captain Henderson, and Dr. Riehl are attached to the Bioastronautics Branch, School of Aviation Medicine, USAF Aerospace Medical Center (ATC), Brooks Air Force Base, Texas. The views of the authors expressed in this paper do not necessarily represent those of the United States Air Force.

objective manner. The tape recorder was included primarily to save time in recording observations and facts of flight, secondarily to permit a semiconfidential record of subjective impressions during flight. Finally, the actual performance and psychological reactions during flight were analyzed after the flight.

Two physiological parameters were telemetered in coded form during the MANHIGH II flight, heart rate and respiratory rate. In both cases mechanical difficulties arose which rendered ambiguous the meaning of the data obtained.

Results. The data obtained on the MANHIGH II flight have been presented previously (1). Summarizing briefly, the readings on thermocomfort remained realistic until noon of the second day. At this time the capsule became hotter and more humid than at any time previously during the flight. Despite this, the reports submitted ranged between comfortable and hot, indicating a situation more satisfactory than that reported late in the afternoon of the first day.

More impressive were the overoptimistic personal condition ratings rendered throughout the flight. At no time during the flight did the ratings drop below 90 percent. The scale was intended to rate 50 percent as an average normal efficiency level under ordinary circumstances. Through the morning and early afternoon of the second day ratings were 95 percent and higher.

The tape recorder proved the most valuable source of information concerning the psychological status and performance efficiency throughout the flight.

Post-flight analysis in retrospect made it clear that between sunset and midnight of the first day (after 24 hours of continuous duty) only a small fraction of the observations which could have been made, and had been carefully planned, were actually accomplished. Throughout the second morning of flight (after 36 hours of continuous duty) the pilot was vaguely aware, but not particularly concerned, about the serious difficulty realized in making relatively simple measurements of the direction of radio stations. It was necessary to report this information to the ground in order to determine the position of the balloon above the clouds.

During descent, in the afternoon of the second day, the capsule passed through a remarkable haze layer at 70,000 feet. This was a phenomenon of the type that would have been fully documented with photographs earlier in the flight. The marked reduction in spread of attention permitted only a mental note to be made of the sight.

The analysis of the tape recordings in terms of the percentage of time spent dictating through different periods of the flight resulted in an impressive record of decreasing initiative and reduced response to observational opportunities. This clearly was a most valuable and objective means of obtaining a quantitative evaluation of initiative and higher-level intellectual performance during the flight.

MANHIGH III FLIGHT

Details of the MANHIGH III flight have also been reported earlier (6, 7). The psychophysiological aspects of this flight have been presented with those of the MANHIGH II flight (4).

In an effort to break through the unrevealing optimism of the personal condition reports of the MANHIGH II flight, the name of the report was changed to *Efficiency* for the MANHIGH III flight, and the 50 percent level was designated the estimated median during the flight, the pilot (Lt. McClure) being exhorted to render as many ratings above the 50 percent level as below. It was reported on a 0–100 percent scale.

In a further effort to distinguish component factors effecting this efficiency rating the pilot was requested to report drive, tension, and alertness, each on a 5-point scale. The original thermocomfort rating (5-point scale) was retained. The addition of pre-flight, in-flight, and post-flight psychiatric interviews to determine changes in affect, motivation, compensation mechanisms, and alertness was considered a major advance in technique.

The tape recorder was retained, but with considerably augmented plans for the analysis to be made of the record following the 24-hour flight. In addition to a simple "percentage of time dictated" analysis, the individual remarks would be further analyzed for their initiative content. New, unsolicited, completely spontaneous observations of aerial phenomena, as well as any questions generated by the pilot, were to be rated as evidence of initiative. Further, spread of attention in terms of the variety of activity and observations would be analyzed. Finally, a camera periodically reported the position of all dials on the flight instrument panel. This record was to be cross-checked against pilot's remarks and performance to detect changes in efficiency of job performance.

Physiological monitoring included effective telemetry of electrocardiogram and respiration rate and depth, with the addition of basal skin resistance, all available on oscillographic write-out in real time during the flight. The pilot read and reported his internal and skin temperatures in order to achieve greater accuracy and simplicity of instrumentation. The flight included an infra-red camera which took pictures of the subject without his being aware of the flash. This was an additional check on his condition throughout the flight. (These pictures were taken approximately every two minutes.)

Results. An entirely unexpected complication of the flight situation led to unanticipated results. The flight was launched several hours after sunrise and reached altitude an hour before noon. By noon the pilot's pulse rate had climbed to 140 beats per minute, unaccountably high even for his characteristically labile pulse rate. Careful enquiry revealed that the pilot felt quite thirsty, warm, and *unaccountably* tired. A steadily increasing pulse rate *demanded* an explanation, so the ground monitors requested a cross-check of the normal temperature readings being received by telemetry. An intolerable and unrelievable hyperthermia within the capsule dictated immediate termination of the flight.

The gradual onset of each stress in the face of enormous motivation to accomplish the flight and its observational objectives permitted the pilot to experience an increasing loss of efficiency and increasing level of discomfort without his ever recognizing for himself the seriousness of his situation. When this was called to his attention he was completely cooperative with the ground monitors. Throughout the following hours, when the steadily rising body temperature of the pilot was threatening his survival in the face of the excruciatingly slow descent of the balloon, the physiological telemetry information available was invaluable. It permitted a rational basis for the decision to permit Lt. McClure to continue the flight in an orderly manner and land using the balloon, the manner most likely to permit his immediate recovery by recovery crews. The alternative was to terminate the flight precipitously by releasing the capsule from the balloon and allow it to come down on a parachute. The

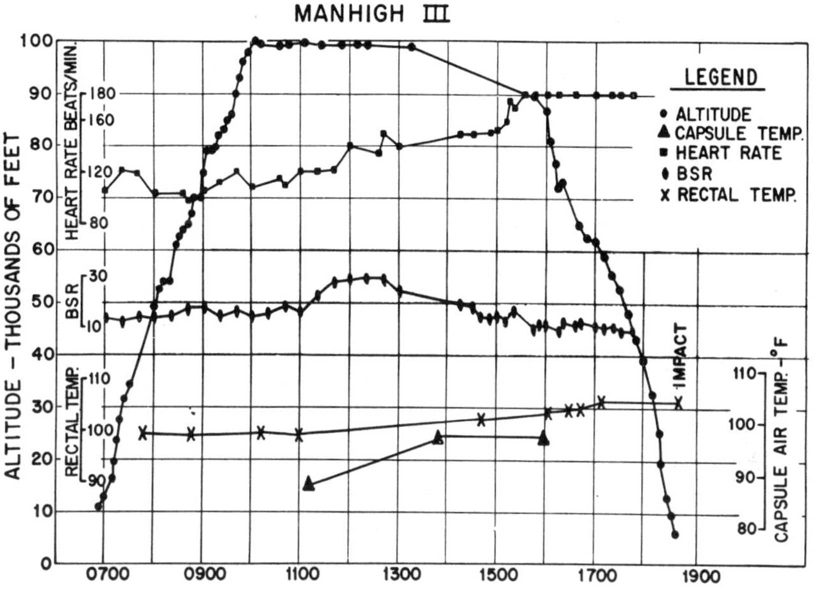

Environmental and Physiological Profile of MANHIGH III

successful outcome of the flight is due in major part to the initial detection of the problem through physiological telemetry.

CHAMBER FLIGHT EXPERIENCE

One 30-hour chamber flight was made with Col. Simons as subject. The chamber itself and the structure of the flight have been described elsewhere (8). There are significant similarities and differences in the conditions and experiences observed in the MANHIGH II flight and in the chamber flight.

Similarities of Conditions. From the point of view of the individual experiencing the flight, five conditions stood out as being comparable. The first was the duration of the flight, 32 hours. I had been awake for approximately 7 hours before the chamber run, and for 12 hours before launching of the MANHIGH flight. The post-flight times were 3 hours in each case.

The degree of physical isolation from other people was similar in each instance. Throughout both flights I was unable to see anyone and communicated on a regular schedule by electronic means only.

During the chamber run no pilot-initiated calls were permitted, and the schedule called for one contact every 1½ hours. The MANHIGH schedule was every half hour, with intermediate calls permitted if desired.

The physical space available was comparable in each case, approximately 50 cubic feet for working and living.

The environmental circumstances with respect to pressure, oxygen tension, humidity, carbon dioxide tension, and the like, were quite similar on both flights.

Although the diet on the MANHIGH flight was *ad libitum*, the total calories consumed on each flight were comparable. The caloric intake was forceably restricted in the case of the chamber run.

Differences in Conditions. From the pilot's point of view, the outstanding difference in the two experiences was the sense of challenge to be alert to detect new phenomena and available observations throughout the MANHIGH flight. The stimulus of the flight opportunity and the sense of accomplishment was of a different magnitude.

Likewise the depth of demands on my alertness and attention was of a different order of magnitude. The "for keeps" nature of the balloon flight was inescapably present. During the chamber run the only demand made of me that required a serious effort was to stay awake. By contrast, there was hardly a time during the balloon flight that I did not feel a sense of pressure and urgency in accomplishment.

The variety of activities and responsibilities could hardly have differed more widely. I never had, nor expect to have, a busier 32 hours than those of the balloon flight. Except for the last 6 or 8 hours of the chamber flight, I was constantly aware of restlessness and impatience with the lack of activity and any form of mental challenge. Vigilance was a task that required constant attention but only rare responses in the unrelieved monotony.

All portholes of the chamber were covered during the run, whereas the portholes of the capsule had provided an inspiring view of a new world.

Uninterrupted vigilance was required during the chamber run. Short naps were permitted during the balloon flight whenever desired. These were indulged to a total of approximately 2 hours of sleep during the flight.

Because of the careful temperature and humidity control, and the fact that no pressure suit was required during the chamber run, there was a marked difference in the comfort experienced. The wide range of temperature fluctuations and the presence of the pressure suit frequently imposed a burden of personal discomfort that was inescapable during the balloon flight.

During the chamber run, classical music was available on demand for diversion, and free use was made of it. No such facility was available or desired during the balloon flight.

Similarities Observed. Two significant similarities were noted. In the course of the 30-hour operation, performance declined with the accumulation of fatigue. In both cases a definite decrease in performance was observed after 24 hours of continuous duty. Only during the last 6 hours of the chamber run did I feel "saturated" with activity by the demands of the vigilance operator system. This loss in vigilance and psychomotor performance after 24 hours of continuous duty was noted in the other two non-pilot Air Force subjects completing a similar chamber flight.

On the MANHIGH II and MANHIGH III balloon flights and on the three completed chamber flights the loss of insight as to performance efficiency after 24 hours of continuous duty was most apparent. This is considered the most significant observation in these experiences.

Differences Observed. Eight significant differences were observed between the MANHIGH II balloon flight and the chamber run. The most notable to me was the sense of frustration experienced early in the chamber run because of insufficient activity demands.

During the balloon flight I experienced a strong emotional reaction to the communication situation. During the first day I resented the necessity to take time from observations in order to report them and to communicate with the ground team. During the night, when physically threatened by external conditions around the capsule, I just as strongly appreciated the opportunity to make radio contact. During the chamber flight I anticipated the change of activity, but felt neither strong desire nor resentment toward the communications *per se.*

Physical discomfort was characteristic of the MANHIGH II flight only.

The availability of external visibility on the MANHIGH II flight gave me a sense of not only being "out" of this world, as I felt during the chamber run, but literally "in" another during the balloon flight.

During the balloon flight I never battled sleep in the sense that I was required to during the night of the chamber run and occasionally during the day. If I felt too tired to go on during the balloon flight, I simply notified the ground and took a "cat nap."

The hallucinations previously described during the chamber run (5) were completely absent during the balloon flight. Which of the other condition or conditions in the flight situation was responsible for this fact has not yet been established.

Following the chamber run, I experienced a post-flight disorientation that was unique. Several days following the chamber flight I described it as follows:

Upon leaving the chamber I felt unsteady in the legs both in standing and walking, although in walking it seemed much more severe. Especially when walking I had difficulty defining mentally the exact position of the walls and different objects within the room. This same phenomenon was present to a lesser degree when standing still. I closed my eyes while doing a Romberg test to check the integrity of proprioceptive sensations and interpretations. I could even lean from one side or to the other with no difficulty in maintaining equilibrium. This suggests that I was having difficulty formulating spatial concepts. I was unable to define clearly in my mind the distance to the walls and to objects in the room. I could distinguish and recognize everything clearly but was unable accurately to relate myself in terms of position and distance to these objects.

One can wonder here whether this relates to the fact that for 33 hours my visual environment was restricted to a space which I could reach within my own span. When this was suddenly expanded to many times that volume, was I simply unable to readjust to this new dimension? On the other hand, was it an impairment of central nervous system function due primarily to degradation of general cerebral function from excessive fatigue? [Following the MANHIGH II flight I simply felt stiff and sore.]

Effects of the chamber run were noticeable for several days. My comments dictated several days after the run were as follows:

During the day following the run I felt physically weak such that it was difficult to sit up, walk upstairs, etc., requiring markedly more effort than usual. I was particularly aware of a shortness of breath on mild exertion such as going up a flight of stairs. A somewhat annoying feature was the marked emotional lability so that rather minor irritations were prone to evoke major emotional reaction and resentment. It was typical that a little exercise would quickly make me feel tired, and that after a short rest I would again feel rejuvenated, having a strong desire to be active and doing things.

Although the physical aspects were noticed following the MANHIGH II flight, the presence of emotional lability was not noted at the time. This, too, may have been a lack of insight.

In conclusion, we have seen that during space flight situations or their equivalent a number of cerebral processes are markedly altered, thereby leading to subjective and objective distortions of function. The problem of hallucinations has never been fully explained on a neurophysiological basis; however, the recent work of Livingston (9) suggests at least one possible mechanism of space or time distortion. Reviewing the original work of Head and Holmes, Livingston emphasizes the central control of peripheral sensory receptors; in that respect Kaada and Granit had already explored the muscle-spindle mechanism (10). The logical extension of their findings is that the peripheral sensory receptors can be made to enhance or suppress a given constant sensory input. The perception can be altered, and aberrations of this controlling mechanism might lead to hallucinations.

The pronounced lowering of the level of performance following prolonged exposure to space-equivalent situations has been observed in all subjects who have been submitted to such an environment. This deficit in psychomotor function is probably quite similar to the "fatigue" seen in crew members in conventional flights of long duration.

The problem of pure "sleepiness" is not unique to the space equivalent environment. The sleep requirements of the human machine are difficult to alter; indeed, the very nature of sleep is poorly understood, although strong evidence exists that identifiable changes occur in the central nervous system during sleep.

The "mood swings," irritability, and "nervousness," which were reported by the participants during the debriefing period and several days after the flights, are difficult to assess by objective neurophysiological criteria. It is possible that autonomic changes accompany these emotional outbursts.

The hazards imposed by alterations in consciousness are apparent. In addition, the decrease in performance efficiency mentioned previously may lead to a poorly formulated appraisal of the "inability to handle the situation," with subsequent anxiety and fear, possibly complete panic and breakdown. It is, therefore, the purpose of the Bioastronautics Branch of the School of Aviation Medicine to study or survey what bioelectric parameters might be useful in the over-all assessment of man in a space situation.

1. It is obvious that gross emotional discharge is usually, if not always, accompanied by autonomic phenomena.

2. The more subtle changes in central nervous system (CNS) reactivity, e.g., "fatigue" and alterations in vigilance, necessitate a new methodology.

Several significant studies have been conducted in recent years, but all methods reported to date have been inadequate to cover the spectrum of CNS reactivity. A method designed to be used under in-flight conditions must of necessity utilize direct bioelectric measurements. The multidimensional approach is motivated by the fact that (a) emotional outbursts will trigger changes in parameters of autonomic functions, and (b) there are good reasons to believe that the subtle CNS changes might also be reflected in alterations in some of the parameters utilized.

The importance of the reticular activating system in relation to "level" of CNS responsiveness was first reported by Magoun and his group in 1949 (11). Since that time there has been considerable data supporting this concept; these were reviewed in two recent symposia (12, 13).

In addition, there are incontrovertible evidences that the limbic system (rhinencephalon) is cross-linked with the reticular activating system and, to a large extent, controls the autonomic display of emotional changes.

It is expected that each bioelectric parameter employed will yield neurophysiological data from the very dimension it measures; but, in addition, we anticipate the cross analysis of two or more of these parameters to yield new "correlates" not detected heretofore.

The most direct means to detect the brain's electrical activity is by definition electroencephalography. If useful information is to be derived, real-time processing of the data becomes of prime importance. A new method of analysis described by Riehl, *et al.* (1960) appears promising (17).

The usefulness of basal and galvanic skin resistance as indices of consciousness and emotional reactions is well documented (14, 15). Burch correlated "fatigue" and changes in nonspecific portions of galvanic skin resistance, which suggested to him a decompensation in the neurophysiological mechanism.

Blood pressure recording is a *sine qua non* condition for significant electroencephalographic recording and, when correlated with heart rate, respiration rate, and skin temperature, may yield additional data to assess CNS reactivity. Baker and Taylor (16) reported significant relationships between skin temperature, skin resistance, and pulse rate, in relation to the arousal response. In addition, the value of muscle tonus as an indicator of activity of the reticular formation should be examined.

REFERENCES

1. Simons, D. G., MANHIGH II. Holloman AFB Technical Report, AFMDC TR-59-28, June, 1959.
2. Simons, D. G., Pilot reactions during MANHIGH II balloon flight, J. Avn. Med., 29:1–14, 1958.
3. Simons, D. G., Observations from the MANHIGH II balloon capsule at 30 kilometers, in *1957 Proceedings*, VIII Int'l Astronautical Congress, Barcelona. Vienna, Spring-Verlag, 1958.
4. Simons, D. G., Psychophysiological aspects of MANHIGH, Astronautics, 4:32–34, 1959.
5. Simons, D. G., Personal experiences in high altitude flight, Am. J. Psychiat., Feb., 1960.
6. Simons, D. G., MANHIGH. Doubleday, 1960.
7. MANHIGH III, Holloman AFB Technical Report, in publication.
8. Hauty, G. T., Psychophysiological problems of manned space flight, in *Lectures in Aerospace Medicine*. School of Aviation Medicine, Brooks Airforce Base, Texas, 1960.
9. Livingston, R., Reticular Formation of the Brain: An International Symposium, Detroit, Mich., Henry Ford Hospital, 1958.
10. Granit, R., and B. Kaada, Influence of stimulation of central nervous structures on muscle spindle in cats, Acta physiol. Scandinav., 27:130–160, 1952.
11. Magoun, H. W., and G. Moruzzi, Brain stem reticular formation and activation of the EEG, Electroenceph. Clin. Neurophysiol., 1:455–473, 1949.
12. Delafresnaye, J. F., ed., Brain Mechanisms and Consciousness. Chas. Dumas Co., 1954.
13. Jasper, H., ed., Reticular Formation of the Brain. Little, Brown Pub. Co., 1958.
14. Burch, N. R., and J. H. Greiner, Drugs and human fatigue: GSR parameters, J. Psychol. 45:3–10, 1958.
15. Burch, N. R., and J. H. Greiner, A bioelectric scale of human alertness: concurrent recordings of the EEG and GSR, Psychiat. Res. Rep., 12:103–193, 1960.
16. Baker, L. M., and W. M. Taylor, The relationship under stress between changes in skin temperature, electrical skin resistance and pulse rate, J. Exper. Psychol., 48:361–366, 1954.
17. Riehl, J. L., *et al.*, Quantification of the EEG-activation response: effects of atropine, Acta psychopharm., 1:200–209, 1960.

Project Excelsior: Personal Experiences in High Altitude Escape Situations

JOSEPH KITTINGER

Project Excelsior was commenced in November of 1959 at Holloman Air Force Base, sponsored by the Aerospace Medical Laboratory, Dayton, Ohio, and directed by Colonel John Paul Stapp. The purpose of the project was to conduct research concerning the physiological actions and reactions of a man from a high-altitude escape situation.

For this project we were required first to solve the problem of a protective device—an adequate pressure suit. The selection that we made was the standard Air Force MC3 partial pressure suit. The reason was that this pressure suit then afforded, and still does, the highest degree of mobility for the subject, which is a problem area in itself. The pressure suit tests that were conducted in the chamber at Wright Air Development Division were conducted with all of the present pressure suits, and the highest degree of mobility and protection for the duration of the mission was obtained by using this partial pressure suit. The clothing was necessarily bulky because of prolonged exposure to cold temperatures. The ascent takes between one and one-half and two hours, and the temperatures, of course, decrease considerably. We hoped originally that we would not have to heat electrically any part of the equipment that the man would wear. We soon found out that, since the man was inactive, we had to add heated gloves and socks in order to protect him against the cold. The cut-off point, I might add, for the extremities was plus 40° Fahrenheit, so we did have electrically heated gloves and electrically heated socks. The rest of the body clothing remained unheated.

Captain Kittinger is attached to the Aerospace Medical Laboratory, WADC, Wright-Patterson Air Force Base, Dayton, Ohio.

The total weight of the equipment was 155 pounds. The cables were collected into a neat bundle on the side, and all in all, considering the job we had to do, I feel that the rig was fairly clean. The kit contained physiological monitoring, a fourteen-channel recorder for heart rate, respiratory rate, accelerometers, etc. One of the problems that we ran into, and I think it still exists, was the need for sensors, physiological sensors, for the man. They work in a laboratory or with a subject in a dormant state, but if you have a subject who is moving about doing any exercise at all, there go the physiological monitors, sensors. If you get a sensor that is effective, then it is uncomfortable for the subject. For prolonged duration this is certainly an area in which we had some difficulty. The sensors were on the man, with this information being recorded in the kit, and of course we had the oxygen equipment, batteries, etc., mounted in the kit.

Some unexpected problems were encountered on our first jump, and we have a most interesting record in the moving pictures taken by the kit camera during the free fall. Because of a procedural malfunction after stepping out of the gondola, the parachute prematurely deployed. Because of inadequate velocity, the parachute wrapped around my neck and, instead of being a stabilized free fall, it became unstabilized chaos. The device that eventually achieved stabilization was the full, free multistage parachute that was designed to get a man down safely from a high altitude. We already knew that free fall from a high altitude presented a serious problem because of auto-rotation, and we had recorded rates as high as 200 RPM on dummies falling from altitudes of 70,000 feet. The physiological limit for humans is generally assumed to be around 140 RPM through a horizontal axis. My fall took a total of three minutes, and the maximum velocity obtained was 623 feet per second at about 40,000 feet. We used two hours of brief reading, 100 percent oxygen, and this was used for all of our chamber flights and of course for the actual flight as well.

We did not use a vent suit with this pressure suit device, so you can well imagine the heat problem that we had on the ground. The serious heat problem begins when you put the helmet on, so we deferred putting the helmet on until about 20 minutes before takeoff. Because one begins to sweat after the helmet is placed on the head, there was a minimum of activity. The stopwatch and altimeter were mounted on my left wrist, so that I could watch the rate of progress down.

The balloon was the lifting device, and I might point out that it greatly complicated the program because of the inherent problems associated with a balloon launch. If we could have done it with an aircraft, it would have saved us an awful lot of trouble. This gondola was an open gondola which Colonel Simons had built out at Holloman. Several years ago we used it for manned balloon flights at low altitude for training, and we just took it and cut a side out of it to make a high-altitude fighter out of it for our jump program. The rate of ascent was about 1,000 feet per minute. Dr. Blanchard was our medical monitor on the ground, and I talked to him every 5,000 feet and gave him my progress as I was going up. He was monitoring my heart and respiratory rates during the ascent, and they remained fairly steady. The heating for hands and feet was used continuously above 20,000 feet; there was also automatically controlled face-plate heat with an exhalation valve. My knees became cold, particularly on the second jump, and we discovered that when the legs were stretched out and were not compressed the cold spot around the legs and knees disappeared. My right hand, which was used continually on the button of the kit transmitter, got very cold. My left hand was in a little muff, and when the heated glove was kept in the muff there was no difficulty with cold, even though the outside temperature gets rather cold at that altitude.

On the second jump, in contrast to the first, I had stability, and it was a much more interesting and enjoyable way down. On the first jump, the first 'chute was set to open 16 seconds after I stepped out of the balloon, but it actually opened after two and one-half seconds and, as a result, I had no velocity. On the second jump I had a free-fall time of about 17 seconds, so that when it came time for the multistage first 'chute to open I had a velocity of about 512 feet per second—enough to keep the 'chute deployed on the second jump. This time the auto-rotation was around through the vertical axis at a very slow rate. I was able to control this by sticking my arms and legs out, and it was rather like riding a motorcycle down the road for four minutes, which was the time of the free fall.

On that hazardous first jump I was quite fortunate in that, when I stepped out of the gondola, I ended up facing squarely down to the earth. Of course, by stepping off I had zero velocity, and it was a most odd sensation. I want to assure you I have never felt anything quite like it—and I flew for four years at Holloman on the zero gravity program in T-33's, 89's, and 94's, so I have had a bit of experience in zero gravity. But when I was looking down at the earth, facing straight down at it, it was a very odd sensation; I was weightless, we will say, but I felt as if I were in a state of suspended animation. "What in the world is happening? I'm sitting up here, but I'm not falling." That was the sensation I had. I had no acceleration, no movement, heard no noise, nothing. It was absolutely quiet, absolutely still, and absolutely horrifying. This rapidly changed, of course, as I picked up speed and started turning.

After I had stepped out, looked down, gone through this transition period of being face down to the earth, and then started accelerating, I felt a pop. I said, "This isn't supposed to be, because my time has just started." I knew that the parachute would open or that something would happen. I ended up, on my back, head down to the earth, tumbling pretty rapidly. Then I started turning a little bit, and I stopped it by kicking my feet down and dropping my arm. This wasn't so bad, but then I went a little bit further and started turning again. I stuck my arm down, stopped it. This was easy, but about that time the boom was lowered and I started spinning very rapidly. I looked down at the rip cord of my parachute. I was tempted to pull it, but I didn't. If I had, I wouldn't be here now. I was at a very high altitude, and the shock of opening a 'chute at high altitude keeps it from being habit forming. Here my previous training was invaluable. Through this, and through a lot of luck and the great White Father looking over me, I was able to resist the temptation to pull that rip cord to stop my fantastic turning.

By this time, I had come to the point where I couldn't even pull my arm in to get the rip cord. The auto-rotation, with a CG right through the pelvic region, literally pulled my arms from me. I couldn't move my legs at all, and very rapidly I got black—gray first, lost peripheral vision, and then the shades came down. It was identically the same sensation to me as was a blackout in an aircraft. Everybody tells me I redout, but to me there was no difference in sensation. It was black. It got just as black as it does in an airplane when you're pulling g's.

I remained in this condition until the parachute opened—the automatic parachute which was reserve. I feel quite sure that the reason Colonel Boynton was killed 17 years ago in a drop was because he was probably unconscious at the time when he should have been pulling the rip cord. I'm sure of this because I was completely confused, disorientated, out of this system when it came time for me to pull that rip cord, and if I had not had an automatic reserve I wouldn't be here today.

Project Excelsior is half through. We have a couple more jumps scheduled, these from about 100,000 feet. I am confident that we can recover a man from above 100,000 feet, using this kind of closed pressure suit system.

Biotechnological Problems and Achievements

PAUL A. CAMPBELL

When one examines progress curves, chronologically plotted, of almost any of the parameters of space flight, one cannot help but notice that in many, many instances the curves are exponential in character. As is well known, such curves are attributed to accumulations of bits and pieces of knowledge piled one upon the other in time sequence; then, in the same time sequence, the accumulations pile upon accumulations. Still later new facilities, better communications between the people involved, new knowledge from other disciplines, and other factors join rapidly to increase the size of the rising pyramid.

One has to examine only a few such curves to gain the impression that we are in the early stages of a new scientific renaissance, comparable possibly to the historical periods of the late 1400s to the early 1600s, during which the achievements of Columbus and his contemporaries, and the thinking of Copernicus, Kepler, Galileo, and others initiated an era of very great change, adventure, discovery, invention, and accomplishment. As proven historically, these events rapidly changed the course of the affairs of the world and changed the Dark Ages into an era of enlightenment.

Among the scientific advances which are spearheading man's rapid progress toward space flight are those of biotechnology—the technics by which the processes of biological life and their interactions with their environment are assessed and necessary protection afforded. Included in the biotechnological sciences are: bioinstrumentation, recording technics, telemetry, monitoring, data processing, and the developments or alterations of the required environments or other situations which occur.

Thus a new science has developed and has been fitted to the needs

Colonel Campbell is Assistant to the Commander (Advanced Studies), USAF Aerospace Medical Center, Brooks Air Force Base, Texas.

of the man-in-space program. The contingencies of the miniaturized environment of the vehicles has required miniaturization of the components of the systems. The inherent difficulty of resupply and maintenance of man in space have required a degree of reliability never before achieved. The hostility of the new environment and the magnitude of the stresses to which the occupant of a space vehicle is subjected require new methods and greater degrees of protection than considered necessary in the past.

Of interest, much of the new knowledge has application outside the space sciences and will not only benefit the man in space but will also make better the life of the mundane creatures who must stay behind. When the cost of the man-in-space effort in terms of resources and energy are finally tabulated against the record achieved, the balance will be on the credit side of the ledger and will be in terms of knowledge—the greatest and most permanent of all resources.

The studies which follow point out some of the knowledge which has been gained by progress, thus far, and some of the problems of the future.

Sensory-Physiological Aspects of the Space Flight Situation

HUBERTUS STRUGHOLD

The situation encountered in space by man is the result of the strange physical environment, per se, and the process of movement to, through, and return from this environment. In my discussion I would like to confine myself to a sensory physiological analysis of human performance during the state of weightlessness, the most characteristic feature in motion dynamics in space. This has been studied in a free fall (1; see also the paper presented by J. Kittinger at this symposium), on a zero-gravity tower (11), and, especially, during parabolic flight maneuvers, a method suggested ten years ago (6, 9).

Thousands of such parabolic flight maneuvers in two-seated jet aircraft and in larger aircraft, during which the state of weightlessness can be produced for maximally one minute, have shown that sensory motor performance is not noticeably disturbed (7, 8, 15, 20). At first glance this seems to be surprising, since weightlessness is an extraterrestrial, exotic condition; a detailed examination of the various sense organs involved or not involved in sensory motor performance gives the answer.

The human body is equipped with several sense organs which inform us about, and exert reflex control upon, the equilibrium of our body as a whole, at rest and in motion; they also inform us about the position and movement of the limbs. The nerve endings in question react to mechanical forces or stimuli; they are therefore referred to as mechanoreceptors. Those mechanoreceptors responding to stimuli, which are related to the gravitational force of Earth, are called gravireceptors or graviceptors, in the physiological

Dr. Strughold is Professor of Space Medicine and Advisor for Research, USAF Aerospace Medical Center, Brooks Air Force Base, Texas.

literature (19). This term is acceptable, not in that we are able to sense gravitational field forces, but rather in that we can perceive weight, a physical attribute of matter resulting from gravitational forces. In the publications dealing with this kind of sensory nerve endings, the gravireceptors of the centrally located labyrinth, or, more precisely, of the otolithic portion of the vestibular organ (contained in the bony cavity of the inner ear), are discussed primarily. In contrast, little attention is given to those mechanoreceptors or gravireceptors which are found in the skin, in the skeletal muscles, and in the connective tissue (2, 3, 13, 16, 17).

These three peripheral (extralabyrinthine) gravireceptors, their physiological function under normal gravitational conditions, and, finally, their function under the condition of zero gravity as it is encountered in space flight, therefore, will be the center of this discussion.

1. The best known peripheral mechanical sense organ is that of the pressure or touch sense of the skin, responsible for the so-called tactile and pressure sensations. The nerve endings are nervous plexuses around the hair follicles and the Meissner corpuscles in the skin of the tactile surfaces such as the palms and the soles. The density of these presso- or tangoreceptors is about 20 per cm^2 on the hairy skin and more than 100 per cm^2 on the palms and soles, totaling altogether more than half a million (5).

The adequate stimulus for these sensory nerve endings is not pressure as such, but rather a change in pressure resulting from a mechanical deformation of the skin.

The pressure sense nerves show rapid adaptation; after fractions of a second or a few seconds, the sensation fades, so that slight changes in the pressure at the same skin area will elicit new sensations.

With a reaction time of about 160 milliseconds the pressoreceptors play an important role in the perception of the position and movement of our limbs and of the whole body (walking, etc.). During swimming, water resistance evokes pressure sensations in the skin. In flying an aircraft, the importance of the pressure sense lies in the sensations produced in the skin contact with the seat, giving information about accelerations in curves and up-and-down movements to which the body is passively subjected. Its importance for active movement lies primarily in handling the controls of the aircraft. In most of these functions the pressure sense is associated with two other sensory mechanisms, the muscle sense and the posture sense.

2. The receptors of the so-called tension sensation of the muscles perceived during passive and, especially, active movements are the so-called muscle spindles, found in all those muscles which fixate and move body masses, especially in those of the limbs. They are not found in the diaphragma or the eye muscles, the functions of which have nothing to do with gravity. The muscle spindles inform us of our body weight and of the weight of objects resulting from gravitation and accelerations. They also serve as receptors of the myotatic reflexes such as the patellar reflex, etc. They are, therefore, the receptors of a gravi-sensory system and, at the same time, of a gravi-reflex system.

3. Besides the pressure sense of the skin and the tension sense of the muscles, there is a third peripheral component in the senso-motoric control of our body and its parts: the so-called posture sense (4, 5), which has probably some relationship to the postural reflexes described by R. Magnus (12). The nerve endings are in all probability the Pacinian corpuscles which are found at strategic places throughout the connective tissue surrounding and penetrating the muscles. They may be stimulated mechanically, when the muscles change their form during the movement. These nerve endings, which are also found in the peritoneum, are large enough to be seen with the naked eye, but their specific function has been somewhat overlooked. The reason may be that, in contrast to the muscle sense and, especially, the pressure sense, the excitations of the posture sense receptors do not fully exceed the threshold of consciousness; they remain more or less subconscious.

Thus the perception of the position and movement of our limbs seems to be thrice secured; namely, by the pressure sense of the skin, the muscle sense, and the posture sense. These three peripheral mechanical sense organs together constitute a functional system in the perception and sensomotoric control of position and movement of body parts. This peripheral, extralabyrinthine system forms, with the labyrinthine otolith organ, a larger functional unit, a statokinetic control system, and is in this way integrated in the process of the perception and sensomotoric control of the position and movement of the whole body.

Table 1. Mechanosensory Statokinetic Control System

Labyrinthine System	*Extralabyrinthine (peripheral) System*
Vestibular organ	Pressure sense
	Muscle sense
	Posture sense

In this latter function it is associated with the eye by nerve connection with the vestibular apparatus. Equilibrium and locomotion, therefore, depend on the coordinated functions of the mechano- or gravireceptors plus photoreceptors (orientation triad; 3, 17).

Not too many comparative histological data about the phylogeny of the peripheral mechanoreceptors are found in the zoological literature; however, what is known demonstrates in an impressive manner their function in the various environmental media.

The dominant creatures in the hydrosphere, the fish, possess on both sides of their body a long nerve, the so-called lateral organ, which is a highly developed mechanoreceptor device. It enables them to sense pressure waves, water currents, etc. This is the sensory part of their biohydrodynamics. Today we observe astounding fish-like performances by deep-sea divers, in which the peripheral mechanosensory nerves play an important role.

Birds possess nerve plexuses around the quills of the flight feathers and muscle spindles and also Pacinian corpuscles in the connective tissue of the wings, by means of which they sense the slightest atmospheric currents and air resistance, and which makes eagles, seagulls, and other birds masters in soaring. We find an approximation to this in human control of a glider plane. Pigeons are unable to fly when the posterior roots of the spinal cord, through which the sensory impulses from the skin and muscles of the wings are transmitted, have been bilaterally dissected, although their motor pathways are intact (19). This illustrates the importance of the sensory parts in their bioaerodynamics.

And now in space flight with no environmental resistance, man enters the realm of the laws of astrodynamics or celestial mechanics. In order to understand his sensomotoric performance during weightlessness let us briefly remember the general fundamental functions of our sense organs. They have an exteroceptive function as they react to external stimuli and inform us of the outer environment.

We speak of interoceptive or proprioceptive functions as they serve to perceive internal conditions, such as pressure, tension, position, etc. The exteroceptive sense organs, *par excellence*, are the eye and ear. Muscle spindles and Pacinian corpuscles are fundamentally proprioceptors. The labyrinth organ and the touch sense lie somewhere between these two extremes.

In the gravity-free state with gravitational stimulation absent, the exteroceptive function of the mechanoreceptors is eliminated; their proprioceptive function is not. Since the peripheral mechanoreceptors are predominantly proprioceptive, there is no reason why precision in performance of hands, arms, and legs should be disturbed. Numerous tests in parabolic flight maneuvers actually have verified this, as mentioned above. It is difficult indeed to see how the muscle sense, for instance, could be affected by zero gravity at all. In contrast, it lies in the nature of the design of the otolith organ, which is primarily responsible for the perception of position and locomotion of the whole body, that its function in both categories is eliminated in the gravity-free state. It follows, then, that its partner in position- and motion-control of the whole body, the eye, has to take over this function alone. Thus the photoreceptors are the only receptors that can furnish the astronaut the information about his position and movement in space. This is in sharp contrast to the life of the blind deep-sea fish which depend, in this respect, exclusively on their mechanoreceptors.

In any geocentric orbit, which is conceivable up to 1.5 million km—the extension of the earth's potential satellite sphere or gravisphere—there is physiologically no gravitational reference point and no gravitational geocentric feeling on the part of the astronaut. This feeling that he belongs gravitationally to the earth will return as soon as the space craft dips below 200 km, i.e., across the mechanical border of the atmosphere. There it gradually receives aerodynamic support, and with this, weight returns. At what fraction of 1g the sensation of body weight becomes noticeable, or what the threshold is for perception of weight, is a question which may some day be answered by returning astronauts.

This whole discussion is based on the assumption that man can tolerate zero gravity over longer periods of time. However, we are not yet sure of this because experimental data on man are still not available.

In case that zero-g cannot be tolerated over longer periods of time, we have to provide for artificial gravitation. The question is: how large or small a fraction of g is needed to overcome any disturbances and to give the occupants of the vehicle the necessary feeling of weight—in other words, to bring about a kind of gravitational normalization of life. This would be an interesting question for astronauts orbiting around the earth. Concerning extended operations; for instance, to the Moon or to Mars, it would be logical and practicable to reproduce, by means of rotation of the vehicle, the gravities found on these target celestial bodies; that is, 17 percent of 1g for the Moon and 38 percent for Mars.

Table 2 shows the period of rotation necessary to produce 1g at radii of 5, 10, and 20 meters (O. L. Ritter), and the respective values concerning Martian and Lunar gravity. It might be that these provisions are not necessary; that is, if zero-g over a longer period of time does not cause disturbances. But we in the medical sector of astronautics must be prepared for all possibilities.

Table 2. Artificial Gravity by Rotation

Gravity	*Radius (in meters)*	*Period of Revolution (in seconds)*
Earth: 1g	5	4.5
	10	6.3
	20	9.0
Mars: .383g	5	7.2
	10	10.0
	20	14.5
Moon: .165g	5	11.0
	10	15.6
	20	22.1

Another way to produce artificial gravity in a space craft is through slight continual linear acceleration by some kind of propulsion. With the present and foreseeable propulsion systems, however, the attainable gravity would be rather small, perhaps below the threshold for the sensation of weight. Yet, it would have great advantages insofar as it would shorten the duration of a trip to the neighboring planets tremendously. For instance, applying 1/100 of 1g continuously would shorten the time of a trip to Mars from about 9 months to 20 days, and the application of 1/10 of 1g would shorten it to 7 days (O. L. Ritter). This is the formula for interplanetary operations; namely, to change from a minimum-energy orbit to a minimum-time orbit which space medicine must suggest to astronautics. In this way many of the neurophysiological problems would be solved.

In conclusion, I would like to touch upon some misconceptions occasionally expressed in conversations and also in the astronautical literature. The first one is this: The orbiting of a vehicle around the earth is often described as a constant falling, and the opinion has been expressed that this might produce the nightmarish sensation of endless falling. If we consider the function of the otolith organ, we must come to the conclusion that this is not so. The astronaut will have the sensation of falling perhaps for only a few seconds when he enters the gravity-free state. Thereafter this sensation should cease, because the otoliths will have attained a new equilibrium. All of this means that falling in the physical sense is not necessarily associated with a lasting physiological fall sensation.

Another misconception is encountered occasionally. If a vehicle is in an elliptic geocentric orbit it increases its velocity coming from the apogee to the perigee. This means the vehicle is accelerated, and the opinion is occasionally expressed that during this phase of the trajectory there should not prevail a condition of zero-g, but rather a certain amount of weight should result. This is not the case, because the sum of all forces (gravitational and inertial) acting upon the vehicle and the body of the astronaut in any phase of the trajectory, outside of the aerodynamically effective atmosphere, is zero (14).

Finally, the state of weightlessness is often compared with floating in water, and the sensory and physiological effects are even identified. It is true that certain features are common to both states, but in other respects they differ. Considered from a sensory physiological point of view, this is the situation: During passive floating in still water, the pressure from the supporting water is evenly distributed over almost the entire surface of the body and, therefore, sensations from the pressoreceptors of the skin do not occur or remain below the threshold of perception. And, if the body has no foothold, tension sensations from the muscles of the legs are more or less absent. In contrast, when standing on solid ground or walking, the cutaneous contact area with the supporting medium is relatively small; the pressure stimulation per unit area of skin resulting from the body's weight is great, and pressure and muscle sensations, therefore, dominate the picture. The absence, during floating in water, of sensations from the peripheral mechanoreceptors may be one of the reasons which induces people to believe that the consequences of this situation are identical with those of the state of zero gravity.

In brief, during immersion in water, the surface forces acting upon the skin of almost the whole body are sensory physiologically ineffective. But (and here is the difference) gravity as a volume force acts, of course, upon the whole body, including the otoliths, a fact which gives the deep-sea diver the capability of orientation. In space flight, all the mechanoreceptors are eliminated, as far as their exteroceptive function is concerned. This is the main sensory physiological difference between weightlessness and floating in water (10).

REFERENCES

1. Armstrong, H. G., Subjective mental and physical reactions to a free fall in space, J.A.M.A., 105:1107–1110, 1935.
2. Bourbon, B., La Perception des Mouvements de nos Membres, L'Anée psychol., 18:33, 1912.
3. Campbell, P. A., Orientation in space, in *Space Medicine*, J. P. Marbarger, ed., Urbana, Univ. of Ill. Press, 1951.
4. Du Mesnil de Rochemont, R., Ueber eine dritte Komponente für die Wahrnehmung von Gliederbewegungen. Ztschr. f. Biol., 84:522, 1926.
5. Frey, M. von., Ueber die sinnlichen Grundlagen für die Wahrnehmung der Gliederbewegungen. Ztschr. f. Biol., Heft 5, 1926.
6. Gauer, O., and F. Haber, Man under gravity-free conditions, in *German Aviation Medicine World War II*, Vol. 1, Part VI, chap. G, pp. 641–644. Washington, D. C., U.S. Government Printing Office, 1950.
7. Gerathewohl, S. J., *et al.*, Sensomotoric performance during weightlessness, Astronautica Acta, 1:203, 1956.
8. Gerathewohl, S. J., and J. E. Ward, Psychophysiologic and medical studies of weightlessness, in *Physics and Medicine of the Atmosphere and Space*, Benson and Strughold, eds., pp. 422–434. New York, John Wiley & Sons, Inc., 1960.
9. Haber, H., and F. Haber, Possible methods of producing the gravity-free state for medical research, J. Avn. Med., 21:395–400, 1950.
10. Knight, L. A., An approach to the physiologic simulation of the null-gravity state, J. Avn. Med., 29:283–286, 1958.
11. Lomonaco, T., A. Scano, M. Strollo, and F. Rossanigo, Alcuni dati sperimentali fisio-psichici effetti delle accelerazioni e della sub-gravita previsti nell'uomo lanciato nello spazio, Riv. Med. Aeronaut., 20:363–393, 1957.
12. Mangus, R., Körperstellung. Berlin, Verlag J. Springer, 1924.

13. Ranson, S. W., and B. L. Clark. The Anatomy of the Nervous System. Philadelphia & London, W. B. Sanders Co., 1953.
14. Ritter, O. L., and S. J. Gerathewohl, The Concepts of Weight and Stress in Human Flight. USAF School of Aviation Medicine Report 58-154, Jan., 1959.
15. Simons, D. G., Review of biological effects of subgravity and weightlessness, Jet Propulsion, 25:209, 1955.
16. Skramlik, E. von, Psychophysiologie der Tastsinne. Leipzig, Akad. Verlagsgesellschaft, 1937.
17. Strughold, H., The mechanoreceptors of skin and muscles under flying conditions, in *German Aviation Medicine World War II*, Vol. 2, p. 994. Washington, D.C., U.S. Government Printing Office, 1950.
18. Trendelenburg, W., Pluegers Archiv für Physiologie, 1906, p. 1.
19. Tschermach-Seysenegg, A. von, Physiological Optics, Charles C. Thomas, trans. Springfield, Ill., 1952.
20. Von Beckh, J. J. A., Experiments with animals and human subjects under sub- and zero-gravity conditions during the dive and parabolic flight, J. Avn. Med., 25:235–241, 1954.

Psychomotor Performance and Nystagmus of a Macaca Mulatta during Missile Flight

CLOID D. GREEN *and* PEI CHIN TANG

Little Joe Number 1B provided data concerning certain aspects of the escape system proposed for use on the capsule in which a human will ride. A seven-pound female Macaca mulatta monkey, 13X, was a passenger in a bio-pack contained within the nose cone of the missile that was fired at 9:23 A.M. on 21 January 1960. It is the purpose of this paper to consider two particular physiologic parameters which were recorded during the flight. These are the psychomotor performance of the animal and the oculomotor movements.

The psychomotor test utilized was a shock avoidance task. The animal was required to monitor a cue light and break an electrical circuit by means of a switch when the cue light came on. Failure to perform this task produced a mild shock through electrodes applied to the ankles of the animal. In the event that the animal broke the electrical circuit by pulling the switch but did not then release the lever, which was spring-loaded, the animal was again stimulated. The subject was not shocked for overperformance. The requirements for a test of this type are detailed by Melching. Animals under physiological stress or suffering various impairments will frequently fail to work for a food reward and a negative-incentive apparatus becomes necessary. It was our belief that a similar situation might exist during missile flight.

The effects of different types of acceleration upon the vestibular apparatus of man and animals have been the subject of considerable

Dr. Green is Assistant Professor of Anesthesiology, University of Virginia, Charlottesville, Virginia. Dr. Tang is at the Civil Aeromedical Research Institute, Oklahoma City, Oklahoma.

investigation; however, the multiple factors present in a missile are not easily simulated in laboratory tests and since the occurrence of motion sickness or failure of visual tracking ability due to nystagmus would seriously impair a man's ability to function aboard a space capsule, this opportunity was used to record the animal's oculomotor movements during flight.

Surgically implanted electrodes consisting of stainless steel wire insulated with teflon were used. For the purposes of recording the vertical movements of the eye a bared portion of the stainless steel wire was sutured into the periosteum of the superior and inferior margins of the right orbital fossa. The insulated portion of the wire was then led subcutaneously to the occipital region where it was anchored to a buried teflon plate and then brought to the surface. Horizontal movements of the eye were recorded by the use of similar electrodes implanted at the lateral margins of the right and left orbital fossae and a single electrode implanted on the bridge of the nose which was used as a common ground. These leads were also anchored to the teflon plate and brought to the skin surface in the occipital region. The electrode pairs from each oculomotor parameters were capacitance coupled to a Taber 202G-4 transistorized A.C. amplifier. By the use of this system clearly diagnostic patterns of nystagmus could be produced by rotating the animal at .5 to 3 revolutions per second on a spin table. This system did not, of course, give us information as to eye position.

The records obtained on the Little Joe flight may be divided into the phases described below. First, the pre-flight period, starting with the first monitoring following final sealing of the bio-pack up to the time of launch. Second, the launch phase, occupying 29.8 seconds from the moment of ignition of the rocket motors up until the activation of the escape system. Third, the escape phase, from the moment of escape rocket ignition to the time of drogue chute cover release, a period of 28 seconds and containing the event of tower separation 21.9 seconds from the start of this phase. The final period can be termed the flight completion phase and covers that period of drogue parachute controlled fall and main chute deployment at 183.35 seconds or 125.55 seconds from the beginning of this phase. Impact on the ocean 456.88 seconds after the beginning of this phase completes the flight. Data is also available after impact.

The first requirement for psychomotor performance began at minus two minutes when the bio-pack equipment was turned on for approximately 10 seconds. The record clearly shows one cue light, followed by shock for nonresponse and response. After an additional $4\frac{1}{2}$ seconds, the cue light again came on. At this point the equipment was turned off. This short period of activity was placed here to awaken and alert the animal and give her time to become oriented before the regular workload started.

Sixty seconds prior to launch the bio-pack equipment was again turned on. The animal's performance during the following minute was erratic and considerably below the standard during training periods. The cue light came on 12 times, and the animal was shocked 10 times for nonresponse. In each instance she reacted in less than .5 seconds with a lever-pull response, and in 8 instances she responded by lever pull at least once in the absence of cue light. In one instance she responded to shock by holding the lever down, and after $1\frac{3}{4}$ seconds she was stimulated for this by an additional shock. On only two occasions did she respond to the cue light by lever pull before shock was applied.

This animal, 13X, had been prepared by psychomotor training over approximately a one-year period. This had included prolonged restraint with periods of performance and also training on the centrifuge. On the centrifuge, the animal was enclosed in a flight type bio-pack; the g loading was increased in successive runs until the animal was performing through a five-minute run to 8g without missing a single cue light. That is, during the run the animal was never stimulated for failure to perform or for hold down of the switch. Although it is possible that the 21 hours of restraint, the atmospheric and temperature alterations, had impaired the psycho-physiological aspects of the animal, I feel, in view of the high level of performance during the latter part of the flight, that the animal was simply inattentive and perhaps quite sleepy. Further, the last 20 seconds prior to launch show a higher level of performance than the 40 seconds at the beginning of our one-minute pre-flight period. The last 20 seconds prior to launch contained both of the responses to cue light without shock, and the three shocks which occurred are of an average of .26 seconds duration. In addition, the first 40 seconds contained the instance of stimulation for holding down the lever.

It is not the purpose of this paper to discuss the acceleration forces generated by the missile, but to consider the sum total of influences on the animal's performance and, particularly, to discuss the correlation of nystagmus with performance decrement. We will, therefore, summarize the events of acceleration by stating that the animal was subjected to an initial positive 10g force followed by a decrease to about 3.5g in 2.5 seconds of flight. Acceleration then decreased gradually, reaching 1g at 25.7 seconds of flight and becoming negative at 26 seconds. The g forces dropped to approximately minus 2 just prior to the activation of the escape system at 29.8 seconds.

During this half-minute period of acceleration there is evidence that the animal's performance was seriously impaired. The cue light came on just at the moment of lift off and was immediately cancelled by lever pull. The construction of the lever was such that a loading of positive 10g would not automatically trip it, however, it is likely that the weight of the animal's hands resting lightly on the lever and suddenly increased in weight by ten times was responsible for the lever pull rather than a meaningful response by the animal. The record further indicates that the lever was held down because stimulation for lever hold down begins $1\frac{1}{2}$ seconds later and continues for nearly $1\frac{3}{4}$ second. Release of the lever at this time, that is, at approximately $3\frac{1}{4}$ seconds, corresponds to a fairly steady acceleration of about 3g. The lever was again pulled however in just .13 seconds and in approximately $1\frac{1}{2}$ seconds the animal was again stimulated for lever hold down. This series of events was repeated until the animal had been stimulated a total of eight times for lever hold down during the first 27 seconds of flight. The shortest period of shock was approximately one-third of one second, which occurred just prior to the longest period of shock, 7 seconds. The termination of the 7-second stimulation period was coincidental with the termination of positive gravity loading as acceleration moved from positive to negative. At $28\frac{1}{2}$ seconds, $1\frac{1}{4}$ seconds before the escape phase of the flight, the cue light came on for the first time since lift off. The loading at this time varied from a negative 1g to negative 2g. Since this phase of the flight terminated here, it is impossible to state whether the animal was becoming adjusted and ready to start an organized type of work or whether the release of the lever long enough to allow the operation of the cue light occurred purely because of the disappearance of positive g. It does, however, seem significant that during this period of stress, 13X retained her grip on the performance lever and was not so disorganized or panicked as to lose this final tie to her conditioned reflex pattern.

If we now consider the oculomotor movements, we see that there was no evidence of nystagmus during the pre-flight period. The eyes were very stable except at the moment when the animal was performing the psychomotor response. There is moderate vibration evident in all leads during the acceleration phase. However, horizontal eye movements, it can be determined, were practically lacking. There were vertical eye movements during the entire accelerative phase but none of these movements appear to have been of a nystagmic type. It is likely that the animal would have been able to perform visual tracking during the entire accelerative phase of flight.

Immediately upon activation of the escape rocket, the record of the oculomotor movements becomes unreadable for 2 to 3 seconds, probably due to violent motion or vibration of the capsule. Thereafter, from plus 32 to plus 66 seconds, the record contains definite evidence of nystagmic eye movements in both the horizontal and vertical planes at rates varying from 2 to 4 seconds. Pylon separation and opening of the drogue chute at 57.8 seconds appeared to increase the rate of nystagmus.

At the beginning of this period the animal was subjected to a positive 11g in the longitudinal axis of the capsule. This dropped in less than 1.5 seconds to a negative 6g. Simultaneously, 13X was undergoing a positive 4.5 to negative 3.5g variation in the transverse axis. Ten seconds from the time of escape-rocket firing the capsule is at less than one g loading in any parameter, and this condition persists for approximately 20 seconds.

The nystagmus then persists until after the opening of the drogue chute, when some g loading in the longitudinal axis of the capsule returns. The increase of nystagmus at the time of drogue chute deployment which ended the period of uncontrolled flight might be compared to the sudden increase of nystagmus which accompanies sudden stopping of a spin table.

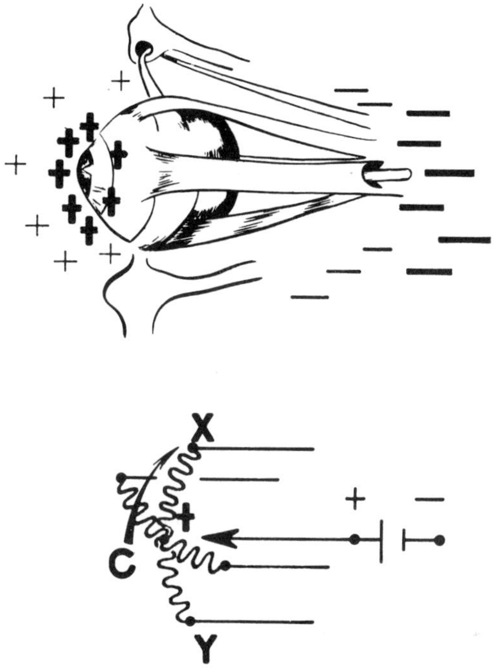

Figure 1. A: Distribution of Eye Polarity Potentials; B: Two-Directional Potentiometer Analogue

The distribution of eye polarity potentials can be compared to a two directional potentiometer. Movement of the midpoint C (the most positive point) toward a peripheral point, X, will cause X to become positive in relation to Y. Appropriately placed electrodes can detect these alterations.

The cue light was on at the time the escape rocket was activated and shock begins .15 seconds later. The switch was thrown in approximately one second, but shock for hold down of lever began $1\frac{1}{2}$ seconds later. The lever was held down for an additional $1\frac{3}{4}$ seconds and then released. The animal now apparently relinquished her hold on the psychomotor performance lever $35\frac{1}{2}$ seconds after flight started and did not take up performance again for 29.5 seconds.

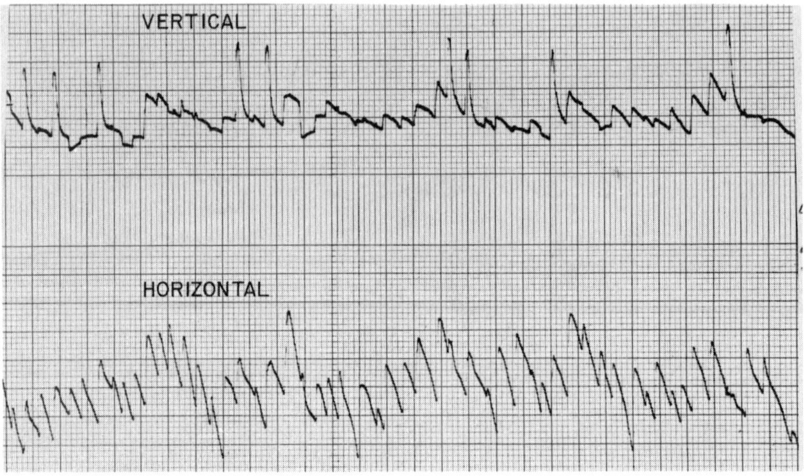

Figure 2. Record of Oculomotor Movements of Macaca Mulatta during Spinning

Pattern diagnostic of nystagmus, i.e. rapid movement of the eyes in one direction followed by a slow recovery in the opposite direction.

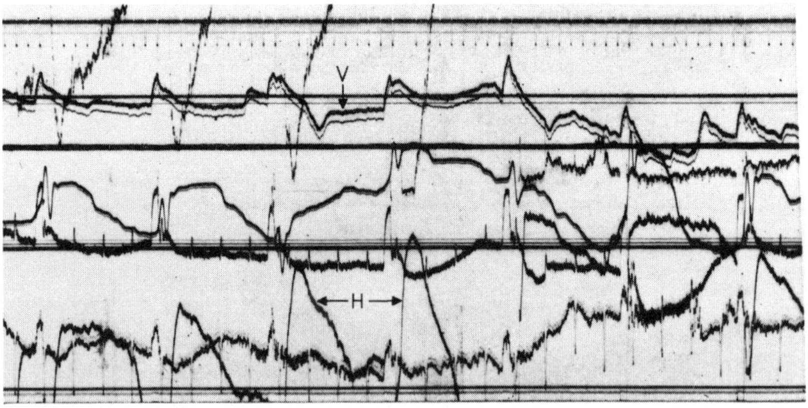

Figure 3. Pattern Diagnostic of Horizontal (H) and Vertical (V) Nystagmus in a Macaca Mulatta; Record Obtained during Missile Flight

It may be coincidental that the animal simultaneously regained the ability to return to psychomotor performance work at the same time that nystagmic eye movements disappear from the record. As stated above, this is approximately 6 seconds after opening of the drogue chute.

At 66 seconds, the animal took up performance and worked rapidly for 17 seconds when she was again shocked for lever hold down. In the next 10 seconds she was shocked twice for lever hold down, and then once for nonperformance. The oculomotor record indicated that the eye movements for the most part were of a slow rotary motion; however, nystagmus did occur at 77, 80, 90, 114, and 132 seconds. It was not until the complete disappearance of nystagmus that the animal's performance record improved to a level close to that ordinarily seen in the laboratory. By 135 seconds she appeared well adjusted to the workload and began to perform on signal from the cue light or slightly faster. At the moment of main parachute opening the performance again deteriorated for approximately 10 seconds, as shown by three occasions of stimulation for lever hold down. Thereafter, her performance was maintained at a high level.

At the time of capsule impact on the water at 521 seconds, the record was obscured for one second. From 522 seconds on, nystagmic eye movements were very marked for approximately 7 seconds and then were superseded by rotary eye movements. These rotary eye motions diminished gradually in amplitude and rate until the eyes became stable. During this period of nystagmic eye movement at the time of capsule impact, the animal increased her rate of performance. She did not lose her grip on the bar as she had done previously; she did not give way to panic. There is no information available to us concerning the force of water impact. The records suggest that the animal probably was momentarily stunned. However, like a well-trained boxer, her performance actually improved during this period of blurred cerebral function.

During the 516 seconds of equipment operation following impact 13X performed rapidly and well, usually on light signal, and received only eight very brief shocks. The high level of performance during this 8.6 minutes indicates that the animal suffered no persistent physiological deterioration as a result of the flight. We can conclude, however, that the multiple stresses led to performance decrement during the flight. No final conclusions can be drawn, but it would seem likely, from the record, that the animal would not have been able to perform a visual tracking test for at least the half-minute period following "escape." This period comprised the uncontrolled, near weightless portion of the flight, and during this time the only complete failure of psychomotor performance training occurred.

Simulated Space Flights

GEORGE R. STEINKAMP *and* GEORGE T. HAUTY

The psychophysiological aspects to be encountered in manned space flight are still subject to much conjecture. While it is true that some of the conditions of flight in this environment must await the actual performance in space, many valuable clues to the ability of crew members to adapt to these circumstances and retain their integrity as a vital element in the system can be gained with the use of laboratory vehicles. With some of these test vehicles, it is possible to achieve reasonable approximations of certain conditions likely to be encountered in manned space vehicles, particularly those designed for extended military missions.

Many of these measurements of the adaptability of the human organism to such situations can then be made, to serve the purpose of extrapolation to the actual flight profile. Experimental data have been collected under such test situations, and these indicate that, while he is a highly adaptable component in the manned space vehicle environment, the human presents certain limitations and expressions of individual capacity, which demand certain refinements and adaptations of purely mechanical construction such as to warrant special consideration of the design of the vehicle and the profile of the flight.

To test such a thesis, a group of experimental subjects has been exposed to certain of these simulated space environmental conditions in a laboratory vehicle called a space cabin simulator. In this, the degree of physical confinement is approximately 46 cubic feet, a constant exposure to one-half atmosphere pressure but with ground-level equivalent oxygen tension, deprivation of the usually accepted

Colonel Steinkamp is Chief, Environmental Health Division, Bureau of Aviation Medicine (FAA), Washington, D.C. Dr. Hauty is Chief, Psychology Branch, Civil Aeromedical Research Institute (FAA), Oklahoma City, Okla. The research described in this paper was conducted in the Space Cabin Simulator, Department of Astroecology, USAF School of Aviation Medicine, Brooks Air Force Base, Texas.

diet, experimental control of the diurnal cycling of work and sleep, and commitment to a schedule of attentive and meaningful work patterns that might be reasonably expected to be demanded in flight for true space vehicles.

The group of test subjects was selected on the basis of several factors:

(1) physical testing for good general health;
(2) psychiatric and psychological testing for stability and adaptability using present accepted criteria and methods;
(3) ability to become quickly familiar with all equipment;
(4) demonstration of past ability to adapt to stress; and
(5) demonstration of personal motivation to participate in potentially dangerous environmental conditions.

The basis for selection and the basic design of the equipment have been previously reported (1). As a general summary, it can be stated that each member of the group of test subjects was physically and mentally of high caliber. All had either worked for long periods with the equipment or adapted to it quickly by intensive indoctrination. Each of them had a dedicated approach to the experimental situation through his career objectives, and all demonstrated a desire to enhance or achieve added status within their working group or within the Air Force structure.

To simulate certain flight conditions and impose as great a physiological stress as possible, the protocol for the experiments included such things as a minimum of food and water, confinement to a cockpit type of seat allowing only minimum ability to move, and a requirement to attend constantly for 30 hours to a flight task which involved the functions of spatial discrimination, perceptual judgment, vigilance, and problem solving, with proficiency being electrically recorded (2).

The period of 30 hours was selected for two reasons: first, this period of time is required for a rigorous testing of circadian events and their possible sequellae; second, at some point in future time, manned orbital flights of this duration would seem to be inevitable. This schedule called for approximately six hours of pre-flight time during which the subjects were required to participate in instrument and equipment checks. At the end of this period all visual and oral contacts were discontinued; the cabin was placed at one-half atmosphere; a level of 84 decibels of constant noise was created by the equipment; and the subjects began attending intensively to the perceptual field of work presented on a small television screen. Every 90 minutes thereafter they were required to report on their condition to the monitoring crews, to simulate the passage over a tracking station. This test situation can be described as a "maximum effort–minimum support" effort. The subjects had the responsibility of staying awake, and even though all of them experienced short, varying periods of sleep, no attempt was made by the monitor to awaken them. At the conclusion of the experiment each subject was interviewed. Their evaluations of certain incidents and experiences are revealing:

1. On sleep: "I found that I was fighting boredom more than anything else. I went 'out' two or three times momentarily, but I was not conscious of being real sleepy, but I would catch myself coming out of these spells. Actually, it was a funny feeling because I wasn't aware of the fact that I was sleepy. Then I would seem to come out of a daze even though I didn't have the sensation of sleep." Another subject reported: "For the first day I tried to relax and conserve my energy for the next day, and I believe it did help. In the middle of the night I noticed that I sort of dozed. I closed my eyes and then looked up. It didn't seem that I had been sleeping. And then I still don't know what happened the next day about noon or afternoon. I missed a report. I don't know whether or not you tried to call me, but it seemed like I should have been doing something but I couldn't realize what. I don't know if I was asleep. I can't remember at all. I am just a blank." (The interval of sleep experienced by this subject was approximately 30 minutes duration.)

2. On aberrations: "The meters at times seemed to be something else. There were any number of things I could see in them. One time it would be an Indian face and the next time it would look like the face of a pig. Once the three meters became a wooden man with one meter his head, another his body and the other seemed to be his foot. The knobs that face the meters became the ears. Sometimes I could look at the meter and not see it, but at others I couldn't get rid of the image. For a while I noticed that the television screen seemed yellow with a brownish tint. I was pretty tired then and thought my eyes were deceiving me. When I became more awake,

I could see it but didn't look for it, and didn't pay any more attention to it. It did bother me at first." Another subject reported: "Possibly the first thing I noticed that was abnormal was the cavitation behind the main section of the cabin where I sat. It was somewhat deeper than I actually knew it was, and I realized this. The next thing I noticed was the dials. I could never really get them into focus and was never quite sure whether or not they were fluctuating. These three, I thought, resembled faces. At one time I thought it was the face of an Indian with a buffalo hood over him. I purposely forced my attention away from them because I realized that it was possibly a hallucination. But I remember looking back many times and thinking they were faces. The next thing I noticed was my feet. I looked down at my toes and thought they were probably six inches longer than I thought they were. But I noticed, too, that when I pulled them up to me they were the right size." A third subject reported: "On the radar pattern, I didn't see things there, but I would lose the presentation every now and then. If I stared at it too long, the only thing I got was a black and white contrast rather than having a clear presentation of the figures. But if I moved about and looked away from it, then when I looked back, I would have the clear presentation. On the dials, for some reason, it looked like it might be some type of savage all painted up on the face." A fourth subject reported: "There was a time when I heard voices. I believe that these voices that I thought I heard were singing voices. I felt there was someone in the cabin with me. I remember turning around once sharply and I thought somebody was perhaps moving there. I thought maybe it was a boat going by me." Still another subject reported: "I knew I was in my right mind except now and then I sort of let myself start daydreaming when I knew I should be at work. I remember I thought I was up in the barracks and it just seemed that I wasn't confined to the chamber." One subject had the sensation that a deep hole had opened up just beyond his feet. While he doubted his senses, he got down and felt the floor to make sure.

3. When asked about the validity of utilizing simulated flights as training devices, one subject made these comments: "I would definitely recommend the exposure to simulated conditions for prospective space candidates. I would ask for both this short and

also a longer exposure. There are a lot of people who do not know how they would react to such confined quarters for an extended length of time and being by themselves in a remote area. I realized that a lot of thoughts went through my mind but I feel better for it. I know that I can take confined quarters, and even though I might have irrational moments, I am stable enough so that I can think it out and rationalize as to what is going on and then make myself stable enough again before I start doing anything, rather than jumping at the first conclusion."

The physiological responses were similar in all subjects and appear to be the result of the combination of accumulative fatigue, sleep deprivation, lowered caloric intake, and mild dehydration. In general, their immediate condition following exposure to the test situation resembled the pattern found among convalescent patients. However, with adequate rest, and within a minimum of twenty-four hours, there was complete return to a normal sense of well-being (3).

Psychologically, all of the subjects experienced aberrations of some kind and in varying degree. It would be difficult to label these as true hallucinations as seen in psychotic states. The subjects recognized the illusions, visual, auditory, and proprioceptive, as being the product of their own minds. Despite this, however, these illusory experiences were deleterious for certain of the subjects as judged from changes in their operator proficiency. In fact, in the most extreme instance, one subject had to be removed from the simulator.

From findings such as these and from other data obtained from simulated space flights, certain implications can be drawn:

1. Pre-flight exposure to conditions provided by space flight simulators would appear to be a prudent and certainly a highly economical precautionary measure.

2. Of equal value are the gains to be realized from continued research with space cabin simulators.

Initially, the etiology of behavioral changes effected by unique conditions and their interactions can be more fully explored. Following this, the efficacy of indicated mitigative techniques can be appraised. And, from this, there will be realized greater predictability and enhancement of human reliability.

PART 2

Critical Problem Areas

Biomedical Aspects of Manned Orbital Flight

DONALD D. FLICKINGER

Project Mercury is a National Aeronautics and Space Administration project from which we are gaining considerable information which will have application in orbital flight. I think it is worthwhile very briefly to consider why are we attacking the problem of man's first adventure into space by means of a ballistic capsule. People who are not with the project frequently wonder why we do not use other means. For example, why don't we just put a bigger booster on the X-15 and put it up into orbital speed? Basically, the problem is one of accepting fairly severe dynamic loads that are inherent in boosting any kind of a package from zero to orbital velocity of 18,000 feet per second, and even more severe loads bringing it back down in an exchange velocity for heat and dynamic force. Realizing the tremendous gain that is possible in terms of leveling out decelerated forces of reentry with a lifting body, and even more with a winged body, the basic consideration is, what type of reliable vehicle do we have to put a man into orbital velocity speed?

Another problem is, what type of reliable propulsive force do we have for such an operation? Realizing that the only reliable propulsive force that can exert this amount of velocity on an orbital body is the Atlas, one must ask what amount of weight will this particular propulsive force put into a modest circumterrestrial orbit? Allowing for a reasonable margin of safety, in terms of fuel utilization and other aspects of the guiding system that have to do with accuracy of insertion angle, the load this reliable workhorse can put into orbit is in the vicinity of 3,000 pounds. This can be done, with all safety requirements for a single man, only if a ballistic shape is used. If even a slight lifting body were used, or a more exaggerated lifting glider-type of body, then the weight requirement would increase from 3,000 to 10,000 or up to 18,000 pounds. This, in a sense, is fortuitous,

General Flickinger is Assistant for Bioastronautics, ARDC, Andrews Air Force Base, Washington, D.C.

because in the areas that would have to be developed, in terms of a wing body going from what we know of mach 4 and mach 5 up into and through mach 20 and 25, there are tremendous numbers of unknowns that would have to be solved in relation to what we know now about the thermodynamics of ballistic reentry bodies. We have 3,000 pounds of ballistic body; between a quarter and a fifth of this weight is directly assigned to the man and his supporting and projective equipment. A good portion of it, of course, is the stabilization control, the inherent integrity of the structure itself, and ablation material to accept the high heats of reentry.

Project Mercury is an exercise designed to produce a steady progression toward development of the necessary knowledge and techniques. It is, I think, an exceedingly well thought out and well carried out program. It will include many tests of practically every aspect of the final orbital mission through a series of ballistic flights, both Regulus and Atlas, in the different configurations of pre-orbital mechanics and reentry mechanics by bearing the particular trajectory. These will go through a series of instrumented animal and then, finally, manned qualifications. By following this plan, we are able to flight-qualify the entire system, and also to gain something which is exceedingly important, second only to the reliability of the basic system, and that is the reliability of all of the support aspects, personnel, and procedures from the start right on through to search and recovery. Finally, we get to the typical mission profile, with the mechanics of launch, staging, orbital ejection, two to sixteen orbits, track communication, and, finally, landing and recovery. From a consideration of the entire mission profile, all of the energy dynamics and orbital mechanics involved, we can very easily extract the most critical, biomedical areas of this first orbital flight, the reliability of life-support system, questionable performance in weightless state, the problem of data return, safety surveillance in flight, and bioradiation effects.

All of us who have been working in this field are convinced that much of the old data that we developed has to be expanded markedly. In the past we have studied tolerance to g-forces in terms of very short-time emergency events—ejections, crash landings, and so on. This means that we predominantly were simply estimating to what degree we could shock the body and still have it show no irreversible injuries or, almost worse than that, how much we could submit the body to this kind of trauma and still have the body live. In space flight there is an entirely different situation in which we are not only worrying about irreversible injury, but we are primarily interested in how the man can perform. We must do a great amount of additional work, construct different types of simulators where we can get into many more translational forces than just a single linear or a single circular force.

The life support system of the Mercury capsule has a considerable amount of redundant safety without paying an excessive penalty in weight. It is a good, simple system, backed up with a pressure suit control system which is really the heart of the safety support. Even this has several areas of redundant safety.

I think a word on the problem of the life-support systems would not be amiss, because I personally think that this is one area where we need an immediate augmentation and expansion of our total efforts from basic research on one side to engineering tests on the other. I see the biomedical field as being the one area where we could very well lag behind the engineering and other physical signs developments that will provide the next jump, the next generation of man-space vehicles. I am very much concerned about this. The logistics in terms of space travel, in terms of the life-support system, are very real and very restrictive. You have to go in one of two directions. If you increase your payload, you have to increase your power supply of energy. (I simply include this to show that we are attempting basically to take an extremely efficient atmospheric energy catalectic system and put this into a hermetically sealed area in space. This, as you well known, is not easy. The other consideration is that when you get away from this infinite capacity of the Earth's atmosphere to accept tremendous variations and not have them have any immediate influence on the organism, when you convert this into all the factors of a capsule—the time, the temperature, the ionizing radiation, the g-stress, weightlessness, and of these intracapsular factors—you really have a major problem.

Accepting the facts that we will go ahead and we will have reliable life-support systems to support the individuals, our next greatest problem is to determine what we can expect from the human component in terms of performance. In the Mercury situation he has been assigned quite an extensive active role. As the project has gone on with the use of new types of simulators to determine how much the individual can do in three dimensional control, in terms of astrogation, and in terms of back-up within the time allocated to take care of the malfunction of an automatic system, I think the consensus of opinion is that the human component has turned out to be one of the most important factors contributing to the eventual success and safety of the total mission.

There are many new instruments and many new considerations from the standpoint of human engineering that have been put into this, and this is almost a separate in itself. Our ability to abstract meaningful data is of great importance from the standpoint of the man's own reaction, his capability to perform, his state of consciousness, his state of response to task requirements and to his environment, both intrinsic and extrinsic, as it is inferential in his particular situation. The task of medical monitoring, crew safety, and data recovery is the single most important aspect, and it is basically for this reason that NASA plans only three orbital flights for this first go-around. To provide the amount of monitoring on an orbital scale that would give the degree of safety required for 18 to 24 orbital flights would require so many more points of communication and control that it would be out of the question from an economic standpoint. These three orbital flights, giving us 90, 180, and 270 minutes away from Earth, will certainly be a tremendous drive forward into this whole area of manned space travel.

When the space age came upon us, much of the data that we had developed as a part of aviation medicine was directly applicable to the problems of the first manned orbital flight. Now, as the age of space exploration dawns, we see the need for the same state of progression of aerospace medicine, space biomedicine, or whatever this new area might be called. It needs to have its share of support, indefinitely into the future. When I say this I am not making a case for the military or civilian or any other type of organizational structure; I am talking about the future of our country. The time has come when we all must realize, those of us who have been in aviation medicine and those who are now joining its ranks, that we have a tremendous job ahead of us. Let's all join hands, exhibit good old American courage, and get on with the job.

Psychiatric Factors in Astronaut Selection

DON E. FLINN

Bring me men to match my mountains,
Bring me men to match my plains,
Men with empires in their purpose
And new eras in their brains.

"The Coming American," by Samuel Walter Foss

New frontiers have always demanded special qualities in the men who explore them. Today, on the brink of the so-called vertical frontier, this verse about our western frontier might be paraphrased—"Bring me men to match my missiles." For technical advances have made it possible for man to venture into regions more alien and hostile than any he has ever known. It does not matter that travel in space may some day be as commonplace as crossing the continent; the psychological demands that will be made upon the astronaut for some time to come can not be minimized. Nor is it sufficient to say that men have always been able to stand up to such challenges. Many have—some have not. In the initial stages of space flight, much will depend upon each mission, and every effort must be made to insure that the astronaut will be able to cope with his pioneering task. Human factors engineering will insure that the skills required in space flight will not be beyond human abilities. In this paper, our concern will be with problems of choosing individuals who can perform the required operations under all varieties of psychological stress that may be encountered.

Attempts to choose men with psychological characteristics which make them suitable for hazardous duty have been of recent origin. Even during the First World War, about the only psychological requirement for the would-be pilot was sufficient courage to fly the flimsy, erratic aircraft of the era. It soon became apparent that men

Colonel Flinn is attached to the Neuropsychiatry Branch, School of Aviation Medicine, USAF Aerospace Medical Center (ATC), Brooks Air Force Base, Texas.

with certain rather hard to define traits, such as practical intelligence, adaptability, and good judgment, were best suited for the occupation, but no attempt at psychologic assessment of pilot applicants was made during the war (1). During the 1920s a clinical psychiatric interview was introduced in the Air Corps as part of the pilot selection procedure, and it has continued in use, with modifications and refinements, until the present. Despite widely held doubts concerning its validity, no more objective substitute has yet appeared which seems able to assess complex personality characteristics such as motivation, attitudes, flexibility, maturity, and level of adjustment. In a recent review of aviation psychology in Western Europe (2), all but one of twelve reporting military and civilian air agencies noted specifically that a similar clinical interview was included in their pilot selection program.

In the circumscribed area of aptitude measurement, much progress has been made. With techniques developed during and since World War II, it is possible to measure the probability that an individual will develop the special skills required for piloting an aircraft. The current USAF selection battery predicts success or failure in primary flight training with a high level of accuracy. However, long-term adaptability to flying depends not only upon technical aptitude, but also upon complex factors such as basic emotional stability, motivation, and chance experiences in the life of the individual. Objective testing aimed at measuring predisposition to maladaptive responses to the stresses of military flying have shown some promise (3), but it is doubtful if a level of accuracy comparable to that achieved in aptitude testing can ever be expected. At present there is no substitute for the clinical psychiatric or psychological evaluation in judging over-all adaptability.

Astronaut selection differs in several important ways from the assessment problem described above. Space flight is so obviously an extension of aviation that, during the developmental phase, it is logical to consider only individuals who have already demonstrated their adaptability in military flying. It is said that submariners, arctic explorers, mountain climbers, and balloonists were considered as a source of candidates for Project Mercury, but it was decided that the skill and tolerance of psychological stress demanded of the test pilot most nearly approached the anticipated requirements of space flight. Test pilots would presumably already have undergone a more valid screening procedure in the course of their careers than any which could be artifically devised. For the present, the number of astronauts required will be small enough that they can be chosen from this select group, any one of whom could probably be expected to perform effectively, provided he had the necessary motivation. This does not mean that psychiatric selection is unnecessary, but only that its emphasis is changed. The task of assessment becomes one of identifying differences in a group of individuals who already possess highly developed skills and who represent the upper level of adaptability. Since the stresses of space flight cannot be fully known during the period when novel missions of increasing complexity are being undertaken, it is necessary to give an extra margin of safety by choosing from among the apparently qualified those who are most outstanding and who seemingly would have the greatest probability of success.

Even when such a select group is considered, it cannot be assumed with certainty that all its members are suitable, for while space flight may be similar to test piloting, it is not identical. The candidate needs to be assessed in terms of some of the differences which have been suggested by research. Further, man's ability to adapt to psychological stress changes with time and varies from one situation to another. Not infrequently flying personnel who have performed effectively under stressful conditions, including combat, develop emotional symptoms or maladaptive behavior at a later date under seemingly less stressful conditions. These situations can be understood only in terms of their meaning to the individual, and it is important to know of any such potentially troublesome areas in the astronaut.

It can be seen from the foregoing that the astronaut assessment program should be one which differentiates between high levels of adaptability to the stresses of military flight, considers the candidate in terms of psychological requirements that are relatively unique to space flight, and assesses basic personality stability in an attempt to predict maladaptive behavior. For convenience, each of these requirements may be considered separately. Reference will be made throughout to the Project Mercury candidate evaluation program, the psychiatric aspect of which was conducted at the Aerospace

Medical Laboratory, Wright Air Development Center (4, 5). To date, this has been the only reported astronaut evaluation program.

Basic personality stability can best be gauged by standard psychiatric interviews and projective psychological testing, which give information about perception of reality, energy level, amount and source of anxiety, prominent defense mechanisms, affective control, concept of self and others, flexibility of adjustment, and other such personality characteristics. During the Project Mercury evaluations, ratings were made on seventeen categories of personality characteristics. Clinical ratings of this sort are considered by many to be a highly unreliable procedure, but they do give an objective description against which later performance can be measured. However, for the purpose of assessing suitability it is not the specific traits themselves that are of primary importance, but rather their interaction, i.e., the "integration" of the personality. For this appraisal there is as yet no substitute for clinical judgment.

If the astronaut is to be fully effective and reliable, he must be free of significant emotional conflicts and anxiety. His task is not merely that of a human guinea pig who, on the appointed day, must tolerate the stress of a brief mission; he must also be able to work productively with others during the long and arduous preparatory phase, and after. Maladjustment in either the occupational, social, or marital sphere might insidiously undermine his morale and motivation for the project. Chronic anxiety from any source could lead to psychosomatic, neurotic, or behavioral symptoms which would mean the loss of the individual to the program. Among flying personnel, emotional symptoms which interfere with performance of flying duty are precipitated by mundane family pressures and disturbed interpersonal relationships far more often than by the stress of flying.

In appraising such complex factors there is no adequate substitute for clinical judgment. It must be acknowledged that brief psychiatric interviews have been disappointing when used to predict military performance under stressful conditions (6). However, the limitation has not been that potential failures could not be identified, but rather that many predicted failures did better than expected. In large scale use, this meant an unacceptable waste of manpower. But this situation is not comparable to the astronaut selection task, where small numbers must be chosen, from a relatively large pool. Here a high rejection rate can be tolerated in order to eliminate potential failures.

With regard to the personality characteristics required in the space traveler, facetious suggestions have been made that he should be a schizoid, a Yogi, an Eskimo, a race-car driver, a jockey, a psychotic, an underweight woman, or a worrier with so many problems with his job and family that one more would not matter. These suggestions seem to express a general attitude that there must be something rather odd about the individual who can tolerate traveling into space. A somewhat related general belief holds that it is the impulsive, mildly psychopathic, or deviant individual who does well in hazardous jobs. This general attitude was expressed by an experienced submarine medical officer who, when asked if he thought submariners should have normal personalities, said "Hell no; anyone who was normal wouldn't have anything to do with submarines." But despite this popular fancy, and certain spectacular exceptions notwithstanding, it is not the impulsive or psychopathic individual who does well under stress (6). Rather, it is the mature, well integrated, realistically motivated man who has a normal self-critical faculty, is capable of forming group identification and loyalty, and who has a minimum of dependency and immature, egocentric self-concern. But, of course, this is not to say that any normal individual could become a satisfactory astronaut. A complex array of innate abilities, developmental experiences, and personality characteristics have gone into moulding the pilot who has the abilities and, of equal importance, the motivation required for such a task.

It is important that a longitudinal study of these factors be carried out in connection with the present assessment program. At present we can afford the luxury of choosing astronauts from a select group with demonstrated adaptability, but eventually larger numbers will be required, and they will need to be chosen before an extensive training program is undertaken. If this is to be done reliably, we will be dependent upon information that can be gained only from a thorough study of the current astronauts, together with observations about future performance.

Given a basically sound individual, we need some measure of his tolerance to psychological stress similar to that encountered in high-performance flight. Some individuals react to sudden threat with disruptive behavior. This can be demonstrated experimentally or studied as it occurs naturally in disasters and emergencies. It is recognized for example, that operation of the aircraft ejection seat must be made as uncomplicated as possible if it is to be properly used during an in-flight emergency. But, even though its operation has been reduced to a few simple steps, fatal errors still occur among experienced pilots as a result of the disruptive psychological impact of an emergency. Some measure of an individual's ability to remain calm and behave appropriately under stress can be obtained by a review of his past flying experience. In addition, candidates can be observed during exposure to stressful experiences. In the Project Mercury program, observation of candidates during psysiological stress testing made such an evaluation possible under controlled conditions. This evaluation of the psychological response was considered to be the main value of stressful physiological tests, as there were no significant differences between those selected and those rejected in physiological response, per se. This type of evaluation should not be a one-shot affair. Some of the indoctrination and training the astronaut receives will combine various stresses and will more closely simulate actual mission requirements. Continuing observation during this time will serve as a further measure of adaptability.

Finally, the candidate must be evaluated with respect to the unique characteristics of space flight for which his past flying experience may not have served as an effective screen. Prior to experience with actual space flight, these remain speculative, but two items of probable significance will be mentioned. The first of these concerns the relative passivity required of the astronaut, compared to the operational pilot. During initial ballistic shots the astronaut will have no direct control over the flight, with the exception of over-ride control of the escape system. In subsequent orbital flights he will have over-ride control of a number of elements, such as capsule attitude and initiation of re-entry from orbit; but, if all goes well, his primary function will be that of monitor. Hence, he will rely upon external agencies, either automatic or human, to a much greater extent than in his past experience. Some pilots deal psychologically with the danger of their occupation by developing an attitude of invulnerability through confidence in their proficiency and ability to cope with any emergency that might arise. This psychological defense will be less available to the astronaut, since he must rely to a greater extent upon the judgment and ability of others. For an individual with an innate tendency to be overly critical or intolerant of the abilities of others, this situation may provoke considerably more anxiety or hostility than would otherwise be the case. Emotional reactions of this sort have been observed in seven-day runs with the SAM Space Cabin Simulator. A number of subjects have been alert to any real or fancied inefficiency or disinterest on the part of support personnel outside the chamber. Some reacted with suppressed resentment, while a few have expressed their anger overtly. These emotions impair motivation and increase the likelihood of intellectual and judgmental errors. Mature, self-confident subjects without projective tendencies should be more resistant to such emotionality, although we do not have sufficient data to support this presumption.

The psychological feature of space flight that has perhaps attracted most attention concerns the possibility that isolation and sensory deprivation may occur to a degree which would cause imagery, hallucinations, and impaired thinking similar to that seen in experimental studies. These studies will be discussed elsewhere in the symposium, and here we will only refer briefly to studies in the SAM Space Cabin Simulator. Under conditions which simulate as closely as possible a thirty-six-hour orbital flight with continuous monitoring required of the operator, many of the perceptual aberrations described experimentally have been seen (7). Under the combined stresses of confinement, restricted perceptual field and fatigue, illusions of body image, distortion of space and time dimensions, and hypnagogic-like imagery have occurred almost routinely. In a few subjects these have required termination of the flight. For example, one volunteer, non-pilot subject experienced severe anxiety which became intolerable after eight hours. Psychiatric evaluation showed how the confinement had interfered with the customary psychologic defenses he employed. Another subject, after twenty-two hours of flight, suddenly shouted that there was a fire inside the chamber, and believed he had seen the flame and smelled the smoke. He could not be reassured that this was not the case, and the flight had to be terminated because of his apprehension.

Emotional reactions and perceptual aberrations such as these would have serious consequences if they occurred during a mission. If man is to be a reliable component of the space vehicle, the extent of his tolerance to this type of psychophysiological stress must be understood, and individual differences in resistance must be appraised. The disruptive behavior shown by the first subject was correlated with unsatisfactory defense mechanisms which required an impulsive, reassuring contact with others. His vulnerability to a feeling of "aloneness" was apparent in his psychiatric evaluation. In the other subject, this aspect of the flight was not stressful. However, with the onset of misperceptions presumably related to the psychophysiologic affect of a restricted sensory input, the situation was restructured in his mind and became threatening. It is of interest that the illusions pertained to a mechanical aspect of the flight system, had a plausible content compared to the weird distortions reported by subjects in sensory deprivation experiments, and involved a potential hazard which he had previously anticipated; hence, the misperceptions were more "believable." This suggests the potential hazard during space flight of hallucinations with a commonplace content, particularly when they involve mechanical aspects of the flight system about which the astronaut may already have been concerned. The relationship of this type of imagery to personality variables has been investigated (8), and is reported elsewhere in the symposium. At present, it seems desirable to include a modified isolation experience simulating the features of the space flight environment as part of the selection process, as well as for its training value.

This survey of psychiatric factors in astronaut evaluation and selection has dealt only with current concerns and has left many problems untouched. The psychological demands of long flights extending into weeks, months, and years will be quite different from those of the early developmental period. While the outer-directed, action-oriented pilot with confidence in his psychomotor skills and a sense of satisfaction when they are challenged may be ideal for developmental missions and military operations, the tedium of longer, routine exploratory flights may be more tolerable to the individual with a higher potential for fantasy and inner satisfactions. The introduction of additional crew members poses interesting questions about interaction in small groups and the personality characteristics required for cooperative endeavors under such restrictive conditions. These and other related problems will be investigated in the SAM two-man Space Cabin Simulator. A sound research program must also include validation of present assumptions and of experimental data through observation of performance when actual space flights are made. Such a program will help insure that the men chosen have the best possible chance of coping with their demanding task—that they are indeed men to match their missiles.

REFERENCES

1. Burwell, R. R., Historical review of aircrew selection, in School of Aviation Medicine Aeromedical Review 1–58, pp. 4–7, Randolph AFB, Texas, 1957.
2. Parry, J. B., and S. D. Fokkema, eds., Aviation Psychology in Western Europe, Amsterdam, Swets and Zeitlinger, 1958.
3. Sells, S. B., Development of a personality test battery for psychiatric screening of flying personnel, J. Avn. Med., 26:35–45, 1955.
4. Ruff, G. E., and E. Z. Levy, Psychiatric evaluation of candidates for space flight, Am. J. Psychol., 116:385–391, 1959.
5. Wilson, C. L., ed., Project Mercury Candidate Evaluation Program. WADC Technical Report 59-505, Wright Air Development Center, 1959.
6. Glass, *et al.*, Psychiatric prediction and military effectiveness, U.S. Armed Forces M. J., 7:1427–1443, 1575–1588, 1956.
7. Flaherty, B. E., *et al.*, Psychiatry and Space Flight. Paper read at Detroit Divisional Meeting of American Psychiatric Association, 1959.
8. Goldberger, L., and R. Holt, Experimental Interference with Reality Contact; Individual Differences. Paper read at the Harvard Symposium on Sensory Deprivation, June, 1958.

Project Mercury: Astronaut Training Program

ROBERT B. VOAS

This paper gives a general outline of the NASA Project Mercury astronaut training program. Basic considerations which entered into the development of the program are listed. Six primary training areas are described, together with the training equipment and facilities which have been employed. Problem areas for future training programs are discussed.

INTRODUCTION

Any training program must be based on three factors: the nature of the job for which training is required, the characteristics of the men to be trained, and the facilities and time available in which to do the training. In Project Mercury the astronaut's job involves both flight and nonflight tasks. He is expected to contribute to systems design and to the development of operational procedures through his daily contact with the project engineers. It was considered that by virtue of the selection process the astronaut had the required skills to make these contributions; therefore, no training was attempted for these nonflight tasks. The astronaut's in-flight activities can be broken down into six areas: (1) "programing" or monitoring the sequence of vehicle operations during launch, orbit, and reentry; (2) systems management, the monitoring and operation of the onboard systems such as the environmental control, the electrical systems, the communications systems, and so forth; (3) the vehicle attitude control; (4) navigation; (5) communications; and (6) research and evaluation. In addition to these in-flight activities, the astronaut has a number of ground tasks connected with the flight operations. He has a role in the countdown and preparation of the vehicle, in communications from the

Dr. Voas is Training Officer, National Aeronautics and Space Administration, Space Task Group, Langley Field, Virginia.

ground to the vehicle, and in the recovery program following the flight. It is for these activities associated with the flight itself that a training program was undertaken. More detailed descriptions of the astronaut's tasks are available in papers by Slayton (1) and Jones (2). It should be noted that the astronaut's job is only one of many associated with space flight for which training is required. Brewer (3) has outlined the over-all training requirements for Project Mercury.

The astronaut selection program was designed to select individuals who would require a minimum of training in order to fulfill the Mercury job requirements. Particularly desired were individuals who had sufficient experience in aircraft development operations to make immediate contributions to the Project Mercury program. On this basis, the following criteria were adopted as the minimum requirements for qualification as a Project Mercury astronaut:

1. Age less than 40 years
2. Height less than 5 ft. 11 in.
3. Excellent physical condition
4. Bachelor's degree (or equivalent)
5. Graduate of test-pilot school
6. 1,500 hours flying time
7. Qualified jet pilot

Records of 508 Air Force, Navy, Marine, and Army pilots who had graduated from test-pilot school were reviewed and screened on the basis of these requirements. Of these, 110 met the seven basic requirements. Forty-one of these pilots were eliminated through further screening based on recommendations from instructors at the test-pilot schools. The remaining 69 pilots were interviewed and given an opportunity to volunteer for the Project Mercury program. Of these, 37 pilots either declined or were eliminated as a result of the initial job interviews. The remaining 32 who were considered to be qualified in education and experience were given detailed medical examinations and were exposed to the physical stresses expected in the space flight. The nature of these tests has been described in more detail by Douglas (4) and Wilson (5). On the basis of the medical examination and the stress tests the number of candidates was reduced to 18, from which were selected the 7 who demonstrated the most outstanding professional background and knowledge in relationship to the job requirements. Through this procedure, a group of experienced test pilots with extensive training in engineering, excellent health, and a high motivation in the Mercury Project were selected for the training program. The availability of such individuals makes it possible to utilize to a great extent self-instruction and to minimize the amount of formal group training required.

At the outset, few, if any, facilities were available to support the training program. Both training devices and training manuals have become available in stages throughout the first twelve to fifteen months of the training program. The more elaborate and complete training devices were not placed in operation until over a year after its initiation. As a result, the early part of the training program depended upon review of design drawings in vehicle components and on travel to various Mercury production facilities to attend design briefings. Great dependence was put upon verbal presentations by scientists of the NASA Space Task Group and of the prime contractor. In addition, early in the program, extensive use was made of established Armed Forces aeromedical facilities for familiarizing the astronauts with the conditions of space flight. Thus, the training methods and the order in which topics were presented were, to a great extent, dictated by the resources available at the time the program was initiated.

Since mature, intelligent trainees were selected, and since little if any training equipment was available initially, it might have been argued that the astronauts should be allowed to work completely on their own without any attempt at a group program. There are, however, a number of desirable factors to be gained by such a program. A planned group program facilitates the scheduling of activities with other organizations. In addition, a structured program permits more efficient use of instructor and student time. It also makes possible progress from one aspect of the operation to the next in an appropriate sequence. Sequence in training activities is important, since learning is simplified if material is presented in a logical order. An organized program also insures completeness in that no major training requirement is overlooked. Finally, since this project represents a first effort of its kind, the use of a group program facilitates the collecting of records and the evaluation both of the astronauts' progress and of the various training activities.

The program which has resulted from these considerations has allotted about one half of the time to group activities and the other half to individually planned activities in the astronaut's area of specialization. A review of the astronauts' travel records provides an example of the relative division of their time between group training and other duties associated with the development of the Mercury vehicle. During the 6-month period from July 1 to December 31, 1959, the astronauts were on travel status almost 2 months, or 1 out of every 3 days. Half of this travel time (28 days) was spent on four group-training activities: a centrifuge program; a trip to Air Force Flight Test Center, Air Force Ballistic Missile Division, and Convair; a weightless flying program; and trips to fly high-performance aircraft during a period when the local field was closed. The other half of their travel time (27 days) was devoted to individual trips to attend project coordination meetings at McDonnell and the Atlantic Missile Range, or for pressure-suit fittings, couch moldings, and viewing of qualification tests at McDonnell, B. F. Goodrich Co., and their subcontractors' plants. These individual activities, while providing important training benefits, are primarily dictated by the Project Mercury development program requirements and are not considered part of the group training program.

The extent to which the Mercury crew space area is "customized" to the seven astronauts and the time required to fit the man to the vehicle should be noted. Each man has had to travel to B. F. Goodrich for a pressure-suit fitting and to a subcontractor for helmet fittings; then to the Air Crew Equipment Laboratory for tests in the suit under heat and lowered pressure; then to McDonnell for couch molding. Usually, he has been required to return to the suit manufacturer for a second fitting and to McDonnell for final fittings of the couch and studies of his ability to reach the required instruments and controls in the capsule. While the Mercury vehicle is more limited in size than future spacecraft, the cost of space flight and the limited personnel involved will probably always dictate a certain amount of customizing of the crew space. The time required for this type of activity should not be underestimated.

TRAINING PROGRAM

The astronaut training program can be divided into six major topic areas. The primary requirement, of course, is to train the astronaut to operate the vehicle. In addition, it is desirable that he have a good background knowledge of such scientific areas related to space flight as propulsion, trajectories, astronomy, and astrophysics. He must be exposed to and familiarized with the conditions of space flight such as acceleration, weightlessness, heat, vibration, noise, and disorientation. He must prepare himself physically for those stresses which he will encounter in space flight. Training is also required for his duties at ground stations before and after his own flight and during the flights of other members of the astronaut team. An aspect of the training which might be overlooked is the maintenance of the flying skill which was an important factor in his original selection for the Mercury program.

Training in Vehicle Operation. Seven training procedures or facilities were used in developing skills in the operation of the Mercury capsule. These included lectures on the Mercury systems and operations, field trips to organizations engaged in the Mercury Project, training manuals, specialty study programs by the individual astronaut, mockup inspections, and training devices. To provide the astronaut with a basic understanding of the Mercury system, its components, and its functions, a lecture program was set up. A short trip was made to McDonnell at which time a series of lectures on the capsule systems was presented. These systems lectures were then augmented by lectures on operations areas by Space Task Group scientists. This initial series of lectures provided a basis for later self-study, in which use was made of written descriptive material as it became available. Individual lectures have been repeated as the developments within Project Mercury have required. A series of lectures on capsule systems by both Space Task Group and McDonnell personnel have been scheduled to coincide with the delivery and initial operation of the fixed-base Mercury trainer. In these lectures, the same areas are reviewed in an attempt to bring the astronauts up to date on each of the systems as they begin their primary procedures training program.

In addition to this lecture program, indoctrination trips have been made to the major facilities concerned with the Project Mercury operations. Two days were spent at each of the following facilities: McDonnell, Cape Canaveral, Marshall Space Flight Center, Edwards Flight Test Center, and Space Technology Laboratories and Air Force Ballistic Missile Division. One day was spent at Rocketdyne Division of North American Aviation, and five days were spent at Convair/Astronautics. At each site there was a tour of the general facilities together with a viewing of Mercury capsule or booster hardware and lectures by top-level personnel covering their aspect of the Mercury operation. The astronauts also had an opportunity to hear of related research vehicles such as the X-15 and Discoverer and receive a brief discussion of the technical problems arising in these programs and their significance to Project Mercury.

Obtaining current and comprehensive study materials on a rapidly developing program such as Project Mercury is a major problem. McDonnell has been providing manuals covering Project Mercury systems. The first of these was the *Indoctrination Manual*, and it was delivered at the time of an early astronaut visit in May, 1959. No attempt was made to keep this manual current, and a first edition of a full systems manual (*Familiarization Manual*) was issued in September, 1959. It quickly became out of date, however, and a new manual, a second edition of the *Familiarization Manual*, was issued in December of the same year. A first copy of the capsule operations manual (*Astronauts' Handbook*) was delivered in June of 1960. During initial phases of the program, the astronauts have had to depend primarily on capsule specifications and specification control drawings for written information on capsule systems. Copies of these, however, were not always available and they were too large to compile into a single manual.

Valuable aids to the astronauts in keeping abreast of the status of the development program are the regularly issued reports of the Capsule Coordination Group meetings. At these meetings the status of each of the capsule systems is reported and any changes are discussed. Miscellaneous reports on boosters and on programs conducted by cooperating agencies have also been provided to the astronauts. Maintaining an up-to-date flow of accurate information on vehicle development status is a critical problem not only for the

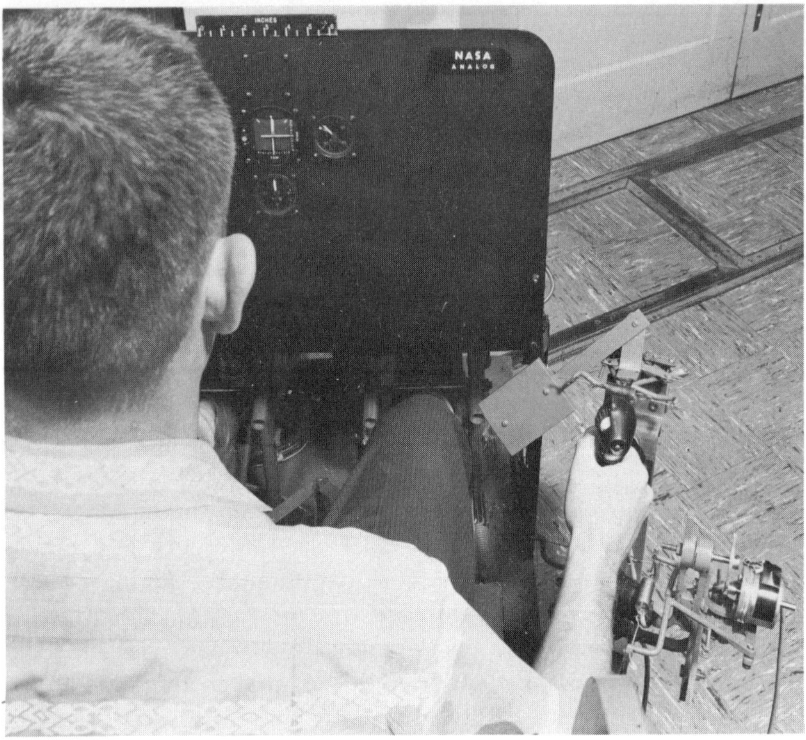

Figure 1. EAAC Simulator

A simulator making use of an analog computer on which astronauts were given initial training in attitude control problems.

Mercury training program but, in all probability, for most near-future space flight applications, since training must proceed during the vehicle development phase.

Another method employed to aid in the dissemination of information to the astronauts was to assign each a specialty area. These assignments were as follows: M. Scott Carpenter, navigation and navigational aids; Leroy G. Cooper, Redstone booster; John H. Glenn, crew space layout; Virgil I. Grissom, automatic and manual attitude control system; Walter M. Schirra, life support system; Alan B. Shepard, range, tracking, and recovery operations; and Donald K. Slayton, Atlas booster. In pursuing these specialty areas, each man attends meetings and study groups at which current information on capsule systems is presented. Regular periods are set aside for

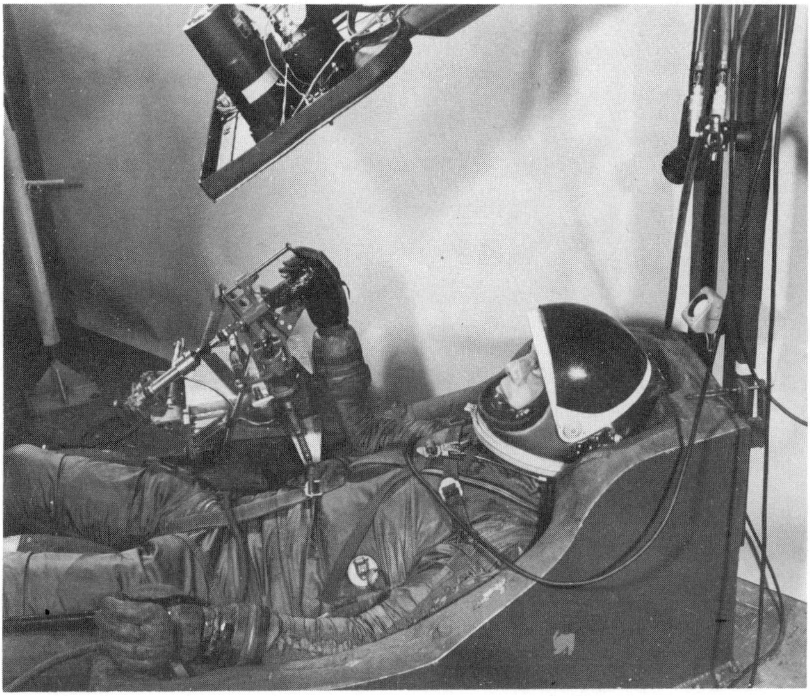

Figure 2. MB-3 Simulator

A second stage of fixed-base attitude control simulation which incorporated the astronaut's couch, pressure suit, and Mercury hand controller.

all the men to meet and report to the group. Another important source of information about the vehicle, particularly in the absence of any elaborate fixed-base trainers, has been the manufacturer's mockup. Each of the men has had an opportunity to familiarize himself with the mockup during visits to McDonnell.

Following the initial familiarization with the Mercury system, the primary training in vehicle operation is being achieved through special training devices developed for the Mercury program. Early training in attitude control was accomplished on the Langley Electronics Associates Computer (Figure 1) which was combined with a simulated Mercury attitude display and hand controller. This device was available during the summer of 1959. Later,

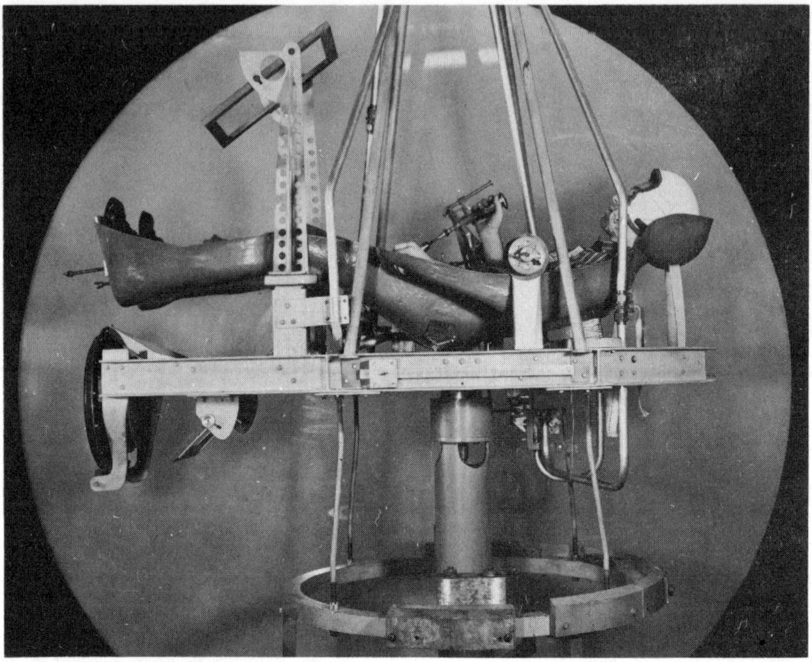

Figure 3. ALFA Simulator

A dynamic simulator making use of an air bearing which provides practice in attitude control during orbit and retrofire phases of mission. External reference is simulated by use of a picture of Earth from orbital altitude projected onto circular screen (seen behind trainer). Astronaut views screen through a set of mirrors and a lens which simulates periscope.

another analog computer was cannibalized from an F-100F simulator and combined with actual Mercury hardware to provide more realistic displays and controls. This MB-3 trainer (Figure 2) also included provision for the Mercury couch and the pressure suit.

In addition to these two fixed-base simulators, three dynamic simulators were used to develop skill in Mercury attitude control. The first of these, the ALFA (Air Lubricated Free Attitude) Simulator (Figure 3) permits the practice of orbit and retrofire attitude control problems by using external reference through simulated periscope and window displays. A simulated ground track is projected on a large screen which is viewed through a reducing lens to provide the periscope display. This simulator also permits training in the use of earth reference for navigation.

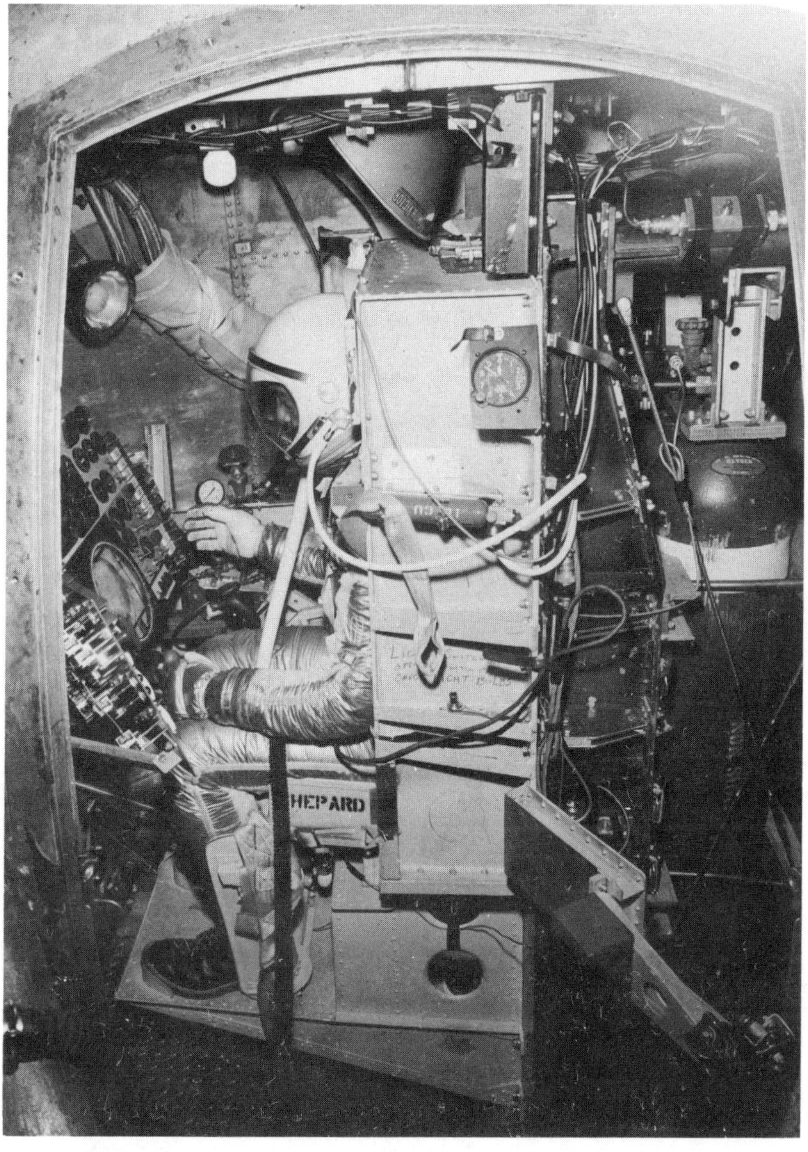

Figure 4. Johnsville Centrifuge

Centrifuge on which astronauts were given experience with launch and reentry acceleration profiles. Note that provisions have been made for use of full pressure suit and for decompression of the gondola. Astronauts are also provided with simulation of Mercury instrument panel and hand controller.

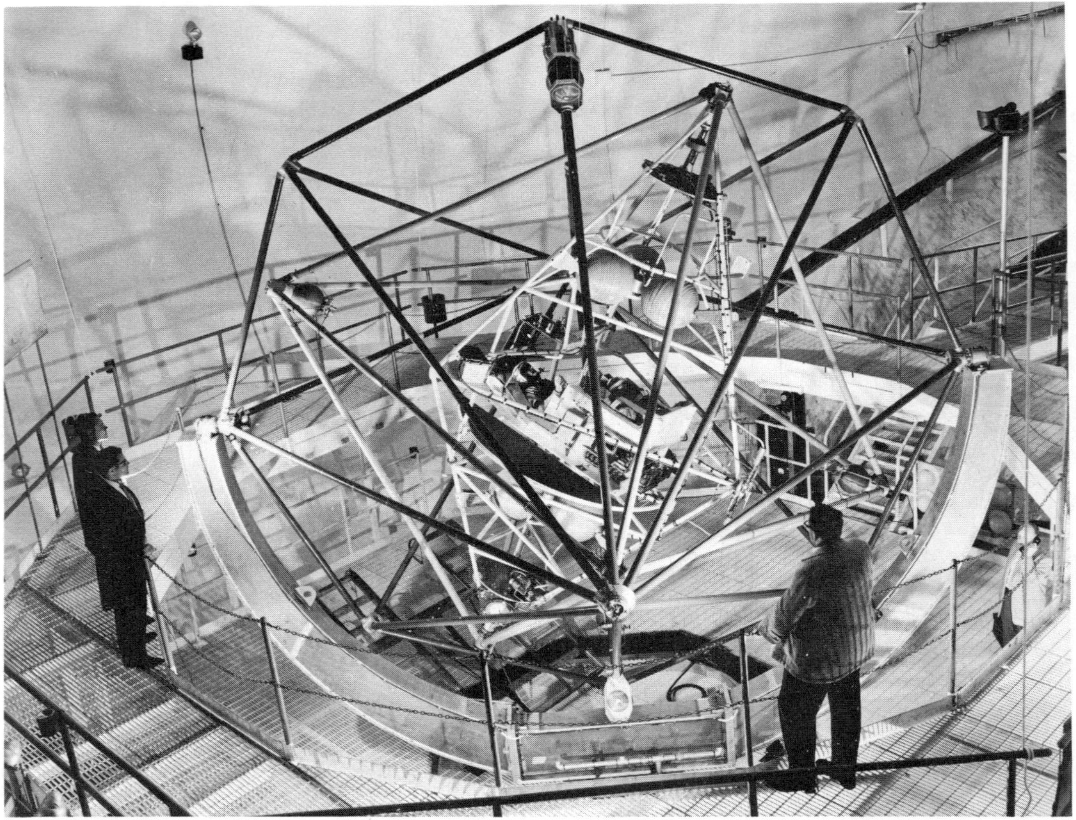

Figure 5. MASTIF Simulator

A tumbling device on which astronauts experienced rotational rates up to 30 r.p.m. in three axes. Once a steady rotational rate is achieved, astronaut assumes control and brings trainer to a stop by using instruments and controls similar to those available in Mercury vehicle.

The Johnsville Centrifuge (Figure 4) was used as a dynamic trainer for the reentry rate damping task because it adds the acceleration cues to the instruments available in the fixed-base trainers. It also provides some opportunity to practice sequence monitoring and emergency procedures during launch and reentry. Another dynamic simulation device used to provide training in recovery from tumbling was the three-gimbaled MASTIF (Multi-Axis Spin Test Inertia Facility) device at the NASA Lewis Laboratory (Figure 5). In this device tumbling rates up to 30 r.p.m. in all three axes were simulated, and the astronaut was given experience with damping these rates and bringing the vehicle to a stationary position by using the Mercury rate indicators and the Mercury-type hand controller.

Two more elaborate trainers became available in the summer of 1960. These trainers provide practice in sequence monitoring and systems management. The McDonnell Procedures trainer (Figure 6) is similar to the fixed-base trainers which have become standard in

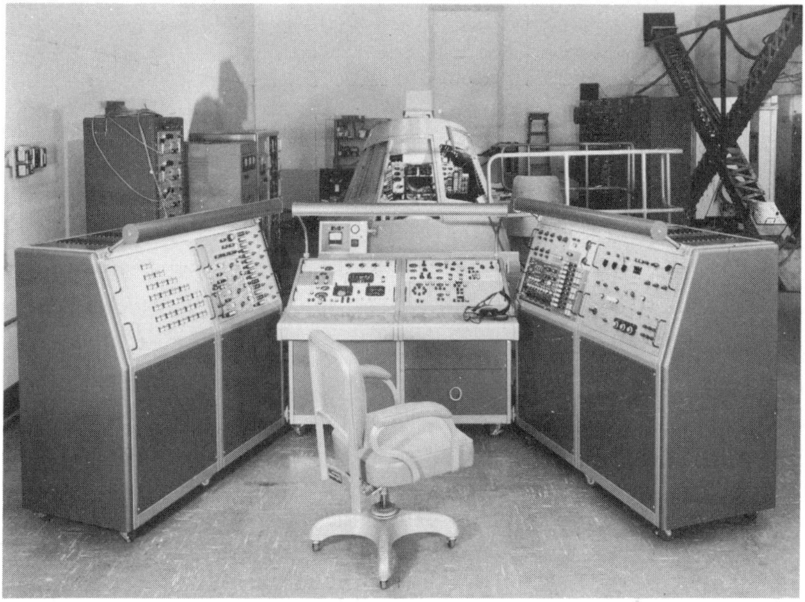

Figure 6. McDonnell Procedures Simulator

A fixed-base trainer which permits practice in management of Mercury systems and attitude control. From instructor's console in foreground, faults can be inserted into any of the Mercury indicators. Astronaut's corrective action is signaled by lights on panel.

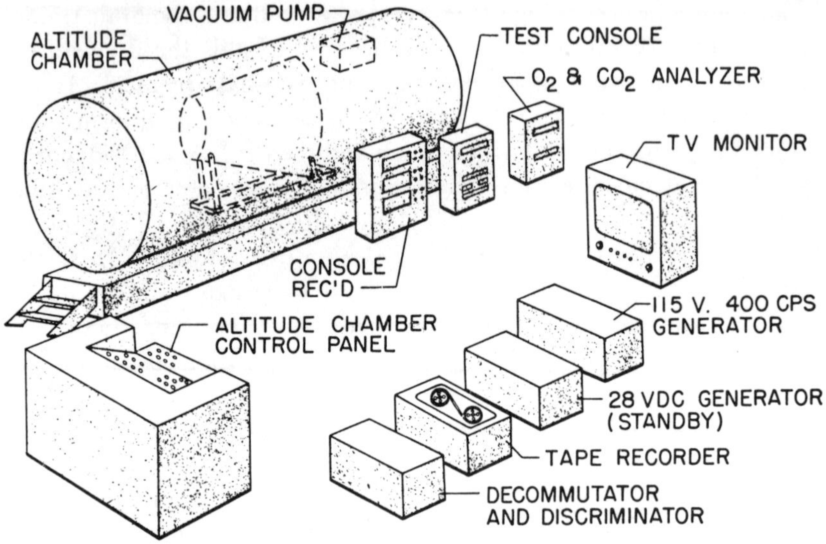

Figure 7. Environmental Control System Simulator

A device consisting of a mock capsule with a flight-type environmental control system which can be placed within a decompression chamber to simulate the operation of the environmental control system during the Mercury flight.

aviation operations. The computer used on the MB-3 has been integrated with this device to provide simulation of the attitude control problem. External reference through the periscope is simulated by using a cathode ray tube with a circle to represent the earth. Provision has been made for pressurizing the suit and for some simulation of heat and noise effects. The environmental control simulator (Figure 7) consists of the actual flight environmental control hardware in the capsule mockup. The whole unit can be placed in a decompression chamber in order to simulate the flight pressure levels. This device provides realistic simulation of the environmental control system functions and failures. Effective use of these two simulators is predicted upon adequate knowledge of the types of vehicle systems malfunctions which can occur. A failure-mode analysis carried out by the manufacturer has provided a basis for determining the types of malfunction which are possible and the requirements for simulating them (2). A record system on which possible malfunctions are listed on cards, together with methods of their simulation, has been set up. On the backs of these cards there is space for noting when and under what conditions this failure has been simulated and what action the astronaut took to correct it. In this way, it is hoped that the experience in the detection and correction of systems malfunctions can be documented.

Training in Space Sciences. In addition to being able to operate the Mercury vehicle, the astronaut will be required to have a good general knowledge of astronomy, astrophysics, meteorology, geophysics, rocket engines, trajectories, and so forth. This basic scientific knowledge will enable him to act as a more acute observer of the new phenomena with which he will come in contact during the flight. It will also provide a basis for better understanding of the detailed information which he must acquire on the Mercury vehicle itself. In order to provide this broad background in sciences related to astronautics, the Training Section of the Langley Research Center set up a lecture program which included the following topics: Elementary Mechanics and Aerodynamics (10 hours), Principles of Guidance and Control (4 hours), Navigation in Space (6 hours), Elements of Communication (2 hours), Space Physics (12 hours). In addition, Dr. W. K. Douglas, Flight Surgeon on the Space Task Group staff, gave 8 hours of lectures on physiology.

Following this initial lecture program, training in specific observational techniques is planned. The first activity of this program was training in the recognition of the primary constellations of the zodiac at the Morehead Planetarium in Chapel Hill, North Carolina. A Link trainer body was modified with a window and headrest to simulate the capsule external viewing conditions. Using this device, the astronauts were able to practice the recognition of constellations while the Planetarium was programed to simulate orbital flight. Future plans call for further training in star recognition together with methods of observing solar and meteorological events, earth and lunar terrain, and psychological and physiological reactions. These activities will be in support of a primary objective of the Project Mercury program, which is to determine man's capability in a space environment. The training program contributes to this objective in three ways:

1. It establishes base lines for both the astronaut's performance and his physiological reactions. These base lines can then be compared with psychological and physiological factors in the space environment.

2. Through the program in basic sciences described above, the astronaut is given sufficient background with which to appreciate the importance of the observations which he can make in the space environment.

3. Specific training in observational techniques and the use of scientific equipment arms the astronaut with the skills with which to collect data of value to science.

Thus, the training program attempts to lay the groundwork for the scientific activities of the astronauts, as well as to provide the specific skills which are required to fly the Mercury vehicle.

Familiarization with Conditions of Space Flight. An essential requirement of the training program is to familiarize the astronaut with the novel conditions which man will encounter in space flight. An important part of the astronaut training program has been to provide the trainees with an opportunity to experience eight types of conditions associated with Mercury flights: high acceleration, weightlessness, reduced atmospheric pressures, heat, disorientation, tumbling, high concentration of CO_2, and noise and vibration.

The astronauts first experienced acceleration patterns similar to those associated with the launch and reentry of the Mercury at the Wright Air Development Division (WADD) in Dayton, Ohio, and later at the Aviation Medical Acceleration Laboratory at Johnsville, Pennsylvania. During this training they were able to develop straining techniques which reduced the problem of blackout and chest pain. It was generally the opinion of the astronauts that the centrifuge activity was one of the most valuable parts of the training program.

The astronauts were given an opportunity to experience weightless flying both in a free-floating condition in C-131 and C-135 aircraft and strapped down in the rear cockpit of a F-100F fighter. While the latter is more similar to the Mercury operation, the astronauts, being experienced pilots, felt that there was little or no difference between this experience and their normal flying activities. The free-floating state, however, they felt was a novel and enjoyable experience. Since the longer period of weightlessness available in the F-100F aircraft is valuable for collecting medical data, while the C-131 aircraft appears to give the most interesting experiential training, both types of operations appear to be desirable in a training program. The fact that the pilots experienced no unusual sensations during weightlessness when fully restrained was an encouraging finding for the Mercury operation and supports the desirability of selecting flying personnel for this type of operation.

The astronauts experienced reduced atmospheric pressure while wearing full pressure suits first at WADD and later at Air Crew Equipment Laboratory (ACEL); in addition to reduced pressure, they also experienced thermal conditions similar to those expected during the Mercury reentry while wearing a full pressure suit. At the Naval Medical Research Institute (NMRI) they were given an opportunity to become familiar with the body's thermal response, and the effect of moderate heat loads on the body's regulatory mechanisms was demonstrated. At the end of March, 1960, the astronauts experienced disorientation in the U.S. Naval School of Aviation Medicine Slowly Revolving Room. As already mentioned, they have also experienced angular rotation up to 30 r.p.m. in all three axes on a gimbaled device with three degrees of freedom at the NASA Lewis Laboratory.

In order to indicate the effects of the high concentration of CO_2 which might result from a failure of the environmental control system, the astronauts were given a 3-hour indoctrination period in a sealed chamber at NMRI. In this chamber they experienced a slow buildup of CO_2 similar to that which they would encounter in the event of failure of the environmental system. None of the men showed any adverse effects of symptoms from this training. As part of the selection program, the astronauts experienced high noise and vibration levels at WADD. During the second Johnsville centrifuge program, noise recorded of the Mercury test flight was played back into the gondola. Further opportunities to adapt to the high noise levels associated with the Mercury launch will be provided by a sound system connected to the McDonnell Procedures Trainer at Langley Field.

Physical Fitness Program. To insure that the astronaut's performance does not deteriorate significantly under the various types of stresses discussed in the previous section, it is important that he be in excellent physical condition. Since most of the trainees entered the Project Mercury program in good physical health, a group physical fitness program, with one exception, has not been instituted.

SCUBA training was undertaken because it appeared to have a number of potential benefits for the Project Mercury, in addition to providing physical conditioning. It provides training in breathing control and analysis of breathing habits, and in swimming skill (desirable in view of the water landing planned in the Mercury program). Finally, there is, in the buoyancy of water, a partial simulation of weightlessness, particularly if vision is reduced. Aside from this one organized activity, each individual has been undertaking a voluntary fitness program tailored to his own needs. This program has included, for most of the astronauts, three basic items. First of all, as of December, 1959, they have reduced or completely stopped smoking. This was an individual, voluntary decision and was not a result of pressure by medical personnel, but a result of their own assessment of the effect of smoking on their tolerance to the stresses to be encountered in the flight, particularly acceleration. Some of the members of the team who have a tendency to be overweight have initiated weight-control programs through proper diet. Nearly all members make it a habit to get some form of daily exercise.

Training in Ground Activities. Frequently overlooked are the extent and the importance of the ground activities of the astronauts. Their knowledge of the vehicle and its operation makes them specially qualified for certain ground operations. The training in ground procedures has fallen into the three main areas; countdown procedures, ground flight monitoring procedures, and recovery and survival. The astronauts are participating in the development of the countdown procedures, and they will be training themselves in their own part of the countdown through observation of countdown procedures for the initial unmanned shots and, finally, by participating in the preparation procedures for the actual manned flights.

An important aspect of the astronaut's activities when not actually flying the vehicle will be to aid in ground communications with the Mercury capsule. Since he is fully familiar with the capsule operation and intimately acquainted with the astronaut who will be in the capsule, he makes a particularly effective ground communicator. Procedures for ground monitoring and communicating personnel are presently being developed with the aid of the astronauts. At Langley Field, a ground monitoring station simulator will be tied in with the McDonnell procedures simulator. By using this device,

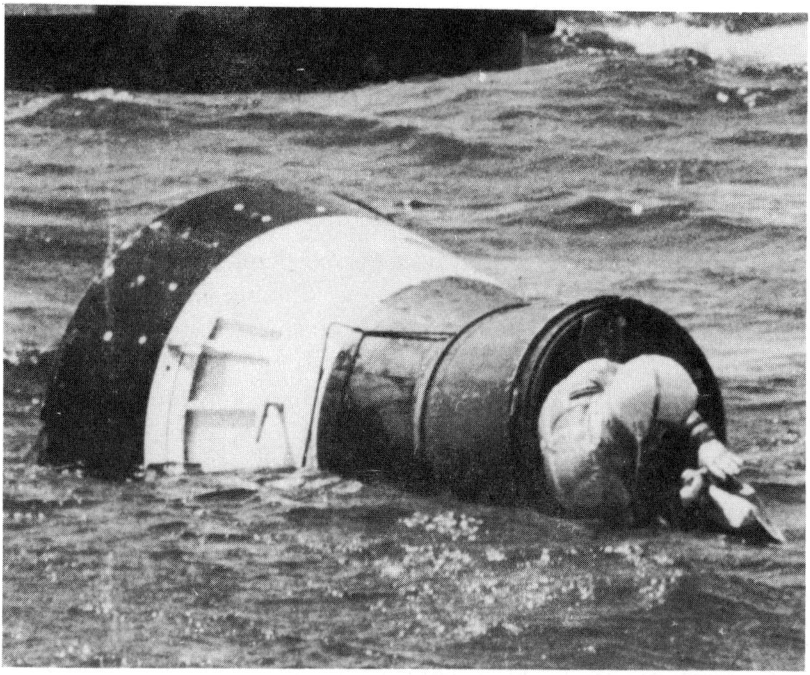

Figure 8. Mercury Egress Trainer

A device accurately simulating internal arrangement and sizes of emergency exits, so that astronaut can practice leaving the capsule in water.

ground station activities can be practiced and coordinated with capsule simulator training. They will also participate in training exercises at the Mercury Control Center at Cape Canaveral. Finally, just prior to manned flights, astronauts not involved in launch activities will be deployed to remote communications stations, at which time they will have an opportunity for some on-site training.

A final area of ground training is in recovery and survival procedures. Study materials such as maps and terrain descriptions of the areas under the Mercury orbits are being obtained. They will be augmented by survival lectures and by field training in survival at sea and in desert areas. Finally, extensive training on egress from the capsule into the water has been given. This activity was accomplished in two stages, using the Mercury egress trainer (Figure 8). Phase I made use of a wave-motion simulation tank at Langley Field for initial training and was followed by a Phase II program in open water in the Gulf of Mexico.

Maintenance of Flight Skills. One of the continuing problems in training for space flight is the limited opportunity for actual flight practice and proficiency training. The total flight time in the Mercury capsule will be no more than four to five hours over a period of three years for each astronaut. The question arises as to whether all the skills required in operating the Mercury vehicle can be maintained purely through ground simulation. One problem with ground simulation relates to its primary benefit. Flying a ground simulator never results in injury to the occupant or damage to the equipment. The penalty for failure is merely the requirement to repeat the exercise. In actual flight operations, failures are penalized far more severely. A major portion of the astronaut's tasks involves high-level decision making. It seems questionable whether skill in making such decisions can be maintained under radically altered motivational conditions. Under the assumption that vigilant decision making is best maintained by experience in flight operations, the Mercury astronauts have been provided with the opportunity to fly high-performance aircraft. The program in this area is a result of their own interest and initiative and is made possible by the loan and maintenance of two F-102 aircraft by the Air Force.

IMPLICATIONS FOR FUTURE PROGRAMS

In conclusion, the problems with implications for future space flight projects which have been encountered in development of the Mercury program can be reviewed. In developing skills in operation of the vehicle, the difficulty of providing up-to-date information on the systems when the training must progress concurrently with the development program has been discussed. Concurrent training and development should tend to be a feature of future space flight programs, since many of these will be experimental in nature rather than operational.

All spacecraft have in common the problem of systems which must be kept functional for long periods without recourse to ground support. Even in the event of emergency termination of the mission with immediate return to earth, prolonged delay may occur before safe conditions within the atmosphere have been achieved. Thus, emphasis on "systems management" will increase in future space operations. Recognition of malfunctions has always been a part of the pilot's task; usually, however, little in-flight maintenance is attempted. Since aborts are dangerous and, in any event, involve greater delay before return, the astronaut must do more detailed diagnoses of malfunctions and more in-flight maintenance. This will require extensive knowledge of the vehicle systems and training in malfunction isolation and correction. In order to provide this training as many as possible of the numerous malfunctions which can occur in even a relatively simple space vehicle must be identified and simulated. Considerable effort has been devoted to this area in the Mercury training and development program and it should become an increasingly important feature of future programs.

The physical conditions (heat, acceleration, and so forth) associated with space flight are simulated to permit the trainees to adapt to these stressors in order that during the actual flight such stimuli may be less disturbing. Present measures of the adaptation process are inadequate to provide criteria for training progress. A second purpose for the familiarization program was to give the trainees an opportunity to learn the specific skills required to minimize the effects of these factors on their performance. However, in many cases the skills required have not been fully identified or validated. For example, in developing straining techniques for meeting increased acceleration, the efficacy of a straining technique has not been fully demonstrated nor has the technique itself been adequately described. As yet, inadequate data are available on the effects of combining physical stress factors. Therefore, it is difficult to determine the extent to which the increased cost and difficulty of providing multiple stress simulation is warranted. In the present program, it has been possible to simulate both reduced atmospheric pressure and acceleration on the centrifuge. Initial experience seems to indicate that this is desirable but not critical. However, further data on the interacting effects of these stresses are required before any final conclusions can be developed.

A factor in space flight not yet adequately simulated for training purposes is weightlessness. Short periods of weightlessness have been used in the present program, as described previously. True weightlessness can be achieved through too short a period to be fully adequate for training purposes. On the other hand, ground simulation methods using water seem to be too cumbersome and unrealistic to be fully acceptable substitutes. At the present time, this lack of adequate simulation does not seem to be critical since the effects of weightlessness on performance appear to be minor and transitory. Should early space flights uncover more significant problems, greater efforts will be justified in developing weightless simulation methods.

Finally, it seems important to reiterate the requirements for reproducing adequate motivational conditions in the training program. The basic task of the astronaut is to make critical decisions under adverse conditions. The results of the decisions he makes involve not just minor discomforts or annoyances, but major loss of equipment and even survival. Performance of this task requires a vigilance and decision-making capability difficult to achieve under the artificial conditions of ground simulation. It appears probable that training in ground devices should be augmented with flight operations to provide realistic operational conditions.

REFERENCES

1. Slayton, Donald K., Paper presented at Annual Meeting of Society of Experimental Test Pilots, Los Angeles, Calif., Oct., 1959.
2. Jones, Edward R., Man's Integration into the Mercury Capsule. Paper [preprint] 982-59, presented at the Am. Rocket Soc. 14th Annual Meeting, Washington, D.C., Nov., 1959.
3. Brewer, Gerald W., Operational Requirements and Training for Project Mercury. Paper presented to Training Advisory Comm. of Nat. Security Ind. Assoc., Los Angeles, Calif., Nov. 17, 1959.
4. Douglas, William K., Selection and training of space crews, in *Lectures in Aerospace Medicine*. School of Aviation Medicine, USAF Aerospace Medical Center, Brooks AFB, Texas, 1960.
5. Wilson, Charles L., Project Mercury Candidate Evaluation Program. WADC Tech. Rep. 59-505, U.S. Air Force, 1959.

The Neurophysiology of Stress

HORACE W. MAGOUN

The background for present thinking concerning stress began a century ago with Claude Bernard's (6) emphasis upon preservation of the stability of the internal environment as a condition for freely changing life, subsequently elaborated by Barcroft (5) and by Cannon (8) in terms of the importance of homeostasis in body functions. Cannon in particular went on to interpret the bodily changes observed in excited behavior as anticipatory of the demands required to reduce, eliminate, or escape from situations evoking pain, hunger, fear, and rage.

More recently Selye (40) has devoted attention to the more prolonged changes which are provoked by chronic environmental conditions of a deleterious nature. He has designated as *stress* the general syndrome of bodily adaptations designed to terminate or overcome evocative stimuli called stressors. If stress is the sum of the changes induced in the body to overcome stressors, it can also be thought of as a negative feedback, in which the animal responds to adversive stimuli by mobilizing reserves which eliminate these initiating alterations, so as to restore the status quo. From this point of view the neurophysiology of stress should concern itself with an analysis of the subjective experience and a determination of the mechanism of objective alterations, which together form the stress state.

Considerable evidence is now available which implicates, in stress, central neural mechanisms called limbic, for their distribution around the hilus of the cerebral hemisphere, bordering its attachment to the cephalic end of the brainstem. It is of interest that this limbic portion of the brain was initially distinguished on anatomical grounds by a contemporary of Bernard, Paul Broca (7). Its implication as a neural mechanism for the integration of

Dr. Magoun is Professor of Anatomy, School of Medicine, University of California at Los Angeles.

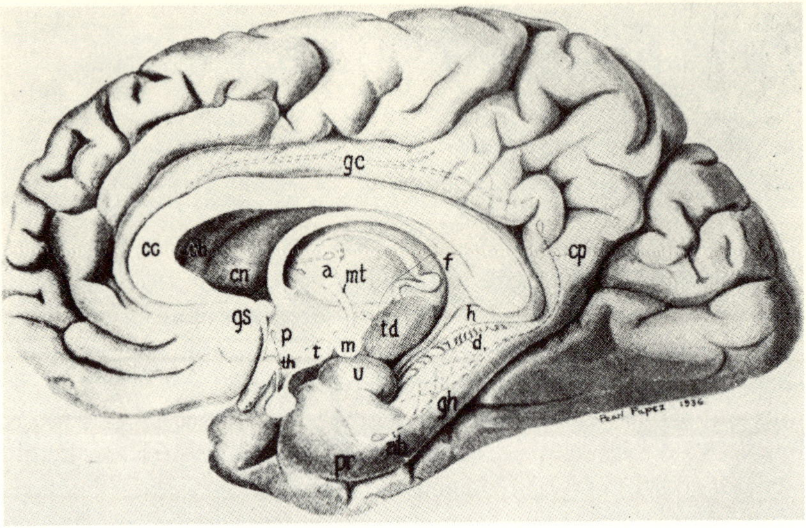

Figure 1. Medial Aspect of the Cerebral Hemisphere of Man

Shows Papez's emotional circuit and the limbic or visceral brain. a: anterior thalamic nucleus; ab: angular bundle; cn: caudate nucleus; cc: corpus callosum; cp: posterior cingulate gyrus; d: dentate gyrus; f: fornix; gc: cingulate gyrus; gh: hippocampal gyrus; gs: subcallosal gyrus; h: hippocampus; m: mammillary body; mt: mammillo-thalamic tract; p: supraoptic hypothalamus; pr: pyriform area; sb: subcallosal bundle; t: tuberal hypothalamus; td: mammillo-tegmental tract; th: hypophyseal stalk; u: uncus. From Papez (34).

emotional experience and expression was, however, first proposed by Papez (34), as recently as 1937 (Figure 1). Succeeding investigations of the Yale School, by Kaada (23), MacLean (27, 28, 29), Pribram and Kruger (37), and Fulton (13), provided physiological substantiation for Papez's proposal of a limbic circuit for emotion.

FUNCTIONAL ORGANIZATION OF THE LIMBIC SYSTEM

The limbic system includes the cingulate and entorhinal cortex of the hemisphere, the paleocortical hippocampus and its basal ganglion, the amygdala, and the interconnections of these structures with the cephalic brainstem. Initial emphasis was placed upon the interrelations of these parts with one another. In Papez's proposal (34), the cingulate → entorhinal → hippocampal → fornix → mammillary body → anterior thalamic nucleus → cingulate circuit formed a feed-back loop, which maintained activity by self-reexcitation, and modulated this activity by resetting the gain at one of the stations in the circuit. In the succeeding neuronographical studies of Pribram and MacLean (38), strychninization of one of these parts led to spiking in all the rest, emphasizing again the existence of major internal connections. In these experiments, delimitation of strychnine spiking to this system pointed also to its relative functional isolation from the remainder of the brain. Similarly, EEG studies of psychomotor epilepsy in man (35), and of experimental hippocampal and amygdaloid seizures in animals (18, 14), have further demonstrated that full-blown electrical seizure discharge may spread widely within the limbic part of the brain, with remarkably little involvement of the remainder of the nervous system. While it has been of great value to have had this feature of internal generalization recognized early, knowledge of the interconnections of limbic structures with the rest of the brain are of equivalent importance for an understanding of its role in the management of stress and emotional behavior.

Recent studies have displayed limbic inputs not simply from olfactory sources, first emphasized by comparative neuroanatomical studies (19), but from contributions by each of the afferent modalities. This generalized sensory input gains the limbic system by way of diffuse ascending connections in the central portion of the brainstem, as well as from the nonspecific thalamic and septal nuclei. Their final path to the hippocampus comprises a major centripetal component of the dorsal fornix, and they reach the amygdala by some still undetermined route. By these means limbic structures can readily be influenced from peripheral afferent sources tuned to changes in the external world (16, 17). Additional inputs to the hippocampus, from the entorhinal and cingulate cortex, provide routes through which the hippocampus can be influenced by activity within the cerebral hemisphere of the brain (3, 4).

A large body of recent information has also accumulated concerning the outputs by which the limbic system can influence the remainder of the nervous system and behavior. Efferent components of the fornix are directed not only into the mammillary feedback of classical comparative neuroanatomy but are distributed more broadly through the medial forebrain bundle to the entire cephalocaudal extent of septum, hypothalamus, and tegmentum of the cephalic brainstem (2). Additionally, a specific projection to Gudden's tegmental nucleus in the pons has been identified by Nauta (30). Outputs from the amygdala, both in the stria terminalis and in more diffuse paths, also reach cephalic brainstem components widely (14). By these routes the limbic system can gain command of the neuroendocrine outflows from the hypothalamus to the pituitary and thence to peripheral target organs. Similarly they can involve the hypothalamic-bulbo-spinal channels for visceral motor innervation, as well as the reticulospinal paths which form the major final relays from the brain for extrapyramidal innervation of skeletal motor function. Indeed, so intimately have the limbic forebrain mechanisms become linked with the cephalic brainstem that functional components of the latter are now often included as parts of the limbic system (2). Some understanding is now possible, therefore, both as to how activity which spins around limbic loops can be initiated either from afferent or central sources, and how its influence can be exerted upon glandular, visceral, and skeletal motor features of behavior. Information is even now accumulating which suggests the possibility of identifying subjective correlates of some of this limbic activity.

LIMBIC ACTIVITY ASSOCIATED WITH SUBJECTIVE EXPERIENCE

In psychomotor epilepsy, with reference to the region of the temporal lobe, the aura with which such seizures begin is typically an affect-laden, usually unpleasant, feeling which colors the disordered perception or recall comprising the aural experience (11, 43). Some of these types of subjective experience have been evoked by direct excitation of the temporal lobe of epileptic patients (35). The question may be raised as to whether the feeling states of psychomotor seizures invariably possess an unpleasant quality or whether some patients may experience pleasurable or enjoyable auras but, having more sense than to seek relief, never get into the medical record (43).

In animals, subjective experience can only be inferred from behavioral manifestations. Application of the techniques of operant psychology by Olds (33) have been exceedingly fruitful. When electrodes are chronically implanted in appropriate parts of the limbic brain and connected to a stimulator with a lever switch, the

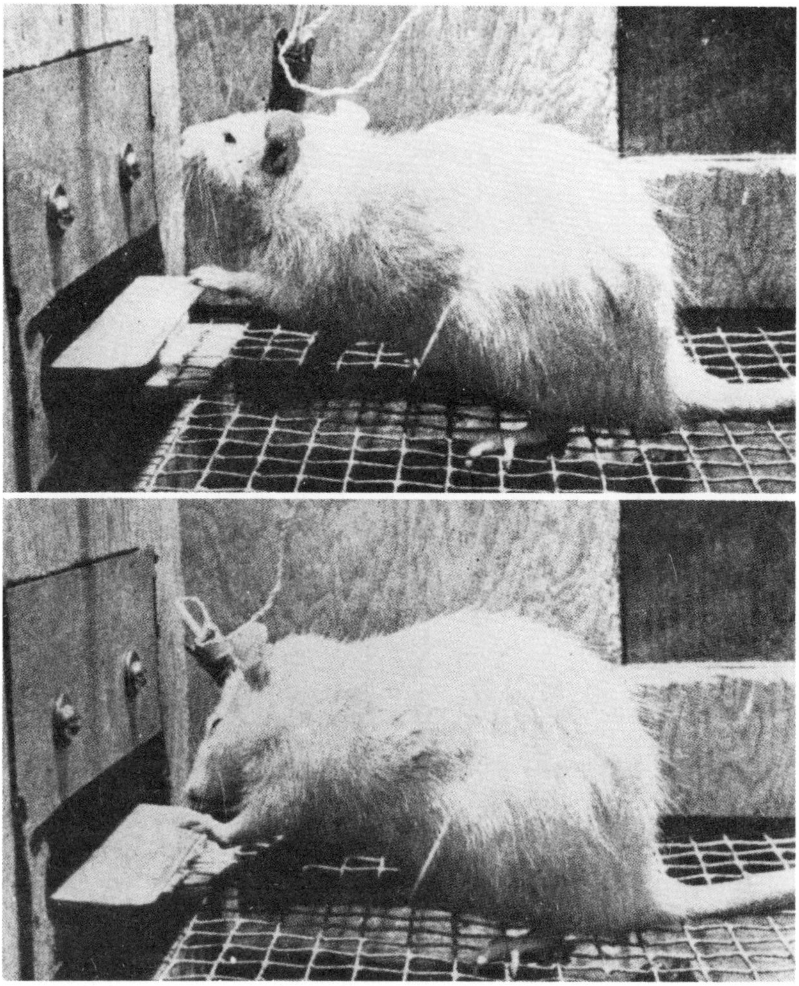

Figure 2. Rat with Electrodes Implanted in Its Limbic System (above), Pushes Lever (below) and Delivers Stimulus to Its Own Brain

From Olds (33)

animal will spend most of its waking time pushing the lever to deliver stimuli to the interior of its own brain (Figure 2; 31). The rate of such self-stimulation can be modified by increasing or reducing internal drives (33). Self-stimulation can serve also as

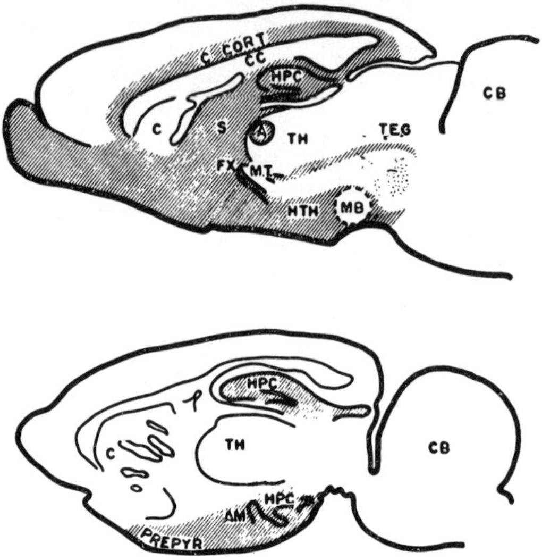

Figure 3. Sagittal Sections of the Rat Brain

Shading marks the area yielding positive reinforcement. C.CORT: cingulum cortex; CC: corpus callosum; S: septum; HPC: hippocampus; A: anterior commissure; TH: thalamus; FX: fornix; MT: mammillo-thalamic fasciculus; HTH: hypothalamus; CB: cerebellar; MB: mammillary body; AM: amygdala; PREPYR: prepyriformis cortex. From Olds (32).

positive reinforcement for maze learning (33). The animal will undertake considerable effort or suffer a surprising amount of punishment to experience it (33). Such self-stimulation gives every impression of being rewarding for the animal, and fragmentary reports of pleasurable experiences have come from stimulating these positively reinforcing regions in the brain of man (41). The effective sites are widely distributed in the limbic forebrain (32), from the cingulate and hippocampal cortex through the septum to the basal diencephalon (Figure 3).

In the diencephalon, an adjacent dorsal zone displays contrasting features, in that once the animal has stimulated this region, it will never do so again (32). Stimulating this zone, extending from the paramedian diencephalon caudalward into the central midbrain, had previously been found to evoke what has been called "affective-defensive behavior," in which the animal displays features of unpleasant emotion (Figures 4 and 5; 20, 21). If the direct excitation of this cephalic brainstem region is associated with a characteristic laboratory setting, the setting alone will soon provoke a general anticipatory unrest (9, 10). With appropriate programming, such stimulation may serve as an unconditional signal in the establishment of a conditional avoidance reflex (9, 10). If such stimulation is undertaken in a social situation, the excited animal may attack its neighbor, further suggesting that activity in this neural mechanism has subjective meaningfulness of an unpleasant type (9, 10). Additionally, if it is taught how to do so, the animal will perform a task, such as turning a wheel or pushing a lever, to avoid having this part of its brain stimulated (Figure 6; 25). Fragmentary reports indicate that unpleasant subjective experience may be induced by exciting this part of the brain in man (41). Modification of affect in the direction of increased subjective unpleasantness, associated with excitation of this negatively reinforcing component of the limbic system, suggests its involvement in stressful states, dominated by tension, anxiety, fear, depression, or less definite types of unpleasant subjective experience.

PATTERNS OF ELECTRICAL ACTIVITY IN THE LIMBIC BRAIN

The only objective measures of brain activity presently available in neurophysiological analysis of limbic function are observations of its electrical activity. In stress, anxiety and other unpleasant emotional experiences in man, EEG records from scalp leads characteristically display low voltage fast activity, the ubiquitous distribution and persistent maintenance of which form its only characteristic features (26). Because of the self-contained nature of limbic activity, electroencephalographic records derived from the external surface of the hemisphere are a most insensitive index of the state of affairs in the basally situated, deep-lying, limbic structures. With deep recording, in the animal brain, two striking patterns of electrical discharge have recently been found to be associated with excited behavior.

The first of these is referable to the hippocampus, in which a smoothly undulating series of high-amplitude slow waves at five to

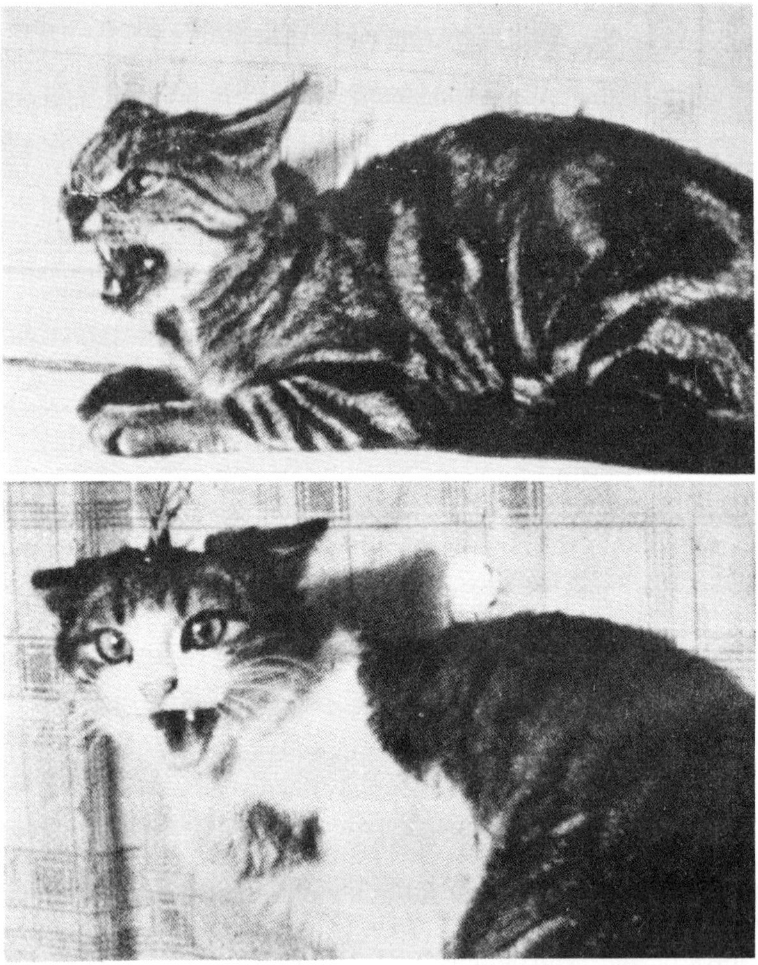

Figure 4. Affective-Defensive Responses

Reaction evoked by stimulating the negative reinforcement area of the cat's brain through implanted electrodes. From Hess (20).

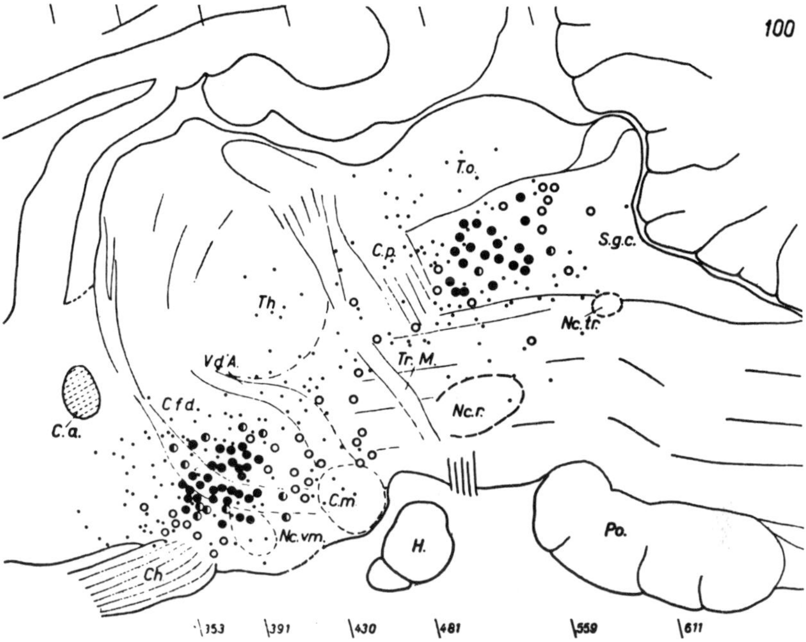

Figure 5. Paramedian Section of Brainstem of the Cat

Solid black circles mark sites where stimulation elicited "affective-defensive" responses, open circles those sites yielding flight reactions, and dots unresponsive sites. C.a.: anterior commusure; C.f.d.: fornix; C.m.: mammillary body; C.p.: posterior commissure; Ch.: chiasma; H.: hypophysis; Nc.r.: red nucleus; Nc.tr.: trochlear nucleus; Nc.vm.: ventromedial hypothalamic nucleus; Po.: pons; S.g.c.: periaqueductal gray; T.o.: superior colliculus; Th.: thalamus; Tr.M.: habenulo-peduncular tract; V.d.A.: mammillo-thalamic tract. From Hunsperger (21).

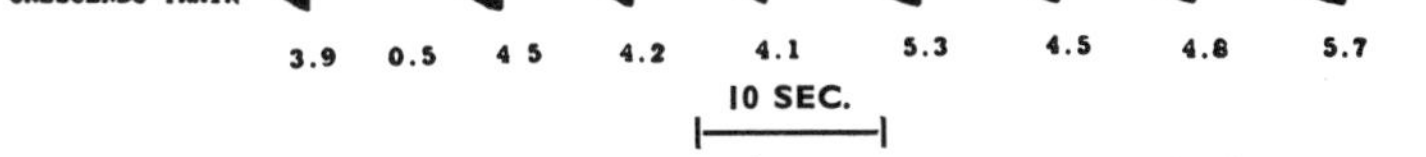

Figure 6. Stop-Capture Record (After Learning)

The lower trace signals recurring, crescendo-like trains of stimuli to a negatively reinforcing area of the monkey's brain. Numbers indicate the highest voltage reached before the animal turned off stimulation by touching and releasing a switch as marked in the upper trace. From Lilly (25).

seven per second, called the theta rhythm, can be recorded widely from the hippocampus whenever any external stimulus or situation arouses the animal (Figures 7 and 8; 17). This theta pattern, best observed in the rodent brain, can be evoked as well by direct excitation of the ascending reticular system in the brainstem, and it

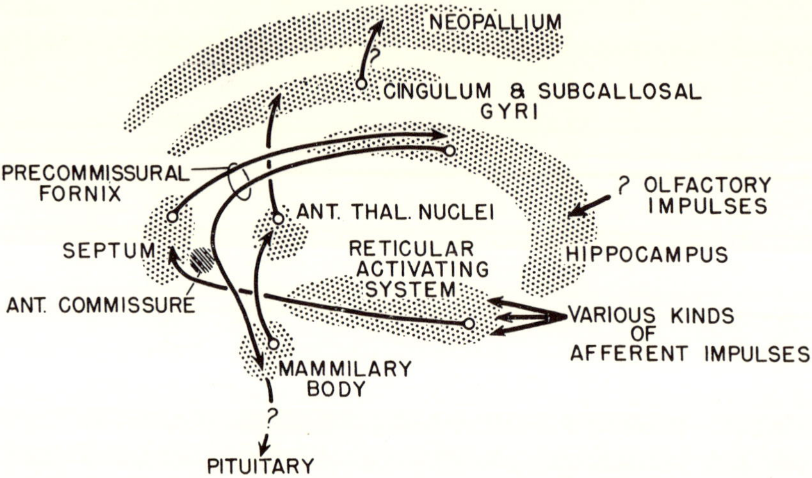

Figure 7. Diagram of Pathways Involved in Hippocampal Arousal Reaction

From Green and Arduini (17).

has been proposed by Green and Arduini (17) to form a characteristic arousal pattern of the paleocortex. Grastyan (15), on the other hand, considers that it forms a conditional response, to which emotional significance is attached, and identifies a low voltage fast discharge, like the EEG arousal response of the neocortex, as the primary, unconditional manifestation of hippocampal arousal (Figure 9). In the rodent brain, the evoked theta pattern is reflected by efferent paths from the hippocampus into Papez's circuit and dominates the activity of the mammillary body, anterior thalamic nucleus, and cingulate cortex. In the cat it is prominently displayed also in the entorhinal cortex (1).

A second pattern of limbic discharge associated with excited behavior consists of recurring bursts of forty-per-second activity which can be recorded in the amygdala (Figures 10 and 11; 24). This activity appears to be the stereotyped concomitant of a variety

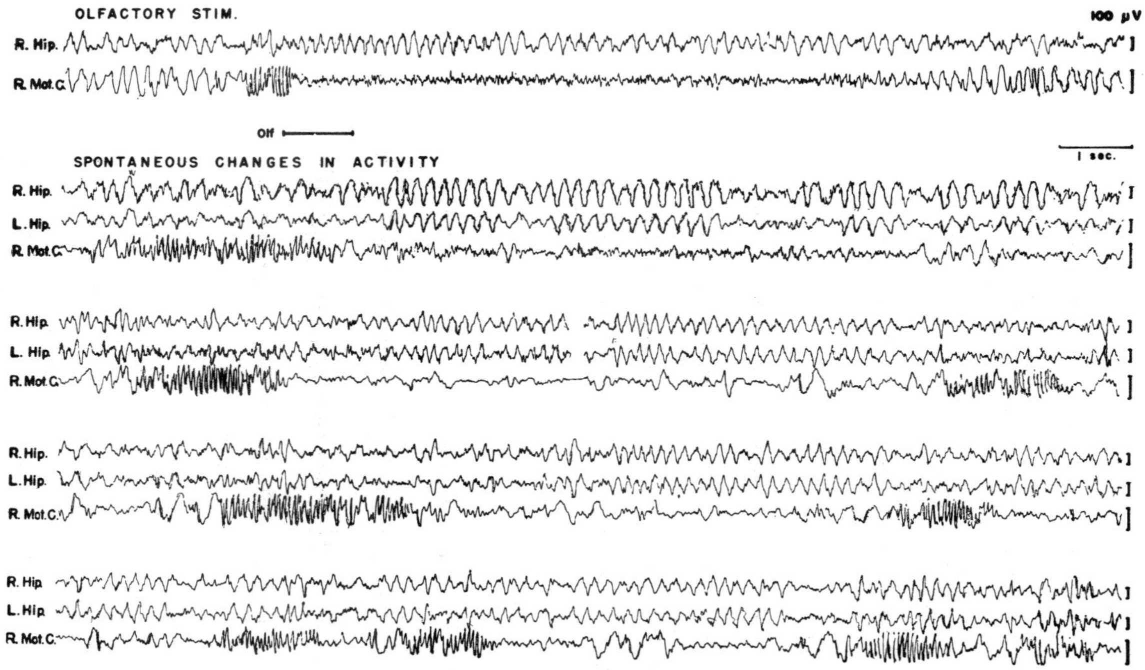

Figure 8. Induced and Spontaneous Hippocampal and Cortical Activity

Upper record shows contrasting pattern of arousal reaction evoked in the hippocampus (upper channel) and motor cortex (lower channel) of the rabbit brain, by olfactory stimulation (signal). Lower records show spontaneous appearance of contrasting discharge patterns in hippocampal (R. Hip.; L. Hip.) and neocortex (R. Mot. C.). From Green and Arduini (17).

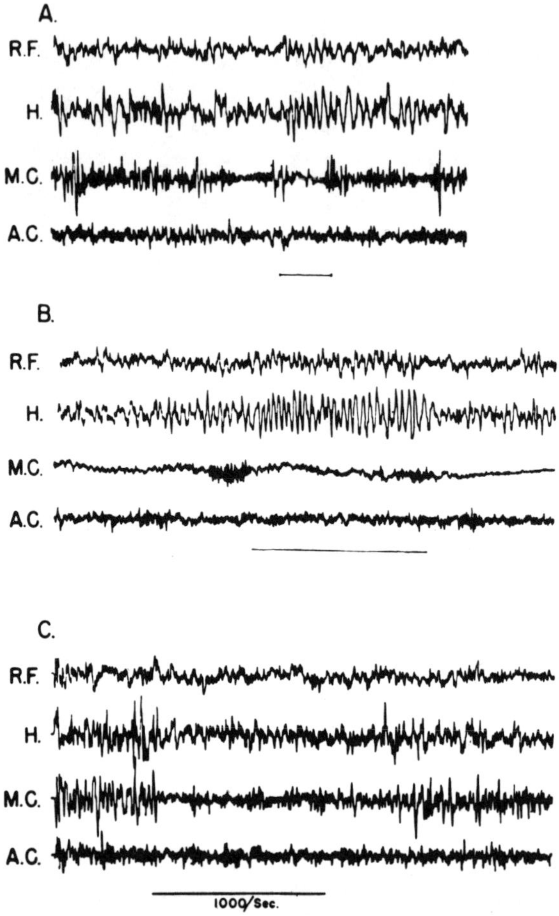

Figure 9. Records of Electrical Activity

R.F.: reticular formation; H.: hippocampus; M.C.: motor cortex; A.C.: auditory cortex. At the signal in A, a familiar sound, "puss," elicits a theta response from the hippocampus of the cat; in B, a similar change is seen when the animal looks at itself in a mirror (signal); in C, the first application of an indifferent 1000/sec. tone (signal) desynchronizes the hippocampal record (H.) and that of the neocortex (M.C.). From Grastyan (15).

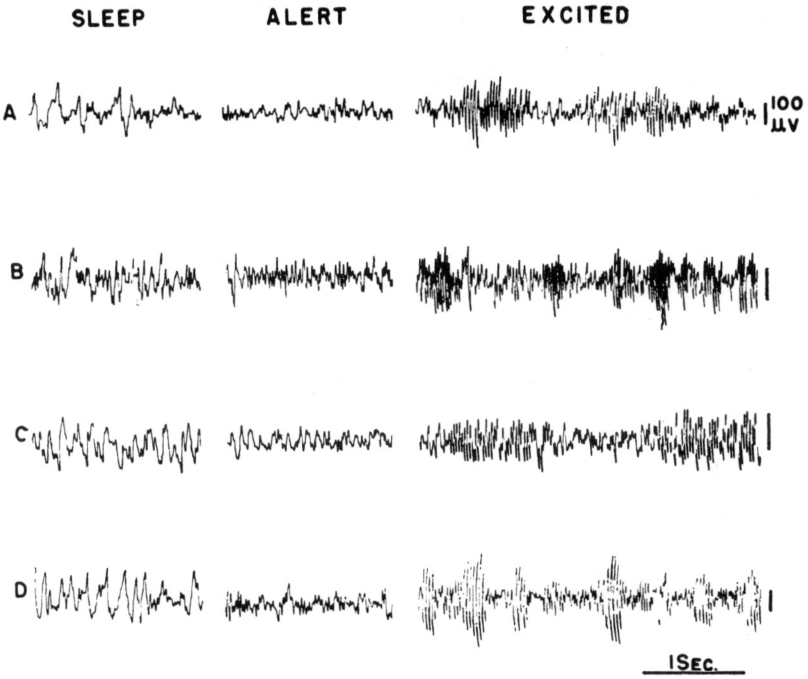

Figure 10. Records of Electrical Activity from the Basal Lateral Nucleus of the Amygdala of Four Cats

Patterns show discharge in sleep (left), alertness (middle), and excitement (right). Note 40/sec. bursts of high voltage activity during excitement. From Lesse (24).

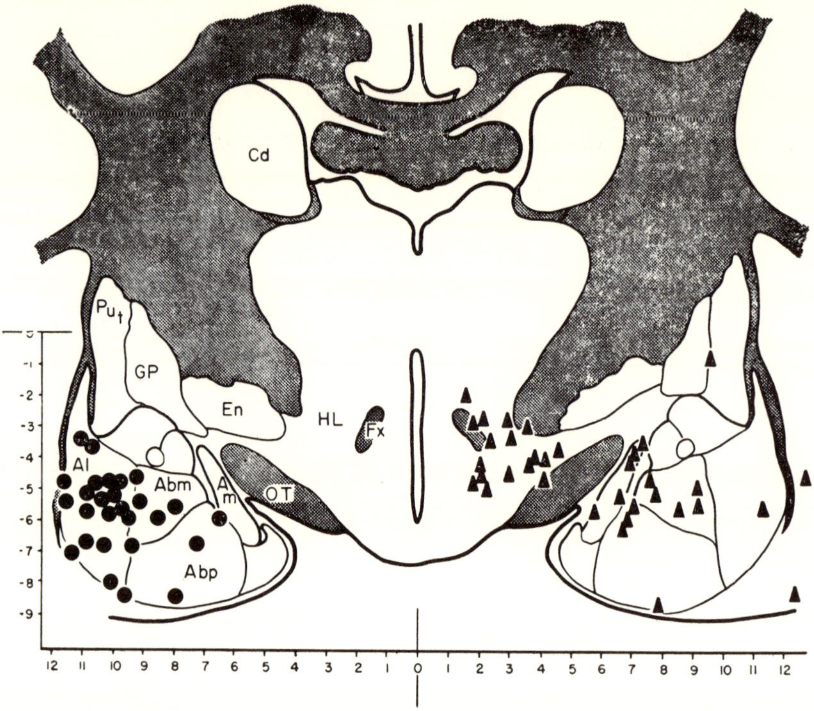

Figure 11. Transverse Section through Forebrain of the Cat

Circles (left) mark sites in the amygdala from which 40/sec. bursts were recorded during excited behavior, and triangles (right) sites from which such activity was not recorded. Abm: basal amygdaloid nucleus (magnocellular); Abp: basal amygdaloid nucleus (parvocellular); Al: lateral amygdaloid nucleus; Am: medial amygdaloid nucleus; Cd: caudate nucleus; En: entopeduncular nucleus; HL: lateral hypothalamus; Fx: fornix; GP: globus pallidus; OT: optic tract; Put: putamen. From Lesse (24).

of situations, the common feature of which is emotional excitement. It is Freeman's view (12) that this burst activity (Figure 12) takes origin in the prepyriform cortex and is transmitted caudalward both

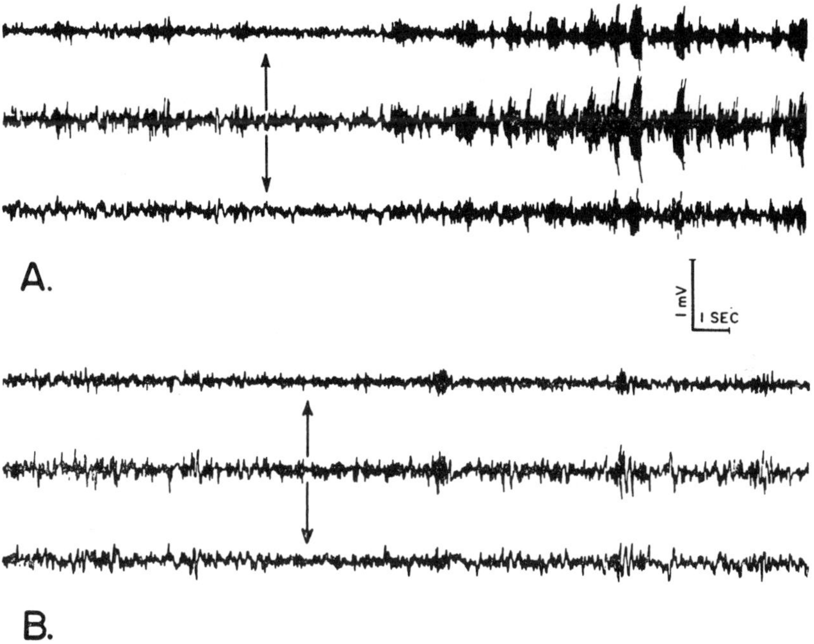

Figure 12. Records of Electrical Activity of Pre-pyriform Cortex of the Cat

High-frequency bursts occurred when fish odors were blown into the cage of the hungry animal (A). After feeding to satiety, the same odors evoked only minimal response (B). From Freeman (12).

to the amygdala and to the septum and hypothalamus. Characteristic patterns of high amplitude fast activity resembling seizure discharge have previously been recorded by Sawyer (39) and by Porter, Cavanaugh, Critchlow, and Sawyer (36) from the lateral preoptic and hypothalamic areas, along the path of the medial forebrain bundle, during sexual excitement in the rabbit and cat (Figures 13 and 14). It is not presently known whether it is displayed during other types of emotional behavior.

It now seems possible, therefore, to distinguish two contrasting patterns of electrical activity in the forebrain of excited animals. One is the four to seven per second, theta rhythm originating in the hippocampus and projecting to the cingulate and entorhinal cortex

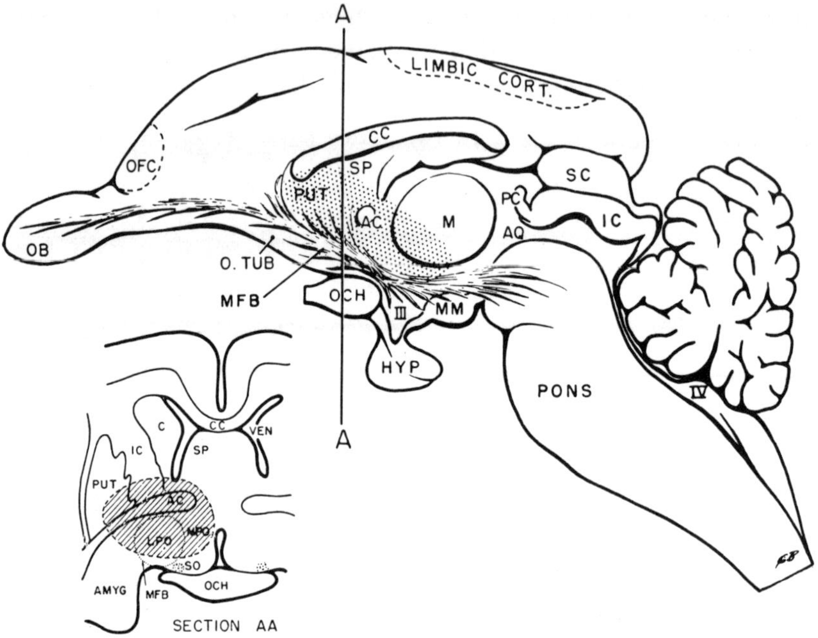

Figure 13. Mid-sagittal View of Rabbit Brain with Section (AA) through Septum and Preoptic Region

Shading marks the area from which high-frequency, large amplitude discharge could be recorded during sexual excitement. AC: anterior commisure; AMYG: amygdala; AQ: aqueduct; C: caudate nucleus; CC: corpus callosum; HYP: hypophysis; IC: internal colliculus or internal capsule; LPO: lateral preoptic area; M: massa intermedia; MFB: medial forebrain bundle; MM: mammillary body; MPO: medial preoptic area; OB: olfactory bulb; OCH: optic chiasma; OFC: orbito-frontal cortex; OTUB: olfactory tubercle; PC: posterior commissure; PUT: putamen; SC: superior colliculus; SO: supraoptic nucleus; SP: septum; VEN: lateral ventricle; III: third ventricle; IV: fourth ventricle. From Sawyer (39).

of the hemisphere. The second is fast, high-amplitude discharge taking origin in the prepyriform cortex or amygdala and projecting to the hypothalamus and lower brainstem. It is tempting to extend Cannon's (8) earlier proposal and suggest that the first of these is concerned in some degree with the subjective features and the second with the expressive manifestations of emotional behavior.

LIMBIC INFLUENCES UPON ACTIVITY OF OTHER PARTS OF THE BRAIN

Beginning insight into the manner in which limbic influences may be exerted upon the performance of other parts of the brain is

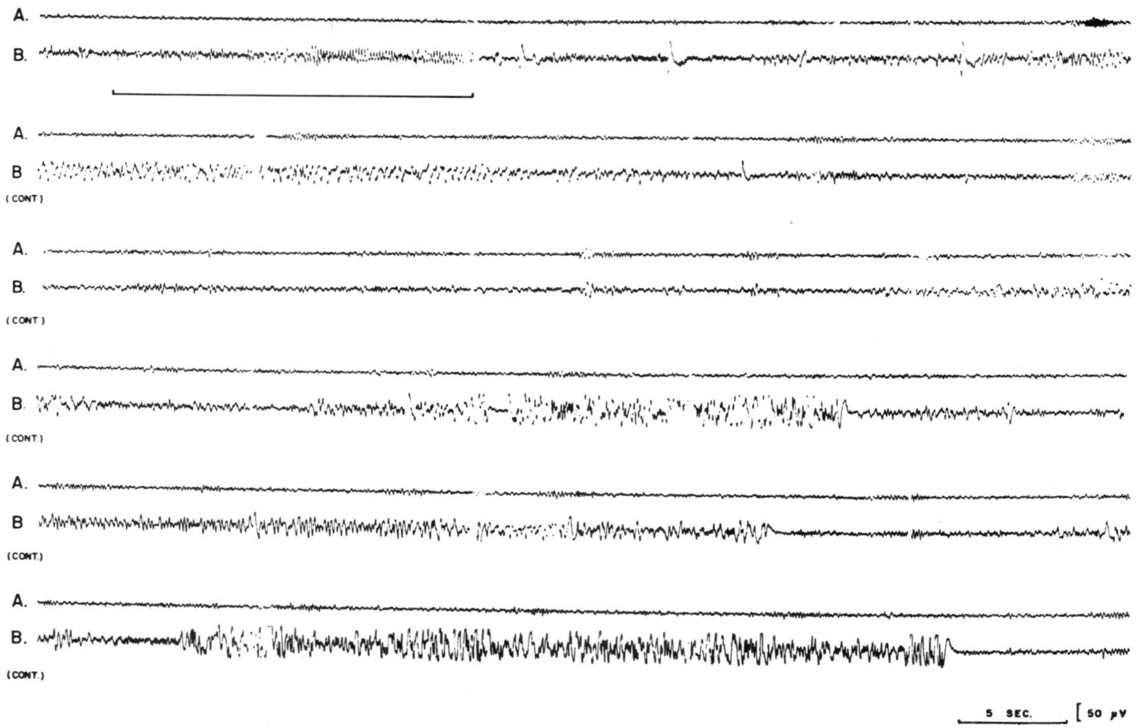

Figure 14. Records of Electrical Activity

The region is that shaded in Figure 13, but from the cat; patterns show high-frequency, large amplitude discharge during vaginal stimulation. Channel A records from the medial and channel B from the lateral hypothalamus. From Porter, Cavanaugh, Critchlow, and Sawyer (36).

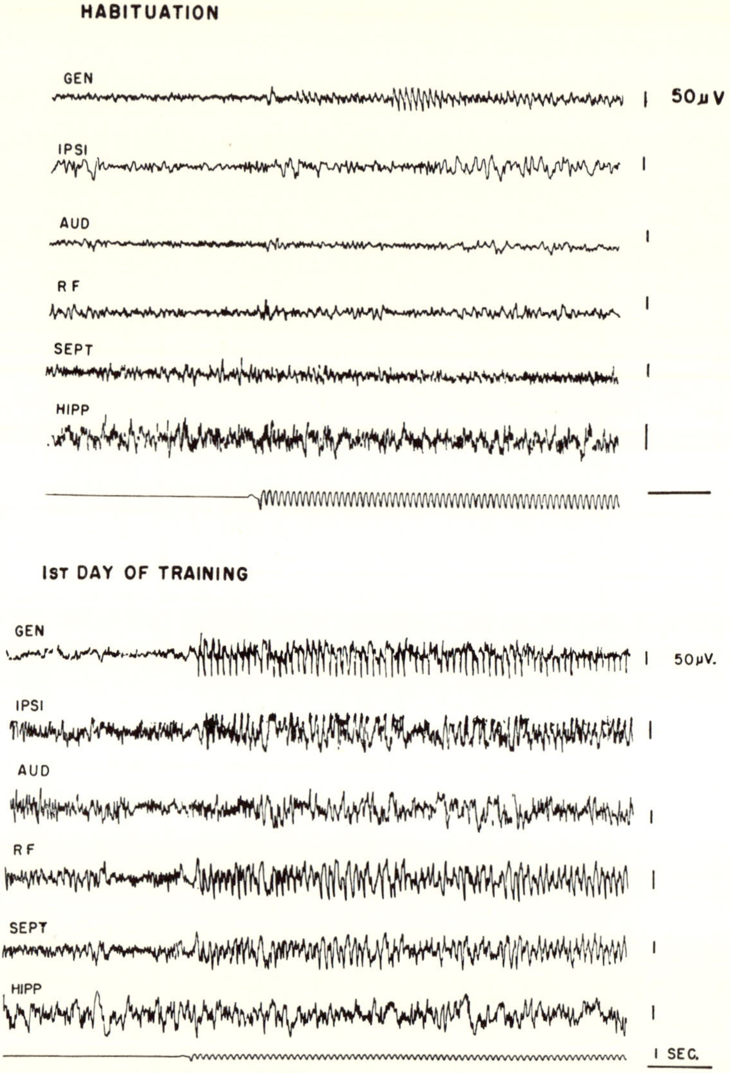

Figure 15. Records of Electrical Activity

Records are from specific (upper three channels) and nonspecific (lower three channels) areas of the cat's brain, showing the minimal and restricted response to photic stimulation (signal) after habituation (above), and the marked increment in amplitude, and the generalization of response with introduction of reinforcement (below). GEN: lateral geniculate body; IPSI: visual cortex; AUD: auditory cortex; RF: midbrain tegmentum; SEPT: septum; HIPP: hippocampus. From John and Killam (22).

afforded by monitoring tracer responses evoked in central neural stations by afferent stimulation before and during reinforcement. In the experiments of John and Killam (22) novel photic stimuli,

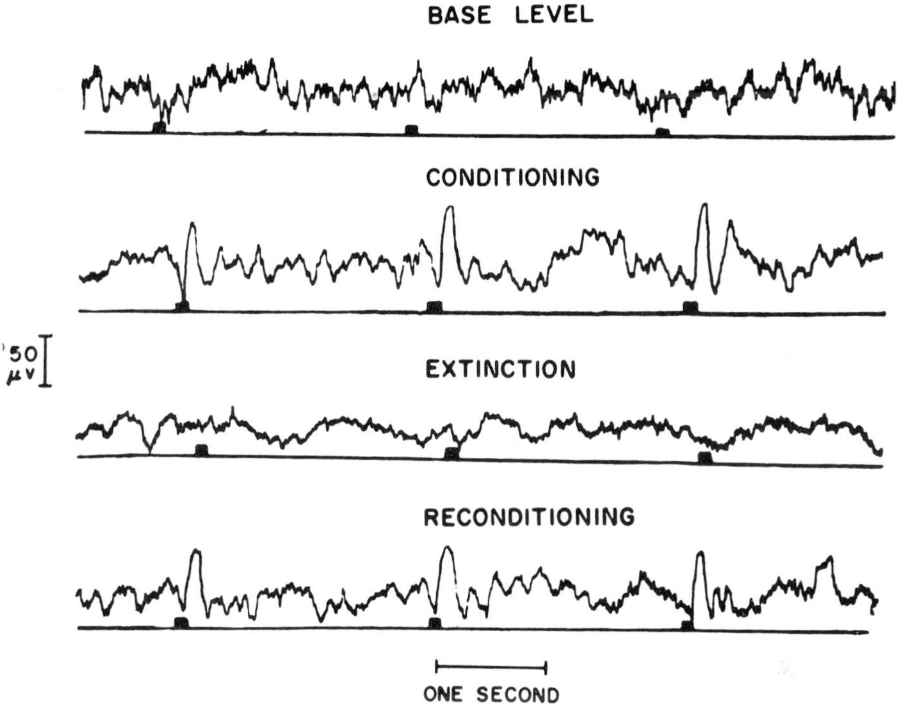

Figure 16. Records of Electrical Activity from Hippocampus of the Monkey

Records show potentials evoked by tone stimuli from above downward: in the control period, during reinforcement in conditioning (note marked increase in amplitude and duration of response), during extinction (note disappearance of response), and during reconditioning (note return of response with increased amplitude and duration). From Hearst, Beer, Sheatz and Galambos (42).

which initially evoked widespread high-amplitude activity, were repeatedly presented, unpaired with any consequence, until their amplitude became reduced and their distribution confined to the visual pathway (Figure 15). Immediately thereafter, when avoidance training was begun, by pairing shocks to the feet with the tracer stimuli, responses again became widely generalized and exhibited a marked increase in amplitude (Figure 15). In similar experiments of Hearst *et al.* (42) tone-evoked responses in the hippocampal cortex were conspicuously augmented when reinforcement was introduced during conditioning (Figure 16). A wide generalization of evoked activity and a pronounced increment in its excursion are thus conspicuous influences exerted by reinforcement mechanisms upon the remainder of the brain.

SUMMARY

In man, the state called stress usually involves unpleasant subjective experience, together with objective features which include patterns of EEG activity and categories of endocrine, visceral, and somatic performance. There is indication from the study of experimental animals that neural mechanisms called limbic, distributed around the hilus of the cerebral hemisphere, bordering its attachment to the cephalic brainstem, are importantly involved.

Recent investigations of limbic function in experimental animals have identified positive and negative reinforcement systems which can be set into play by direct electrical stimulation. Recording the electrical activity of limbic structures has distinguished two patterns of electrical discharge associated with excited behavior. One of these is the high-amplitude, four to seven per second, theta activity distributed from the hippocampus to the cingulate and entorhinal cortex. The second is a forty-per-second burst discharge distributed from the prepyriform cortex and amygdala to the hypothalamus and brainstem. Involvement of the reinforcement mechanisms of the limbic brain has been found to increase the amplitude and to generalize the distribution of activity in other parts of the brain.

These developments of the last twenty years, following Papez's fertile hypothesis, provide most of what we know currently about the neurophysiology of stress.

REFERENCES

1. Adey, W. R., Studies of hippocampal electrical activity during approach learning, in *Brain Mechanisms and Learning*. Montevideo, CIOMS Symposium, 1959.
2. Adey, W. R., C. W. Dunlop, and S. Sunderland, A survey of rhinencephalic interconnections with the brain stem, J. Comp. Neurol., 110:173–203, 1958.
3. Adey, W. R., C. R. Merrillees, and S. Sunderland, The entorhinal area: behavioral, evoked potential and histological studies of its relationships with brain-stem regions, Brain, 79:414–439, 1956.
4. Adey, W. R., S. Sunderland, and C. W. Dunlop, The entorhinal area: electrophysiological studies of its interrelations with rhinencephalic structures and the brain stem, EEG Clin. Neurophysiol. 9:309–324, 1957.

5. Barcroft, J., Features in the Architecture of Physiological Function. Cambridge, The University Press, 1934.
6. Bernard, C., Leçons sur les Propriétés Physiologiques et les Altérations Pathologiques des Liquides de l'Organisme. 2 vols., Paris, 1859.
7. Broca, P., Anatomie comparée des circonvolutions cérébrales: Le grand lobe limbique et la scissure limbique dans la série des mammiferes, Rev. anthrop., 1:385–498, 1878.
8. Cannon, W. B., Bodily Changes in Pain, Hunger, Fear and Rage. New York, D. Appleton & Co., 1929.
9. Delgado, J. M. R., W. W. Roberts, and N. E. Miller, Learning motivated by electrical stimulation of the brain, Am. J. Physiol., 179:587–593, 1954.
10. Delgado, J. M. R., H. E. Rosvold, and E. Looney, Evoking conditioned fear by electrical stimulation of subcortical structures in the monkey brain, J. Comp. & Physiol. Psychol., 49:373–380, 1956.
11. Feindel, W., and W. Penfield, Localization of discharge in temporal lobe automatism, Arch. Neurol. & Psychiat., 72:605–630, 1954.
12. Freeman, W. J., Correlation of electrical activity of prepyriform cortex and behavior in cat, J. Neurophysiol., 23:111–131, 1960.
13. Fulton, J. F., The limbic system: a study of the visceral brain in primates and man, Yale J. Biol. Med., 26:107–118, 1953.
14. Gloor, P., The pattern of conduction of amygdaloid seizure discharge, Arch. Neurol. & Psychiat., 77:247–258, 1957.
15. Grastyan, E., The hippocampus and higher nervous activity, in M. A. B. Brazier, ed., *CNS and Behavior*. New York, Josiah Macy Jr. Foundation, 1959.
16. Green, J. D., and W. R. Adey, Electrophysiological studies of hippocampal connections and excitability, EEG Clin. Neurophysiol., 8:245–262, 1956.
17. Green, J. D., and A. Arduini, Hippocampal electrical activity in arousal, J. Neurophysiol., 17:533–557, 1954.
18. Green, J. D., and T. Shimamoto, Hippocampal seizures and their propagation, Arch. Neurol. & Psychiat., 70:687–702, 1953.
19. Herrick, C. J., The Brain of the Tiger Salamander. Chicago, Univ. of Chicago Press, 1948.
20. Hess, W. R., Diencephalon, Autonomic and Extrapyramidal Functions. New York, Grune & Stratton, 1954.
21. Hunsperger, R. W., Affektreaktionen auf elektrische Reizung im Hirnstamm der Katze, Helvet. physiol. acta, 14:70–92, 1956.
22. John, E. R., and K. F. Killam, Electrophysiological correlates of avoidance conditioning in the cat, J. Pharmacol. & Exper. Therap., 125:252–274, 1959.
23. Kaada, B. R., Somato-motor, autonomic and electrocorticographic responses to electrical stimulation of "rhinencephalic" and other structures in primates, cat and dog, Acta physiol. Scandinav. (Suppl. 83), 24:285, 1951.
24. Lesse, H., Rhinencephalic electrophysiological activity during "emotional behavior" in cats, Psychiat. Res. Rep., 12:224–237, 1960.
25. Lilly, J. C., Learning motivated by subcortical stimulation: the "start" and "stop" patterns of behavior, in H. H. Jasper, ed., *Reticular Formation of the Brain*. Boston, Little, Brown & Co., 1958.
26. Lindsley, D. B., Emotion, in S. S. Stevens, ed., *Handbook of Experimental Psychology*. New York, Wiley, 1951.
27. MacLean, P. D., Psychosomatic disease and the "visceral brain": Recent developments bearing on the Papez theory of emotion, Psychosom. Med., 11:338–353, 1949.
28. MacLean, P. D., Contrasting functions of limbic and neocortical systems of the brain and their relevance to psychophysiological aspects of medicine, Am. J. Med., 25:611–626, 1958.
29. MacLean, P. D., The limbic system with reference to two life principles, in M. A. B. Brazier, ed., CNS and Behavior. New York, Josiah Macy Jr. Foundation, 1959.

30. Nauta, W. J. H., Hippocampal projections and related neural pathways to the midbrain in the cat, Brain, in press.
31. Olds, J., and P. Milner, Positive reinforcement produced by electrical stimulation of septal and other regions of the rat brain, J. Comp. & Physiol. Psychol., 47:419–427, 1954.
32. Olds, J., A preliminary mapping of electrical reinforcement effects in the rat brain, J. Comp. & Physiol. Psychol., 49:281–285, 1956.
33. Olds, J., Self-stimulation of the brain, Science, 127:315–324, 1958.
34. Papez, J. W., A proposed mechanism of emotion. Arch. Neurol. & Psychiat., 38:725–745, 1937.
35. Penfield, W., and H. H. Jasper, Epilepsy and the Functional Anatomy of the Human Brain. Boston, Little, Brown & Co., 1954.
36. Porter, R. W., E. B. Cavanaugh, B. V. Critchlow, and C. H. Sawyer, Localized changes in electrical activity of the hypothalamus in estrous cats following vaginal stimulation, Am. J. Physiol., 189:145–151, 1957.
37. Pribram, K. H., and L. Kruger, Functions of the olfactory brain. Ann. N. Y. Acad. Sci., 58:109–138, 1954.
38. Pibram, K. H., and P. D. MacLean, Neuronographic analysis of medial and basal cerebral cortex: II, Monkey, J. Neurophysiol., 16:324–340, 1953.
39. Sawyer, C. H., Nervous control of ovulation, in C. W. Lloyd, ed., *The Endocrinology of Reproduction*. New York, Academic Press, 1959.
40. Selye, H., and G. Heuser, Fifth Annual Report on Stress, 1955–56. New York, M.D. Publications, 1956.
41. Sem-Jacobsen, C. W., in H. H. Jasper, ed., *Reticular Formation of the Brain*, pp. 725–726. Boston, Little Brown & Co., 1958.
42. Hearst, E., B. Beer, G. Sheatz, and R. Galambos, Some electrophysiological correlates of conditioning in the monkey, EEG Clin. Neurophysiol., 12:137–152, 1960.
43. Williams, D., The structure of emotions reflected in epileptic experiences, Brain, 79:29–67, 1956.

Neuroendocrine Aspects of Stress

MORTIMER H. APPLEZWEIG

Some interesting parallels can be drawn between space and neuroendocrine stress research. Both have captivated man's imagination from early times, and yet man has lacked adequate philosophic and practical tools to explore either directly. In the past several decades, however, both fields have shown markedly accelerated activity curves.

Both have seen the introduction of new languages, new technological procedures, and new theoretical concepts. With regard to language, at least in the field of endocrinology, reading a summary of research is like reading a directory of federal agencies (e.g., ACTH, STH, TTH, DOC, LH, LSD, APS, ADH, FSH, NSM, F-COL). At the technological level, both fields have benefited immensely from the same types of advances in miniaturization, improved electronic signalling and recording devices, and precision computation and data analysis equipment. We have been able to observe, to store, and to integrate more things, and more varied things, more rapidly.

At the conceptual level, both areas have arrived—admittedly through mutual stimulation—at identical frames of reference, revolving around the same single fascinating idea, the feed-back loop (1, 2, 3). And finally, as a footnote to this list of parallels, one may note that both areas have been significantly stimulated by the theoretical and technical advances made and being made by our opposite numbers in Russia.

PROGRESS IN NEUROENDOCRINOLOGY

The tracing of hidden relations within the body is as exciting an adventure as any past expedition to unknown lands or even the

Dr. Applezweig is Professor and Chairman, Department of Psychology, Southern Illinois University, Carbondale, Illinois.

prospective explorations of the great beyond. Progress is being made despite the intrinsic difficulties of working in areas where so much must be learned by inference about systems which are not directly observable. In addition to this major handicap to rapid progress, there are limitations inherent in the circumstances of the different particular laboratories with regard to available means, methods, and species of subjects. Thus, one laboratory studies rats exclusively, another rabbits, a third monkeys or men. One laboratory relies on blood plasma evaluations primarily, a second uses histology, a third population decimation, or clinical evaluation of subjective states. One laboratory straps its subjects into special "conditioning chairs," a second flies its investigators to field locations, a third uses naturally diseased patients in hospitals, or artificially incubates "disease models," or studies *in vitro* preparations, and so it goes. Generalizations from each of these situations must be carefully checked against comparable studies elsewhere; contradictory findings must be evaluated as to species used, method of treatment, method of analysis of effects, and method of testing for significance, etc.

This wide range of differences in methodologies and findings need not be discouraging, however, in light of the sheer volume of work being done and the resultant cross-checking this permits. Through frequent review and evaluation, and through regular unrestricted exchange of information, considerable progress is being made toward clarifying the multitude of problems in the field.

This writer could claim neither the space nor the competence to provide a comprehensive synthesis of this vast and rapidly changing field. Instead, these pages will be devoted to (1) an indication of the sources where attempts have been made to review, synthesize, or summarize relevant topics; (2) an outline of the "stress concept" as it currently stands; and (3) an indication of some of the more active areas of research which seem likely to produce useful new information or integration.

CURRENT RESOURCE MATERIALS

In the neuroendocrine family (including such siblings as neuropharmacology, neurophysiology, neuropsychology, neurochemistry, neuropsychiatry, psychoendocrinology, psychophysiology, psychopharmacology—and close cousins like electroencephalography, bioelectrics, neuroanatomy, etc.), the rate of new findings has outstripped normal publishing channels, giving rise to crowded report meetings, new interdisciplinary journals, and the publication of proceedings of more and more special meetings (such as this). Well over a dozen English-language conferences have been held in the past decade, directly or closely related to the topic of neuroendocrinology and stress (4–15, 25–29).

Probably the most courageous attempts to marshal the burgeoning literature of the field of stress research were made by Hans Selye, who followed his comprehensive volume on the *Physiology and Pathology of Exposure to Stress* (16) with five successive annual reports (17–21), classifying over 40,000 papers and books in the field up to 1956. Our own modest attempt to bring together the references in the more delimited area of psychological stress ran to over 2,600 items in 1957 (22), and one could estimate that over 1,000 papers and books have been published in English alone since then.

Specialized collaborations and reviews continue in selected areas in the *Annual Review of Physiology* (23), the *Recent Progress in Hormone Research* series (24), and in the cumulating Ciba colloquia (25), the Josiah Macy, Jr., Foundation conferences (3, 26, 27), and the Publications of the Association for Research on Nervous and Mental Diseases (28, 29). So much for general source material. There is not, to my knowledge, a thoroughly up-to-date textbook on neuroendocrinology, a fact not difficult to understand in a field so rapidly changing.

THE CONCEPT OF STRESS AND THE GENERAL ADAPTATION SYNDROME

Claude Bernard focused our attention on the importance of balanced states within the "milieu interior" of the organism (30), and Walter Cannon gave us both a name for these balanced states—homeostasis—and some very useful insights into the means by which the body maintains them (31). In particular, Cannon greatly stimulated research on the autonomic nervous system and the adrenal medulla as part of the organism's reaction to emergency requirements imposed on its homeostatic systems (32). Along these same lines, an even more powerful unifying theory and stimulus to research was offered by Hans Selye in his concept of systemic stress and the processes of adaptation. Selye distinguishes between the *specific* effects induced by a particular marked stimulus change and the effects induced by such stimulation which are *not* specific to it. He had observed that whereas one stimulus (e.g., cold) may produce a vasoconstriction, and a second stimulus (e.g., heat) a vasodilation, both (or either), if applied intensely or long enough, produce nonspecific effects in common. Selye described these common changes, taken together, as *systemic stress* (". . . the sum of all non-specifically induced changes in a biologic system" [33, p. 403]). He described any stimulus sufficient to induce such changes as a *stressor agent*. Subsequent investigation has shown that a very large number and variety of stressors exist, as we shall indicate shortly.

Pattern of Adaptation. The common response, or stress syndrome, seems to follows a characteristic adaptive pattern. Selye has labeled this the General-Adaptation-Syndrome (G-A-S). This syndrome has three stages: (1) an *alarm reaction*, including the initial *shock phase* and a *countershock phase*, in which the defensive mechanisms begin to operate; (2) a *stage of resistance*, in which the adaptive responses are optimal; and (3) a *stage of exhaustion*, marking the loss of acquired adaptation. The G-A-S may be short-circuited by an intense or overwhelming stressor, such that no countershock or resistance develops, the organism going from the shock phase into exhaustion and death; or, it may be foreshortened or prolonged, depending upon the intensity and/or duration of the stressor and the state of the organism at the time of exposure. We shall return to these "conditioning" factors a little later.

Specific vs. General Adaptation. As was earlier indicated, specific stimuli elicit specific responses. The stress syndrome refers only to those responses over and beyond the particular local or focal adaptations associated with the type of stressor (e.g., vasodilatation with heat, antibody formation with infection, etc.). The general function of the stress syndrome would appear to be the modification of bodily processes in such a way as to make available energy resources normally kept in reserve or utilized for other functions (such as digestion, anabolism). The excess demands placed upon the organism by the application of a stressor agent appear, then, to arouse local response, where a local stressor has been applied (a tri-phasic Local Adaptation Syndrome has been observed and described by Selye); but when systemic threat is indicated (as by continuous or intense stimulation, or by anticipation of noxious stimulation), the general systemic reaction is invoked, namely, the G-A-S.

The Over-All Pathways of the Stress Syndrome. Figure 1 illustrates the over-all pathways of the stress syndrome. We will hasten to say that not all of the interconnections are shown, that certain alternate pathways are shown where it is not clear which one or more is *the* channel of influence, and that many of the pathways shown may exert inhibitory as well as facilitatory influence. Contributions to general resistance may be direct or mediated through indirect processes.

On the left side of the diagram are shown some of the identified symptoms of stress—those associated with the pituitary-adrenal axis and those which appear in stress responses even in the absence of the adrenals and/or the hypophysis. Between the two we have suggested the likelihood that other somatopsychic and psychosomatic symptoms or disease entities may be expected to be identified as stress phenomena.

In the main diagram, we have tried to show how the stress syndrome operates. Damage or trauma give rise to defensive reaction. Two pathways are shown. The one on the right, labeled neurohumoral defense, runs through the nervous system to the endocrine system (with intermediate feedback loops). Before describing this further, we may note what has been called a possible direct pathway to the anterior pituitary. Fortier (34) and Harris (35) have postulated such a direct pathway for certain systemic (as opposed to neural) stressors in light of the observed release of ACTH from the anterior pituitary in the absence of connection with the hypothalamus. However, Ganong and Forsham (36), in a current review, challenge this idea on the basis of the fact that no pituitary activity has been observed when lesions are placed in the median eminence. The evidence is by no means complete, however, and the possible distinction between systemic and neural or "psychic" stressors as acting through these separate pathways must remain an unsettled question for the time being.

Tracing the main pathways of neurohumoral defense, we come first to the designation "cortex and other higher brain centers." This refers to the complex of interrelated systems above the level of the hypothalamus, including sensory and motor centers in the

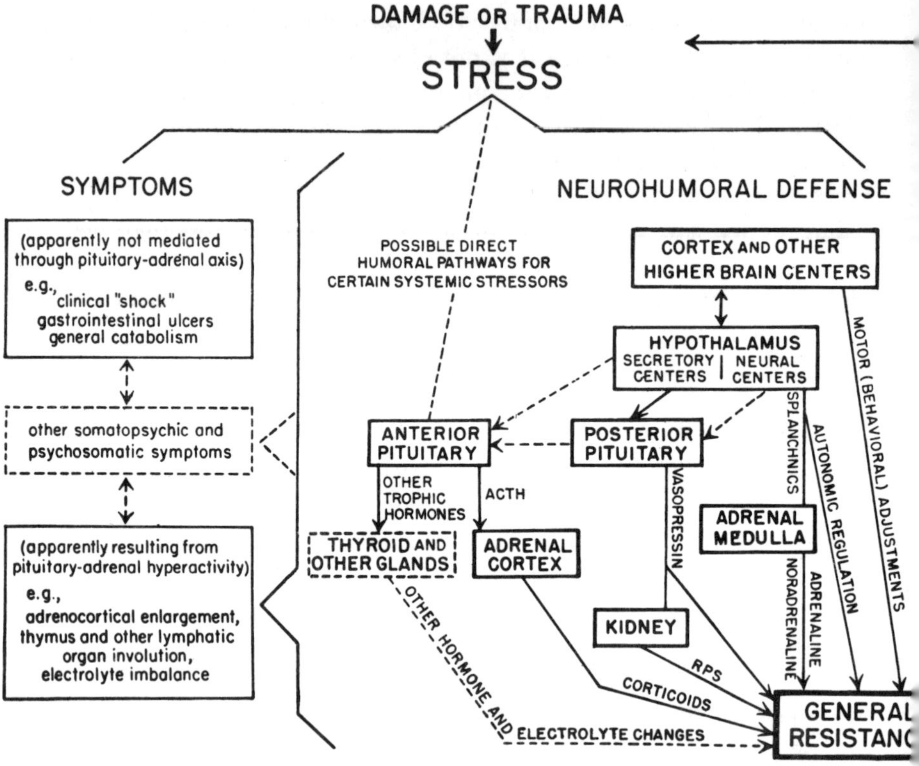

Figure 1. General Schema of Stress Syndrome

Solid lines represent known relations, broken lines suspected relations.

cortex, and the limbic system complex, which is being so carefully explored with new techniques (37, 38), as Professor Magoun has described in this volume. Where stress is communicated through sensory or "psychic" means, the involvement of the central nervous system is obvious. That it may be involved regardless of the source or nature of stimulation is gaining wider acceptance today, by virtue of the possibility of feedback mechanisms through the hypothalamus and the ascending reticular formation.

We have shown the autonomic nervous system as becoming involved via a "neural" center of the hypothalamus, thus to distinguish nervous from humoral stimulation. Whether such a distinction is very meaningful anymore, in light of the discovery of neurohumoral substances and neurosecretory material (15, 39) is an open question. At any rate, autonomic involvement is indicated directly, and also through the release of adrenaline and noradrenaline from the adrenal medulla. The interesting question of the relation of these two catechol-amines, and the quantities released under different circumstances, has occupied a number of investigators recently, (40, 41).

The profusion of arrows from the hypothalamus to the posterior and anterior pituitary reflects this writer's uncertainty as to the latest state of hypothalamic-hypophyseal relationships. For example, it is now fairly well established that vasopressin, and probably oxytocin, the posterior pituitary hormones, are actually neurosecretory materials, produced in the hypothalamus and only stored in the pituitary. Vasopressin, the anti-diuretic substance (ADH), is known to act through the kidney, as well as contributing directly to general resistance. In addition, some claim has been made for vasopressin, or a closely related corticotrophin-releasing-factor (CRF), as a stimulant to ACTH release, although this could not be the only means of ACTH activation. Facilitation and inhibition of ACTH release by the hypothalamus are facts beyond question, though whether these actions occur directly, through the hypophysioportal circulation, indirectly through capillary anastomoses between the hypothalamus and the median eminence, and thence to the anterior pituitary, indirectly through the general circulation, or in some unidentified way through the posterior pituitary, is not yet clearly established (39, 42).

However stimulated, a major pathway of the stress syndrome is through the release of ACTH from the anterior pituitary and its effect on the adrenal cortex. Gluco- and mineralo-corticoids released by the adrenal cortex are known to act upon the stressor (as for example in inflammation) as well as on the catabolic responses of the organism as a whole. A number of other actions are effected by trophic hormones of the anterior pituitary, although it is not known that any of them is directly produced as a result of stress. We have shown these influences by use of a broken line.

Finally, the diagram illustrates the contribution of a number of patterns of response, intricately interrelated, and all contributing to what we have called "general resistance." This in turn acts back upon the stressor, completing the main feedback loop. Intermediate loops, some of which are known, must be traced to account for facilitation and inhibition of (1) manufacture, (2) storage, and (3) rate of release of subsystem products. It is known, for example, that adrenaline may stimulate ACTH release, as can perhaps a drop in the amount of circulating gluco-corticoids, and also vasopressin or others of the posterior pituitary substances. If and how these depend on each other we simply do not know.

In any event, as in a fascinating treasure hunt, the clues are coming in one by one, some confusing and others clarifying the over-all pattern.

Characteristic Changes in Stress. Among other indications, the presence of a stress syndrome can be inferred from a triad of distinct and readily identifiable manifestations: adrenocortical enlargement, thymicolymphatic involution, with associated eosinopenia and lymphopenia, and gastrointestinal ulcers. Figure 2, through the courtesy of Doctor Selye, illustrates the nature of these changes as observed in a rat exposed to a single prolonged session of forced immobilization. These changes are characteristic of an intact organism exposed to stressful stimulation. However, as could be inferred from the multiple pathways of Figure 1, the pituitary-adrenocortical axis is only one of the many pathways of stress. Selye early demonstrated, as have others, that the adrenal glands, and even the pituitary which stimulates the adrenal cortex, are not essential to the occurrence of the stress response. Manifold effects of stressor agents (including the gastric ulcers of Figure 2)

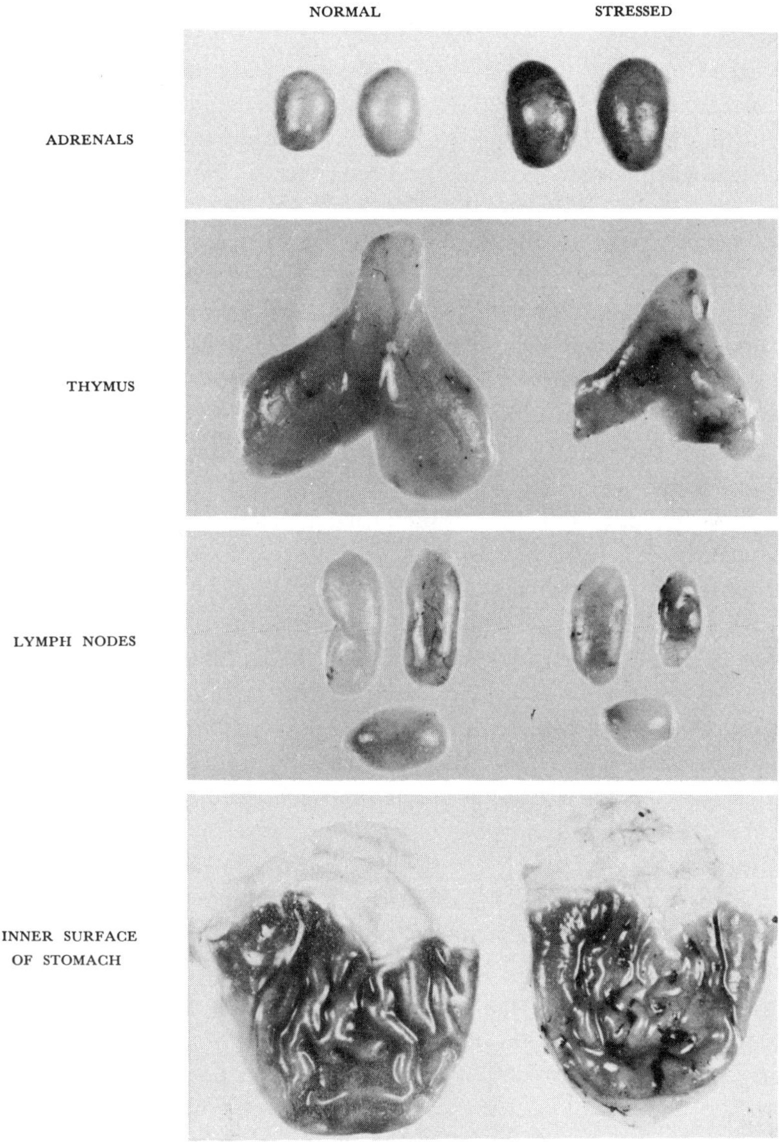

Figure 2. Characteristic Symptoms of Stress Syndrome

Note enlarged and discolored adrenals, involuted thymus and lymph nodes, ulcerated stomach wall. After H. Selye, *The Story of the Adaptation Syndrome* (Montreal, Acta Inc., 1952); reproduced with permission.

can be observed in stressed adrenalectomized and/or hypophysectomized animals. However, the stage of exhaustion is reached much more rapidly in hypophysectomized and/or adrenalectomized organisms, as both experimental and clinical data have shown.

Stress and the "Diseases of Adaptation." A most significant aspect of systemic stress is the fact that initially adaptive changes may themselves become stressful. Thus, research at the Institute in Montreal has produced a large series of "experimental diseases" in animals as a result of prolonged exposure to and/or treatment with large quantities of exogenously administered "adaptive" hormones of the adrenal gland, in combination with other factors. Damage to the heart, the kidney, the liver, the blood vessels, the bones, and the skin have all been produced as a result of normally nonpathogenic factors intensified through stress exposure. Similarly, the flurry of clinical reports on side-effects of ACTH and cortisone treatments reflects this problem. The concept of psychosomatic medicine is predicted on the hypothesis of self-damage through attempts at adaptation (see e.g., 29). The precise mechanisms of somatic compliance are by no means clear, but the production of disease—or its precipitation, at least—is readily predictable.

Stress and Homeostasis. We have already indicated that the stress syndrome is, in a way, a result of the breakdown of homeostatic mechanisms in one or more of the body's systems. The homeostatic processes have been well-conceived as feedback systems, and the failure of a feedback system may be understood in terms of a modification in the amount of input at any point in the system. Automatic invoking of additional feedback loops may follow such quantitative change in input. If the system is complex enough, a very large series of changes can be started by a failure anywhere in the system. Stress may usefully be conceptualized as such a cycle. Stress responses may contribute to re-levelling of the homeostatic system initially in jeopardy. But they may, in addition, start cycles of changes in other systems that can, if prolonged, produce effects unrelated to the source of pathology. They may actually aggravate the pathological changes and, in a general purposive sense, serve no real value to the organism's survival.

It seems to us that a theoretical framework exists in the cybernetic notions of communication nets which appears adequate, descriptively, to account for the multiple interrelationships associated with homeostatic feedback loops and the more widely involved stress syndrome. The diverse input sources and the varied effects of stress may be conceptually linked in terms of such a frame of reference. The current search for linking mechanisms has actually been much stimulated by this concept. The signal systems used by the organism in its vast communication networks are so far identifiable as involving electrical, chemical, and pressure modes. Whether bioelectric and biochemical studies will establish still more significant electromagnetic or other means of passing signals from one system to the next, remains one of the intriguing questions still to be answered.

What Is Stressful? Perhaps the most important reason for the widespread interest in the stress syndrome is that it may be aroused by such varied stressor agents. Selye and his associates have used a large number of systemic stressors to activate the syndrome (16–21): e.g., cold, heat, inflammation, hemorrhage, restraint, muscular exercise, drugs, exogenous hormones, injury, shock, and surgical trauma. From the psychoanalytic literature, and from both clinical and experimental medicine and psychology, we have had a quantity of data suggesting that those conditions which induce anxiety are factors which give rise to a stress syndrome (43–47). Anxiety here referred to has been measured through evaluation of subjective feeling states, projective tests, behavior change, and ratings of "emotionality" in both men and animals. In many instances it has also been shown to be correlated with blood or urine changes indicative of the stress syndrome.

In a review covering only the past year, and that selectively, Ganong and Forsham (36) cite nineteen stressors producing pituitary-adrenocortical response. These include varieties of drug and hormone treatments, use of intense or novel stimuli, "psychic" stressors, and infectious materials. Actually, any stimulus can serve as a stressor, depending on the context of its application. Significant is the fact that not only direct intervention (surgical, pharmacological, or physical) but indirect (neurogenic or psychogenic) stimulation can induce a stress syndrome. Mason (48), for example, has shown that such subtle factors as the presence or absence of persons in a room, the change from one room to another, or the application of previously shock-associated stimuli could produce measurable indices of adrenocortical response. Christian (49) has reported both laboratory and field studies in which what he calls "sociopsychological" stimulation of size of animal colony has produced stress. Such factors are independent of mere physical crowding or space restriction. The preliminary studies of Porter *et al.* (50) suggest that gastric ulcers can be produced in monkeys placed under a decision-making stress. Paired controls, receiving as much shock but having no choice to make as to whether or not the shock would be received, remained ulcer-free.[1]

Basowitz *et al.* (45) using paratroopers, Cook and Wherry (51) studying submariners, Mason (48) with pilots, and Davis *et al.* (52) with combat infantrymen, among others, have demonstrated that life-threat and social-status-threat situations could serve as stressors. The degree of stress depends on the type of threat and certain pre-stress "conditioning" factors (see below). In humans we often include among such factors the so-called "dynamic" variables of personality and motivation. A wide range of clinical data has particularly pointed to such pre-exposure determinants of "stressability" (29, 43, 46).

What appears to emerge, then, is that systemic insults (e.g., injury, injection of foreign substances, drugs) and neuro- and psychogenic stimulation (e.g., anticipation of pain, uncertainty, excess or deficiency of neural input, anxiety-provoking situation, or situations made noxious only as a result of prior conditioning) may both invoke patterns of stress. Depending on the length and severity of exposure, both may lead to similar adaptations or diseases of adaptation—in the form of psychological as well as somatic response; there is an intimate interplay of psychic and somatic factors. Timing, motor, sensory and ideational behavior may become distorted as a result of the multiple metabolic derangements induced by stress exposure (47).

This dual capacity of stress—to serve both adaptive and maladaptive ends, continues to be one of its most fascinating characteristics. Sorting out the conditions which give rise to protective effects from those which lead to disease is an extremely important current area of active research.

[1] Apparently the ulcers are produced only under certain particular temporal patterns. Experimental parameters of these studies are under careful reinvestigation now at the Walter Reed laboratories, where the preliminary results were reported.

THREE DETERMINERS OF STRESSFULNESS

Temporal Factors and Adaptation. One clear clue to stress minimizing is the factor of timing. In the Montreal Institute as elsewhere, studies are showing that "critical periods" exist for the incubation of stress effects as well as for the "readiness" of the system(s) to be exposed to stress. Slow adaptation, through systematically increased exposure to stimulation, may be able to modify stress thresholds, such that stimulus intensities earlier intolerable may be experienced without inducing full-blown stress responses. The parameters of adaptation procedures need careful working out, however.

Actually, one cannot go through life avoiding stress—life and stress are too intimately related. Living "hard" or "fast" may wear out the organism more rapidly—but who is to be the judge of one's life pace? What is indicated from stress research, however, is the need for ordered or systematic living. Selye recently offered the analogy of a driver applying the brake at the same time he steps on the accelerator as an example of inappropriate use of the life vehicle. Certainly both brake and accelerator are to be used—it is only their simultaneous use that is pathogenic.

Hormonal Factors as "Conditioners." A second consideration of major importance is that hormonal changes induced by stress may play not only a direct role in inhibiting or releasing energy, but an even more significant role as "co-operators" with other factors in modifying body metabolism and causing or preventing damage. Selye has described these effects as "conditioning factors" (a term not to be confused with the Pavlovian use). Conditioning here refers to the sensitizing effect of pre-exposure or simultaneous exposure to stress or to adaptive hormones on a particular organ or system. Thus, administration of certain electrolytes in large doses to rats would ordinarily be nonpathogenic. But if a quantity of cortical hormone is administered at the same time, the combination will be effective in producing such pathologies as cardiac necroses, nephroscleroses, etc. More to the point is the further demonstration that nonpathogenic combinations of steroids and electrolytes may become suprathreshold (and thus pathogenic) upon exposure to stress. On the other hand, damage can be prevented by gradual adaptation to stress prior to exposure (53). Why these interactions occur, and what their mechanisms are, remain unknown, but the fact of their occurrence has been established beyond doubt.

Neuroendocrine and Neurovisceral Conditioning. The term conditioning, in the sense used by psychologists (after Pavlov and Bechterov), describes the effects of pairing a neutral stimulus with one capable of eliciting a given response. Under appropriate conditions, a series of such pairings would lead to the elicitation of the response by the previously neutral stimulus alone. Extensive research has shown that conditioning is possible not only of motor and exocrine reactions, but of endocrine and visceral responses as well. Bykov, recently edited and translated by Gantt (54), has summarized a vast Russian literature showing the conditionability of a variety of visceral processes through the use of both exteroceptive and interoceptive stimuli. Thus conditioned diuresis was established to a particular room, to a distinct stimulus (horn), to injection of water into the stomach; inhibition of this response was likewise able to be controlled as a result of the systematic pairing of stimuli. Heart and vascular conditioning, splenic conditioning, respiratory conditioning and conditioning of HCl secretion have all been demonstrated in response not only to stimulation via the exteroceptive sensory pathways, but to physiologically neutral solutions after pairing with such hormones as thyroxine (see 54). Further, it has been shown that both chemical and neural stimulation of internal organs can serve as conditioned stimuli to overt responses which are induced through separate means. Finally, a complex system of interrelations has been demonstrated between chemical (i.e., hormonal and metabolic) and neural receptor and response systems—interrelationships which may be modified by experimental conditioning. It is reasonable to assume that these modifications occur quite regularly through what might be called the "circumstantial conditioning" of life.

Two current examples of neurohumoral conditioning appeared in recent issues of *Science*. In one study, Cook *et al.* (55) demonstrated that epinephrine, nor-epinephrine and acetylcholine could serve as conditioned stimuli to a shock avoidance response. Control injections of saline were ineffective as conditioned stimuli.[2] In a

[2] It should be noted that the stimuli were introduced via catheters. Had they been injected directly, one might expect conditioning to the needle, as has elsewhere been observed.

second study, two Czechoslovakian investigators (56) were able to show a significant rise in blood-sugar levels during repeated ten-minute waiting periods in a special cage prior to administration of electric shock to rats. Bilateral lesions of the midline thalamic nuclei—a part of the brain-stem reticular formation—abolished this "metabolic preparatory response." The authors conclude that ". . . afferent pathways from the diencephalic reticular ascending system induce, via hypothalamic centers, neurohumoral mechanisms participating in stress situations . . ." (56, pp. 1097–98).

We have cited these two instances of many recent studies to indicate the consistent nature of findings of neurohumoral interrelations and the usefulness of conditioned responses as measures of experimentally introduced changes (57, 58).

One interesting feature which emerges from the use of avoidance conditioning procedures is the distinction between escape responses from present noxious stimulation and avoidance responses in anticipation of such noxious stimulation. Apparently the two types of processes are different—the anticipatory response being more readily interrupted by a variety of procedures. In a series of studies with rats we found consistently greater difficulty in establishing avoidant responses in hypophysectomized animals as compared with controls, whereas escape responses were learned as quickly (59). A similar distinction was observed by Wenzel in reserpine-treated cats (60), and was reported earlier by Solomon and Wynne for sympathectomized dogs (61). This effect on anticipatory behavior would further affirm a close neurohumoral relation. The fact that varied types of interruptions of neurohumoral circuits produce the same interference with avoidant behavior may be only further evidence that organisms are supplied with alternate adaptive routes, permitting shifts from one to another means of self-regulation.

SUMMARY

It has been demonstrated that organisms exposed to noxious stimulation, or to the threat of noxious stimulation, develop both local and general adaptive responses. The General-Adaptation-Syndrome, or stress response, is a multisystem response, involving neural, humoral, and metabolic mechanisms in complex interrelation with each other.

Early conceptions of static and independent neural and endocrine systems, unresponsive unless stimulated, have given way to the more dynamic idea of an integrated series of neuroendocrine feedback loops in constant activity. In response to stimulation there occur shifts in function, rather than arousal. These functional shifts may lead to reverberations in systems far removed from the initial source of stimulation.

Recent research has established that the pituitary gland, of central significance to the maintenance of endocrine balance through its secretion of regulatory trophic hormones, is itself regulated by hypothalamic and brain-stem reticular areas, which receive and integrate signals from the cortex and from the viscera. Whether these centers are responsive to humoral stimulation directly is not clear. The release of humoral agents from the hypothalamus has now been established, and the suspicion that brain metabolism—and hence brain function—is influenced reciprocally by hormonal activity controlled by brain centers is widespread.

Finally, we have tried to call attention to the value of coordinate examination of neural, humoral, and behavioral data in the pursuit of the elusive mechanisms of control. Why certain agents are stressors and others are not may be determined as a function of three sets of information: (1) the innate toxicity of the agent—that is, its capacity to destroy tissue or function; (2) the unique "readiness" of the organism—its age, tissue state, previous exposure history, metabolic condition, etc.—at the time of exposure; and (3) the personal history of the individual—rat or human—in terms of prior neural, humoral, or neurohumoral conditioning. In man we have been more willing to recognize the importance of such prior conditioning histories. We refer to these generally as personality or motivational variables, but are only on the threshold of serious investigation of the ways in which such variables are established, maintained, and/or extinguished.

As neurochemistry provides more specific "natural" substances, as depth stimulation and recording studies isolate more specific functional connections, and as behavior research develops more precise methods for the quantification and manipulation of psychological variables, we can anticipate exciting, though surely more subtle, means of improving adaptation without the damaging effects of the adaptation diseases.

ACKNOWLEDGMENTS

This paper was prepared during my tenure as a National Science Foundation Science Faculty Fellow at the Institute of Experimental Medicine and Surgery, University of Montreal. I wish to thank Professor Hans Selye, Dr. Eörs Bajusz, and the other members of the Institute staff for their constructive suggestions. I am particularly indebted to Dr. Selye for the excellent opportunities provided me at the Institute[3] to become intimately acquainted with its operation and to participate in its activities. Thanks are likewise due to the National Science Foundation for making this stay possible. Naturally, the writer alone must take responsibility for any errors which appear in the manuscript.

[3] The Institute receives support from the National Institute of Neurological Diseases and Blindness, Grant No. B-2037-C1, U.S. Public Health Service, and from the National Research Council of Canada, Consol. Grant No. 11.

REFERENCES

1. Wiener, N., Cybernetics. New York, John Wiley, 1941.
2. Ashby, W. R., Design for a Brain. New York, John Wiley, 1952.
3. Von Foerster, H., ed., Cybernetics: Circular Casual and Feedback Mechanisms in Biological and Social Systems. New York, Josiah Macy Jr., Foundation, 1951.
4. Jeffrees, L. A., ed., Cerebral Mechanisms in Behavior:. The Hixon Symposium. New York, John Wiley, 1951.
5. Milbank Memorial Fund Symposium, The Biology of Mental Health and Disease. New York, Hoeber, 1952.
6. Army Medical Service Graduate School, Symposium on Stress. Washington, D.C., Walter Reed Army Medical Center, 1953.
7. Delafresnaye, J. F., ed., Brain Mechanisms and Consciousness. Oxford, Blackwell, 1954.
8. Elliott, K. A. C., I. H. Page, and J. H. Quastel, eds., Neurochemistry: The Chemical Dynamics of Brain and Nerve. Springfield, Ill., C.C. Thomas, 1955.
9. Fields, W. S., R. Guillemin, and C. A. Carton, eds., Hypothalamic-Hypophysical Interrelationships. Springfield, Ill., C. C. Thomas, 1956.
10. Korey, S. R., and J. I. Nurnberger, eds., Progress in Neurobiology. Vol. I: Neurochemistry. New York, Hoeber, 1956.
11. Heller, H., ed., The Neurohypophysis. New York, Academic Press, 1957.
12. Harlow, H. F., and C. N. Woolsey, eds., Biological and Biochemical Bases of Behavior. Madison, Univ. of Wisconsin Press, 1958.
13. Jasper, H., *et al.*, ed., Reticular Formation of the Brain. Henry Ford International Symposium. Boston, Little, Brown & Co., 1958.
14. Watterson, R. L., ed., Endocrines in Development. Developmental Biology Conference Series, 1956. Chicago, Univ. of Chicago Press, 1959.
15. Gorbman, A., ed., Comparative Endocrinology. Columbia University Symposium, Cold Spring Harbor. New York, Wiley, 1959.
16. Selye, H., The Physiology and Pathology of Exposure to Stress. Montreal, Acta, Inc., 1950.
17. Selye, H., First Annual Report on Stress. Montreal, Acta, Inc., 1951.

18. Selye, H., and A. Horava, Second Annual Report on Stress. Montreal, Acta, Inc., 1952.
19. Selye, H., and A. Horava, Third Annual Report on Stress. Montreal, Acta, Inc., 1953.
20. Selye, H., and G. Heuser, Fourth Annual Report on Stress. Montreal, Acta, Inc., 1954.
21. Selye, H., and G. Heuser, Fifth Annual Report on Stress. New York, MD Publications, 1955–56.
22. Applezweig, M. H., ed., Psychological Stress and Related Concepts: A Bibliography. Office of Naval Research NR 172–228, Contr. Nonr 996(02). New London, Connecticut College, 1957. Indices, 1958.
23. Hall, V. E., F. A. Fuhrman, and A. C. Giese, eds., Annual Review of Physiology. Palo Alto, Calif., Annual Rev., Inc., 1960.
24. Pincus, G., ed., Recent Progress in Hormone Research. Proceedings of the Laurentian Hormone Conference. Vol. XV. New York, Academic Press, 1959.
25. Wolstenholms, G. E. W., and C. M. O'Connor, eds., Neurological Basis of Behavior. London, Ciba Foundation, 1958.
26. Brazier, Mary A. B., ed., The Central Nervous System and Behavior. New York, Josiah Macy, Jr., Foundation, 1959.
27. Abramson, H. A., ed., Neuropharmacology. New York, Josiah Macy, Jr., Foundation, 1955.
28. Association for Research in N. & M. D., The Brain and Human Behavior. Research Publ. Assoc. Nerv. Mental Disease, Vol. 36. Baltimore, Williams and Wilkins, 1958.
29. Wolff, H. G., ed., Life Stress and Bodily Disease. Research Publ. Assoc. Nerv. Mental Disease, Vol. 29. Philadelphia, Williams and Wilkins, 1950.
30. Bernard, C., Introduction a l'étude de la médecine expérimentale. Paris, Flammarion, 1876.
31. Cannon, W. B., The Wisdom of the Body. New York, W. W. Norton, 1939.
32. Cannon, W. B., Bodily changes in Pain, Hunger, Fear and Rage. New York, Appleton, 1929.
33. Selye, H., Perspectives in stress research, in *Perspectives in Biology and Medicine*, Vol. II, No. 4. Chicago, Univ. of Chicago Press, 1959.
34. Fortier, C., Dual control of adrenocorticotrophin release, Endocrinology, 49:782–788, 1951.
35. Harris, G. W., Neural Control of the Pituitary Gland. London, Arnold, 1955.
36. Ganong, W. F., and P. H. Forsham, Adenohypophysis and adrenal cortex, in Ref. 23, pp. 579–614.
37. Magoun, H. W., The Waking Brain. Springfield, Ill., C. C. Thomas, 1958.
38. Mason, J. W., Limbic System Influences on the Pituitary-Adrenal Cortical System. Paper presented to American Psychosomatic Society meetings, Montreal, March, 1960.
39. Bäjusz, E., Neuroendocrine relationships, in *Progress in Neurology and Psychiatry*, New York, Grune and Stratton (in press).
40. Ax, A. F., The physiological differentiation between fear and anger in humans, Psychosomat. Med., 15:433–442, 1953.
41. Funkenstein, D. H., S. H. King, and M. E. Drolette, Mastery of Stress. Cambridge, Mass., Harvard Univ. Press, 1957.
42. Ham, A. W., Histology. 3d ed. Philadelphia, J. B. Lippincott, 1957.
43. Janis, I. L., Psychological Stress. New York, John Wiley, 1959.
44. Spitz, R. A., Some observations on psychiatric stress in infancy, in Ref. 21., pp. 193–204.
45. Basowitz, H., H. Persky, S. J. Korchin, and R. R. Grinker, Anxiety and Stress. New York, McGraw-Hill, 1955.
46. Applezweig, M. H., Psychological stress. Appendix II in *A Study of Operational Safety Requirements in the Submarine Polaris Missile System.* Groton, Conn., Electric Boat Div., General Dynamics Corp., Feb., 1957, pp. 49 (Dittograph).

47. Applezweig, M. H., Motivation and Psychological Stress. Psi Chi Lecture, U.C.L.A., Los Angeles, June, 1959.
48. Mason, J. W., Psychological influence on the pituitary-adrenal cortical system, in Ref. 24., pp. 345–389.
49. Christian, J. J., The roles of endocrine and behavioral factors in the growth of mammalian populations, in Ref. 15., pp. 71–97.
50. Porter, R. W., J. V. Brady, D. Conrad, J. W. Mason, R. Galambos, and D. McK. Rioch, Some experimental observations on gastrointestinal lesions in behaviorally conditioned monkeys, Psychosomat. Med., 20:379–394, 1958.
51. Cook, E. B., and R. J. Wherry, The urinary 17-ketosteroid output of Naval Submarine enlisted candidates during two stressful situations, Human Biol., 22:104–124, 1950.
52. Davis, S. W., F. Elmadjiann, *et al.*, A Study of Combat Stress: Korea 1952. Chevy Chase, Md., Operations Research Office, Johns Hopkins Univ., 5 Dec. 1952.
53. Selye, H., The Chemical Prevention of Cardiac Damage. New York, Ronald Press, 1958.
54. Bykov, K. M., The Cerebral Cortex and the Internal Organs. Ed. and trans. by W. H. Gantt. New York, Chemical Pub. Co., 1957.
55. Cook, L., A. Davidson, D. L. Davis, and R. T. Kelleher, Epinephrine, nor-epinephrine and acetylcholine as conditioned stimuli for avoidance behavior, Science, 131:990–991, 1960.
56. Gutmann, E., and B. Jakoubek, Nervous regulation of conditional hyperglycemia to nociceptive stimulation, Science, 131:1096–1098, 1960.
57. Miller, N. E. Effects of drugs on motivation: the value of using a variety of measures, Annals N.Y. Acad. Sci., 65:318–333, 1956.
58. Brady, J. V. Comparative Psychopharmacology: Animal Experimental Studies on the Effects of Drugs on Behavior (WRAIR-91-56); A Comparative Approach to the Evaluation of Drug Effects upon Behavior (WRAIR-105-56). Washington, D.C., Walter Reed Army Institute of Research, May, 1956.
59. Applezweig, M. H., and G. Moeller, The pituitary-adrenocortical system and anxiety in avoidance learning, in *Proceedings*, Fifteenth Internat. Congr. Psychol., Brussels, 1957 pp. 602–603. Amsterdam, North Holland Publ. Co., 1959.
60. Wenzel, Bernice, Personal communication.
61. Solomon, R. L., and L. C. Wynne, Avoidance conditioning in normal dogs and in dogs deprived of normal autonomic functioning, *Amer. Psychologist.* 5:264, 1950.

Physiological Cycling

NATHANIEL KLEITMAN

Physiological cycling enters into the critical problems of space flight when (a) the flight is to last one or more days, (b) the occupants of the space vehicle have regular tasks assigned to them in the course of the flight, and (c) the team of monitors carrying out these tasks comprises three or more persons. The period involved is the twenty-four hours of the rotation of the earth around its axis, with the resulting alternation of day and night. Upon this physical periodicity depends the social—family and community—pattern of living, regular hours being given over to work, meals, recreation, and sleep. From birth on, human beings are under the combined influence of the physical and social cycles, and each individual develops and maintains a 24-hour rhythm of sleep and wakefulness. Along with this rhythm there is a concomitant fluctuation in alertness and in efficiency of performance, as well as in several other physiological variables, including body temperature. A 24-hour curve of body temperature can be plotted by the use of an ordinary clinical thermometer at 2-, 3-, or even 4-hour intervals; it runs parallel to, and thus reflects, other physiological changes whose monitoring necessitates the employment of expensive and cumbersome equipment and time-consuming procedures.

The body temperature method of observation owes its inception to two empirical observational findings. The first resulted from a study of the effects of prolonged enforced wakefulness of several days' duration. As expected, the subjects of these experiments became sleepier as time passed and their test performance worsened, but the downward trend was not uniform; rather, it showed a 24-hour oscillation. Alertness was often greater, and test scores better, in the afternoon of the third day than in the middle of the second night of complete sleep deprivation. Body temperature, taken routinely,

Dr. Kleitman is Professor of Physiology, University of Chicago, Chicago, Illinois.

was found to vary in direct relation to the 24-hour fluctuations in alertness and performance. The second finding was made during an attempt to determine the recuperative value of a night's sleep by comparing scores obtained on a number of neuromuscular and mental tests made before and after sleep. Performance appeared to be little better (often worse) immediately on getting up in the morning than it was just prior to going to bed the night before; again, the body temperature levels varied accordingly at the two test hours. These findings led to a systematic investigation of the variation in performing such tests as hand steadiness, reaction time, code transcription, color naming, multiplication of large numbers, etc. (1, 2, 3). The test scores improved from the getting-up time on, along with a rise in body temperature, reached a peak or plateau in the late morning, early or late afternoon, or even early in the evening, but eventually became progressively worse, as the body temperature curve turned downward, until at bedtime they approximated the early morning scores. The negative correlation between body temperature and degree of sleepiness and the positive correlation between body temperature and performance were both confirmed; the first in a study of the effects of 98 hours of sleep deprivation on fifteen subjects at the Walter Reed Army Research Institute (4), the second in around-the-clock tests on a group of recruits following a simulated "dog-watch" schedule of duties at the Naval Medical Research Institute (5; Figure 1). Even the ability to sustain muscular contraction, without overt movement, seemed to be related to body temperature. Thus, fixing an object in binocular vision, to produce a single image, requires a maintained alignment of the visual axes of the two eyes. Subjects were studied photographically by reflecting light spots from the two corneas on moving film, and diplopia equal to that known to occur in alcoholic intoxication was revealed in sleepiness. By means of an ophthalmograph, the fixation ability of the extrinsic eye musculature in sleep-deprived subjects was measured around the clock. This ability was found to become progressively poorer during the night, reach its low point in the early hours of the morning (2:00 to 4:00 A.M.), and improve *spontaneously*, with no intervening sleep or oculomotor rest, later in the morning as the body temperature curve turned upward.

It should be remembered that the 24-hour variation in body

temperature, ranging from 1 to over 2 degrees F., is in no way connected with correctional changes in response to ambient heat or cold, but takes place within the thermostatic band, even if the environmental temperature is kept constant. The "normal" body

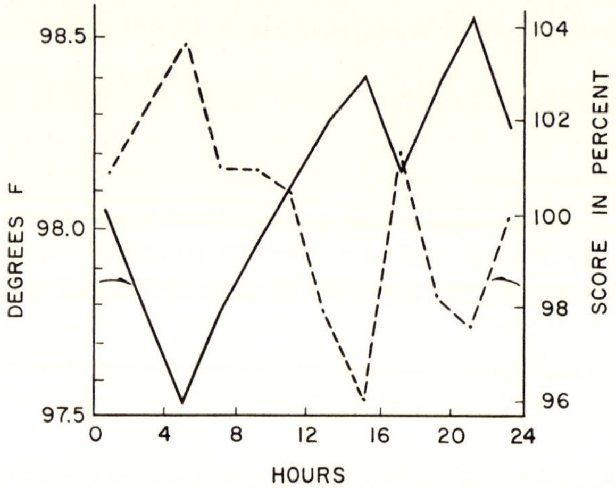

Figure 1. Correlation between Body Temperature and Performance

Variations in group mean oral temperature (solid line) of nine subjects, taken at test hours around the clock, on a staggered "dog-watch" routine, and concomitant variations in the mean time required to name the colors of 600 small squares of paper (broken line), the latter expressed as percentage of total group mean scores, for a period of 18 days, 100 percent equaling 312 seconds. The correlation coefficient between these two variates was —0.8874 (P less than 0.01). Each 24 hours of testing was done in 96 hours of elapsed time, allowing for longer than 8-hour breaks between some successive watches. From 16 to 20 o'clock (because the dogging of the watch was at 18 o'clock) longer tests were omitted, and the subjects were less active, resulting in a dip in the upward sweep of the body temperature curve and poorer performance (5).

temperature is not fixed—at 98.6 degrees F.—any more than are the other physiological "constants". Like the 24-hour sleep-wakefulness rhythm (3, 7), the body temperature curve is absent at birth and is individually established and maintained by being made to follow the customary routine of family and community (3, 8). The immediate cause of noncorrectional body temperature change is probably the amount of muscular activity and, at rest, the degree of muscle tonus. Merely lying down and relaxing results in a measurable drop in body temperature (1), and wakefulness during the hours usually devoted to sleep may raise body temperature as much as 1 degree F. above the sleep level. Excitement may also raise body temperature (9). In any case, the validity of the body temperature method does not depend upon the elucidation of all the factors responsible for the 24-hour body temperature rhythm. The method can therefore be used in an investigation of the relation of body temperature to the watch-standing routine of "4 hours on duty, 8 hours off duty," prevailing on U.S. submarines under way for several days (10). Although this schedule of watch-standing was geared to an artificial 12-hour cycle, life aboard a continuously submerged schnorkel-type submarine was found to run as close to the usual shore routine as the duties of the three watch-standing sections permitted. Games were played mostly in the afternoon and evening, meals were served at 8, 12, and 20 o'clock, and, though sleep was taken perforce in two periods, the two were unequal, no one being up and about during the post-midnight hours unless on watch. The body temperature curves of the members of the crew observed were affected by the combination of 12- and 24-hour cycles of activity, with the exception of the non-watch-standing group of cooks, messmen, and specialists on call at all hours, who had typical 24-hour body-temperature curves. On the basis of these observations, a "close" schedule of watches was proposed, with the eight hours of daily duty divided into three 2- or 3-hour watches. Regular meals were served to each section at the hours appropriate to its schedule, and provision was made for a "long" sleep during an unbroken duty-free period of 12 hours (9). A comparison of the mean group body temperature curves of the three watch-standing sections under the old "4-on, 8-off" and the new experimental "close" schedules of watches (Figure 2) reveals the shallow, often bimodal, curves under the former and the deep monocyclic curves under the latter. The 24-hour body temperature range is increased in the experimental schedule crew; the body temperature levels are above 98° F. at practically all the watch hours, and below 97° F. during sleep, as against temperatures below 98° F. between 4 and 12 o'clock, and sleep temperature levels considerably above 97° F. between 12 and 24 o'clock under the "4-on, 12-off" routine. The day-to-day variations of the mean group body temperature curves (Figure 3) show that the "close" watch schedules not only lead to higher temperature levels during duty hours, but also provide stable,

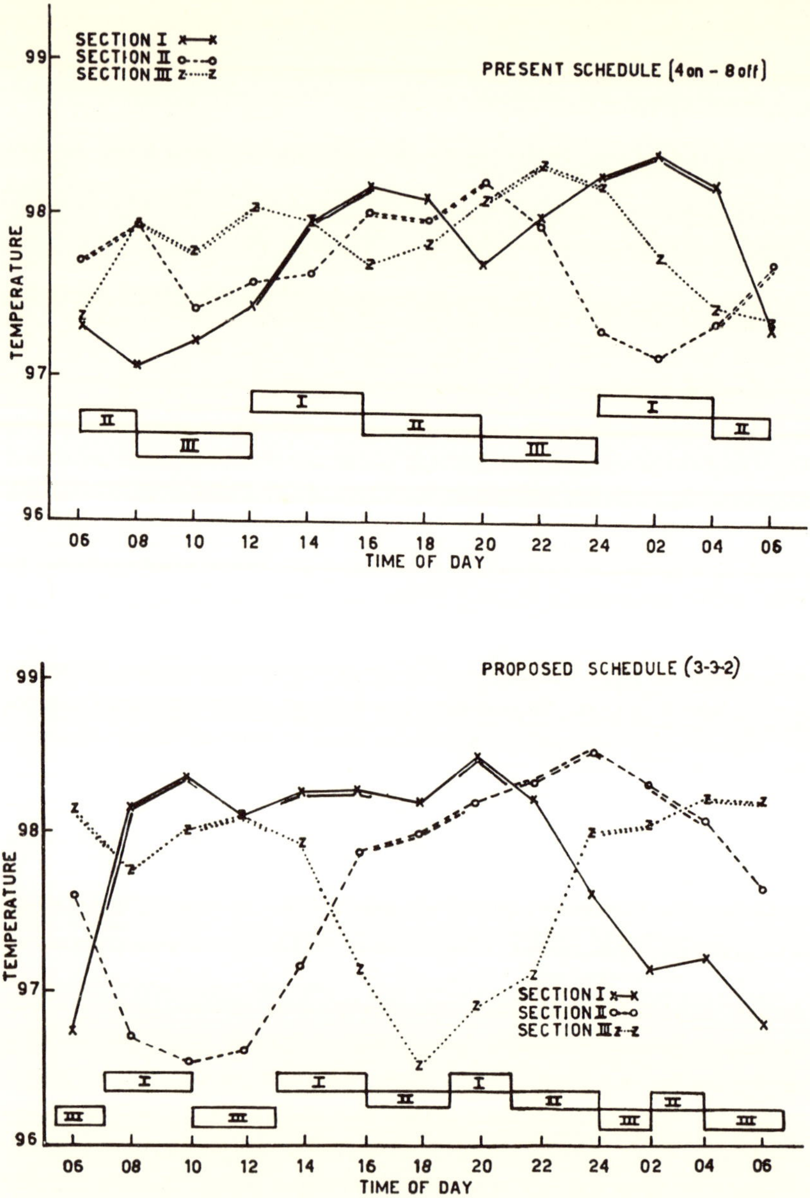

Figure 2. Comparison of Mean Group 24-Hour Body Temperature Curves

Curves are for 29 men from three watch-standing sections of the crew of a cruising submarine, based on seven days of the current "4-on, 8-off" schedule, with those of 28 men from three similar sections, for seven days on the "close" 3-3-2 watch schedule. The watch periods of the three sections are indicated by double lines on the respective body temperature curves and by horizontal blocks under the curves (9).

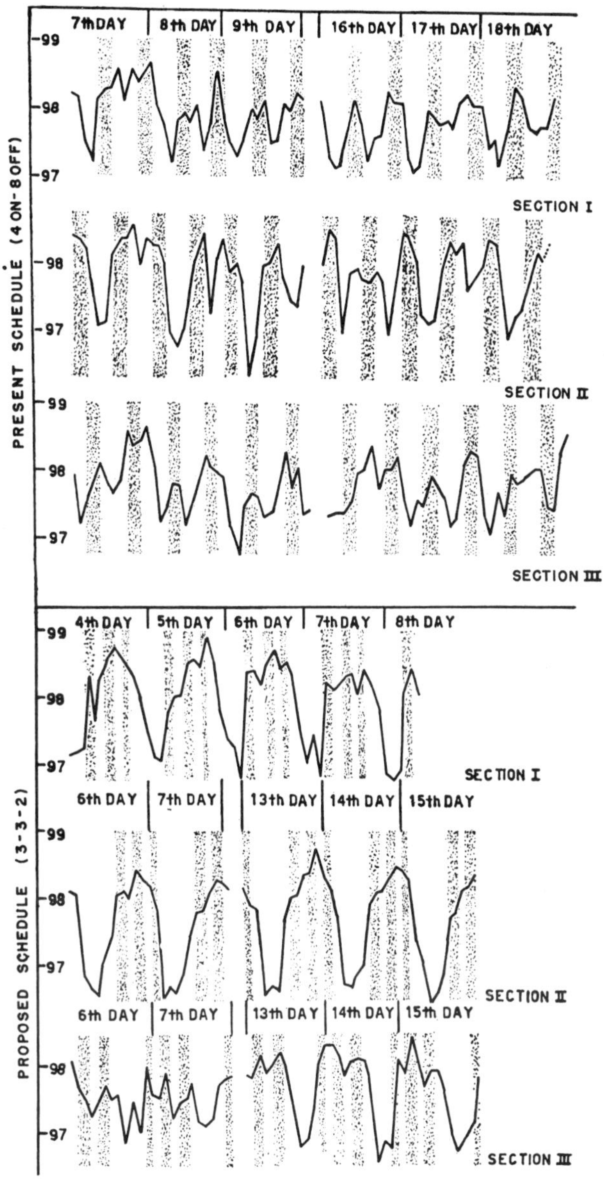

Figure 3. Comparison of Five Successive Mean Group 24-Hour Body Temperature Curves

Curves are for 29 men from three watch-standing sections of the crew of a submarine under way, during a 19-day cruise, on the current "4-on, 8-off" schedule, with those of 28 men from three similar sections, during a 21-day cruise, on the "close" 3-3-2 schedule. The watch periods are indicated by vertical shaded areas (9).

repetitive, 24-hour patterns which are conducive to alertness during watches and to sleepiness during the middle of the free 12-hour period, irrespective of the hours of day and night. Each section of the crew lived (worked, ate, played, slept), as it were, under its own time-zone clock, separated by eight hours from the other two sections. It is interesting to note that members of two sections voted overwhelmingly (26 to 9) for the proposed watch schedule, the only section not favoring it being the one that stood 8 to 12 o'clock and 20 to 24 o'clock watches under the old "4-on, 8-off" routine, which permitted them to sleep between midnight and 8 A.M.

It is this "close" watch schedule that is suggested for trial and possible adoption by the occupants of space vehicles, in order to further alertness and efficiency in performing tasks that are likely to become uninteresting under the monotonous environmental conditions, while, at the same time, encouraging sleep during the free hours. It is obvious that a preliminary period of one to two weeks on the new routine would have to be employed to swing each traveler into his assigned time zones. It will be found that some individuals have a 24-hour rhythm that cannot be shifted with ease. Whether such persons should be barred from participation in space flights should depend upon the abundance or paucity of subjects, as well as upon the weight given to other desirable characteristics which these persons may possess.

Granted that each space traveler should operate on a *fixed* routine, must his schedule of activity and rest be based on a 24-hour periodicity when he is no longer earthbound and thus freed from the alternation of day and night? It has been established that one could develop experimentally non-24-hour rhythms—specifically, rhythms of 18, 21, and 28 hours (3, 11). Such rhythms should be more easily maintained off the earth than on it, and there are reasons for adopting cycles longer than 24 hours. In the studies of artificial rhythms referred to, it was shown that the longer the cycle, the greater the body temperature range. This means that one can expect to reach a greater degree of alertness and a higher level of performance, on the one hand, and a more complete relaxation, perhaps better sleep, on the other. The exact length of the period finally adopted would depend upon the ultimate wakeful capacity of the space travelers, to be determined by actual trial of cycles of varying duration. Even then, since the preliminary findings are arrived at—as they must be—under conditions of terrestrial existence, they may be found not to apply in space travel. This was suggested by reports of the effects of simulated weightlessness on muscular fatigue, with a decreased need for sleep and a greater than expected wakefulness capacity (12).

To summarize, information on physiological cycling available now can be applied to the handling of problems of space travel by (a) preparatory development of fixed rhythms of living for individuals, with staggered schedules for groups, and (b) giving serious consideration to experimenting with longer-than-24-hour cycles of activity and rest.

REFERENCES

1. Kleitman, N., and A. Doktorsky, The effects of the position of the body and of sleep on rectal temperature in man, Am. J. Physiol., 104:340–343, 1933.
2. Kleitman, N., S. Titelbaum, and P. Feiveson, The effect of body temperature on reaction time, Am. J. Physiol., 121:495–501, 1938.
3. Kleitman, N., Sleep and Wakefulness. Pp. 191–234, 249–269. Chicago, University of Chicago Press, 1939.
4. Murray, E. J., H. L. Williams, and A. Lubin, Body temperature and psychological ratings during sleep deprivation, J. Exper. Psychol., 56:271–273, 1958.
5. Kleitman, N., and D. P. Jackson, Body temperature and performance under different routines, J. Appl. Physiol., 3:309–328, 1950.
6. Kleitman, N., and J. E. Schreider, Diurnal variation in oculomotor performance, Année psychol., 50:202–215, 1951.
7. Kleitman, N., and T. G. Engelmann, Sleep characteristics of infants, J. Appl. Physiol., 6:269–282, 1953.
8. Kleitman, N., and A. Ramsaroop, Periodicity of body temperature and heart rate, Endocrinology, 43:1–20, 1948.
9. Utterback, R. A., and G. D. Ludwig, A Comparative Study of Schedules for Standing Watches Aboard Submarines on Body Temperature Cycles. Nav. Med. Res. Inst., Project NM 004 003, Report No. 1, March 1949. 11 pages.
10. Kleitman, N. The sleep-wakefulness cycle of submarine personnel, in *Human Factors In Undersea Warfare*. Pp. 329–341. Baltimore, William & Wilkins, 1949.
11. Kleitman, N., and E. Kleitman, Effect of non-24-hour routines of living on oral temperature and heart rate, J. Appl. Physiol., 6:283–291, 1953.
12. Zylstra, D. Astronauts will require less sleep, Missiles and Rockets, Feb. 29, 1960, pp. 33–34.

Circadian Rhythms: A Basis of Human Engineering for Aerospace

FRANZ HALBERG

Physiologic rhythms with periods of about twenty-four hours, briefly circadian (*circa, dies*) (1–3) rhythms, have been the subject of several recent reviews (4–10). Some of their already known characteristics have a bearing upon aviation and space medicine, particularly if we discuss the organism's ability to withstand damage, as we do at this symposium on psychophysiologic problems.

SOME MISCONCEPTIONS

Study of circadian rhythms involves more than determinations of functions at different clock hours. One may single out the attitude of identifying rhythms with the unqualified effects of certain hours of the day as one of those factors contributing most heavily to the undesirable status of medical research on circadian periodicity. The questionable value of descriptions of "time-of-day effects," unqualified as to routine, other conditions, sampling, etc., seems obvious, since the timing as to a particular clock hour of peaks or troughs in many physiologic rhythms can be shifted by any desired number of hours (4–10; Figure 1).

Another point may be made at the outset. Circadian changes in physiologic functions should not be restricted to the scope of a source of variability, i.e. to that of "another factor," to be kept in mind in dealing with biologic data. Heredity used to be another factor, and so was diet. In these latter instances, however, concern with another factor has developed into basic disciplines, genetics and nutrition, that contribute to our understanding of health and disease. It seems reasonable to expect that rigorous periodicity analysis will ultimately

Dr. Halberg is Elsa U. Pardee Professor of Cancer Biology and Experimental Pathology, University of Minnesota Medical School, and Director of Research, Cambridge State Hospital, Cambridge, Minnesota.

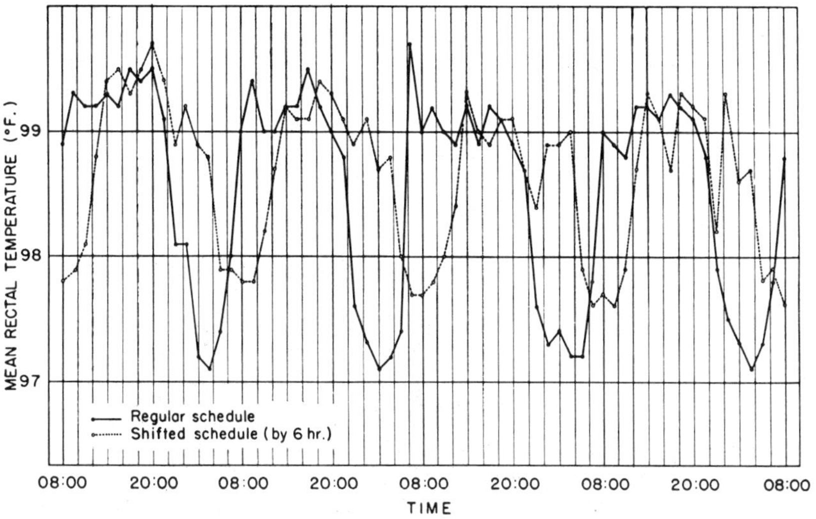

Figure 1a. Shift in Phase of Temperature Rhythm Following a 6-Hour Shift in Daily Routine

12 subjects per group.

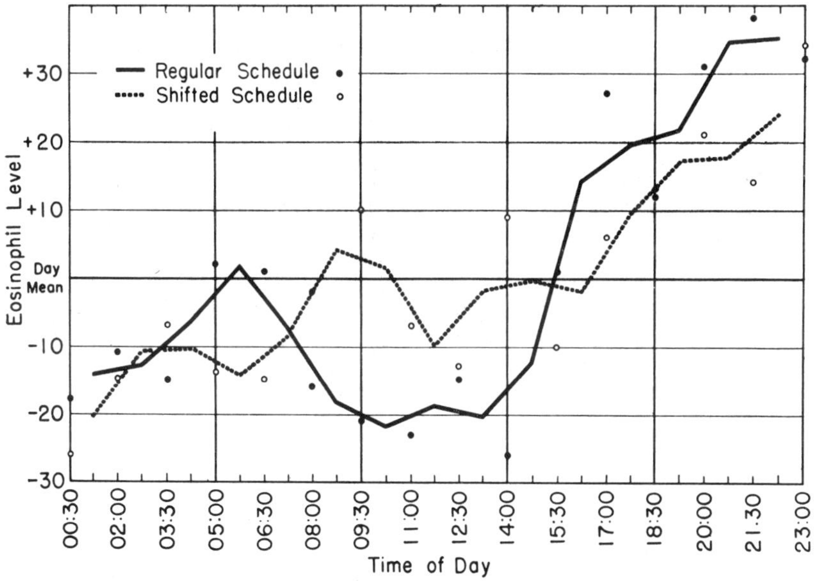

Figure 1b. Six-Hour Shift in Eosinophil Rhythm

12 subjects per group. Second month after initiation of the shifted schedule. Even though curve is smoothed by moving average of two items, relative means for each time and group serve to visualize the original data.

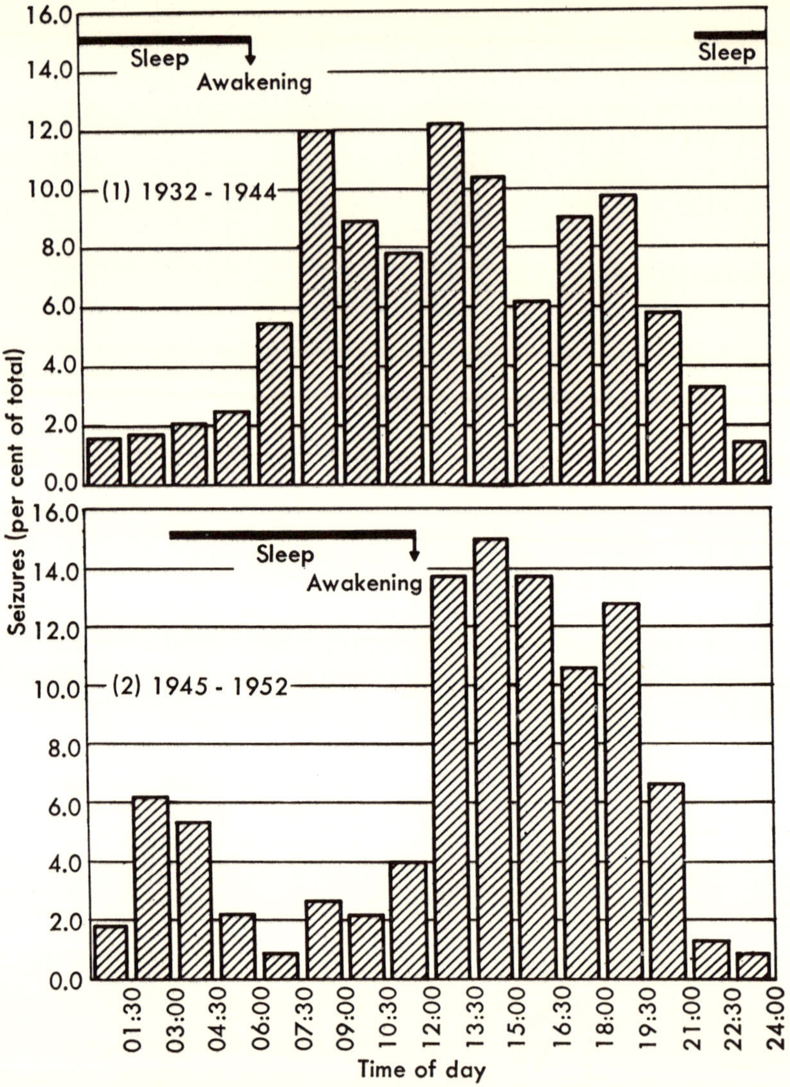

Figure 1c. Unequal Distribution of Epileptic Seizures during the Hours of the Day on Two Routines, Maintained for Many Years

Note change in seizure distribution following change in routine in same subject. Daily routine may be regarded as synchronizer (see text). Clock hour as such does not matter in determining times of occurrence of seizures.

contribute to the same end. Thus, instead of discussing rhythms merely as another factor, we now focus upon them in order to resolve in time the integration of various physiologic functions with each other and the environment.

HOW GENERAL ARE CIRCADIAN RHYTHMS?

Figure 2 depicts several rhythms at different levels of physiologic organization. An intracellular sequence of periodic events in growing

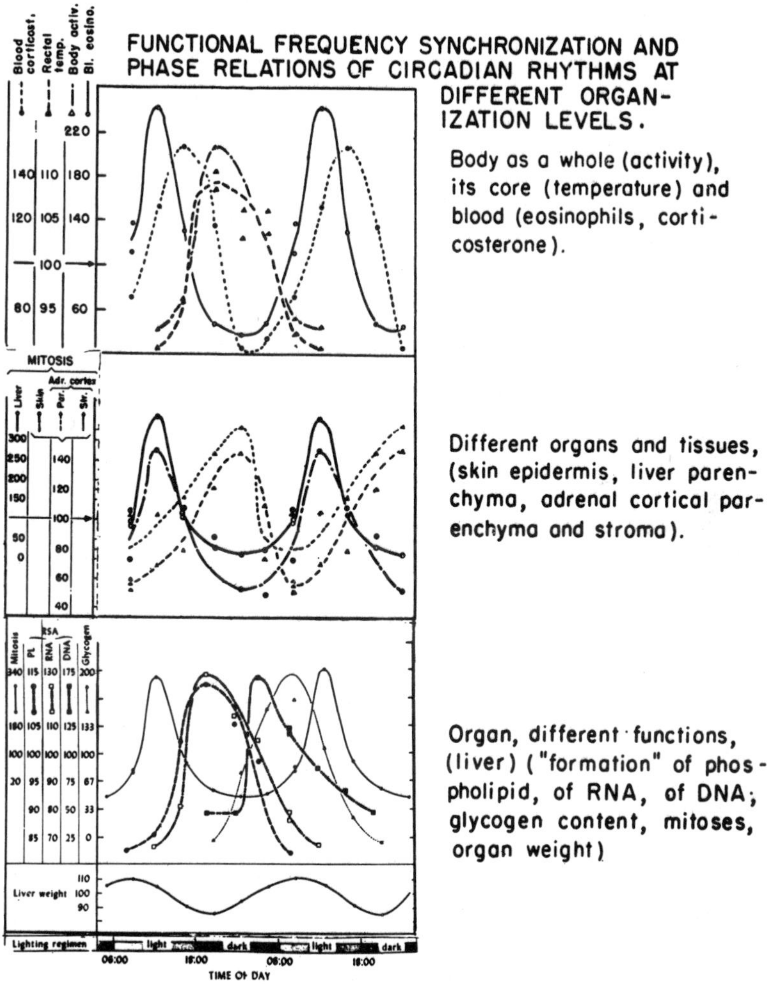

Figure 2. Circadian Synchronization with Differences in Phase (Positive, Zero, or Negative)

liver is shown in the bottom row. Time relations of cell division in different organs are depicted in the middle. Gross motor activity, rectal temperature, blood eosinophils and blood corticosterone are graphed on top. All of the data are on the mouse and are shown as percent of their series-mean. The figure is a circadian map in time (9); the method by which the data were obtained is direct light-synchronized periodicity analysis (1). Similar data, though less extensive in depth, also are available for human beings (9; Figure 3).

CIRCADIAN SYNCHRONIZATION, WITH DIFFERENCES IN PHASE

The lighting regimen used for the study described by Figure 2 involved twelve hours of light, alternating with twelve hours of darkness, among certain other provisions (1). The study documents two temporal characteristics of functional integration. First, it reveals similar periods, i.e. synchronization, among circadian rhythms and an environmental routine (of lighting). (In other words, an organism confronted with an acceptable outside frequency undergoes circadian periodic changes; its circadian rhythms have similar periods, corresponding to that of the routine.) Second, circadian synchronization does not imply synchrony. The characteristic of functional integration along a twenty-four scale is the similar length of the periods involved but not necessarily the occurrence of peaks or troughs at the same time for all physiologic functions. Phase differences among certain circadian rhythms are readily apparent in Figure 2; such differences may be positive or negative, as well as zero.

HOW SIGNIFICANT ARE CIRCADIAN CHANGES IN PHYSIOLOGIC STATE?

Figure 4 shows results of indirect light-synchronized periodicity analysis (1, 10). This method involves the application of an agent under study at different times during twenty-four hours. Separate groups of inbred mice, with comparable past history, are exposed every four hours, for twenty-four hours, e.g., to an endotoxin (11), to noise (12), to ouabain (13) or to ethanol (14). It can readily be seen that the percentage of animals dying from an agent tested is a function of the phase relations among circadian rhythms. Moreover, these hours of diminished resistance to one agent can coincide with peak resistance to another agent (Figure 4). Again we find that

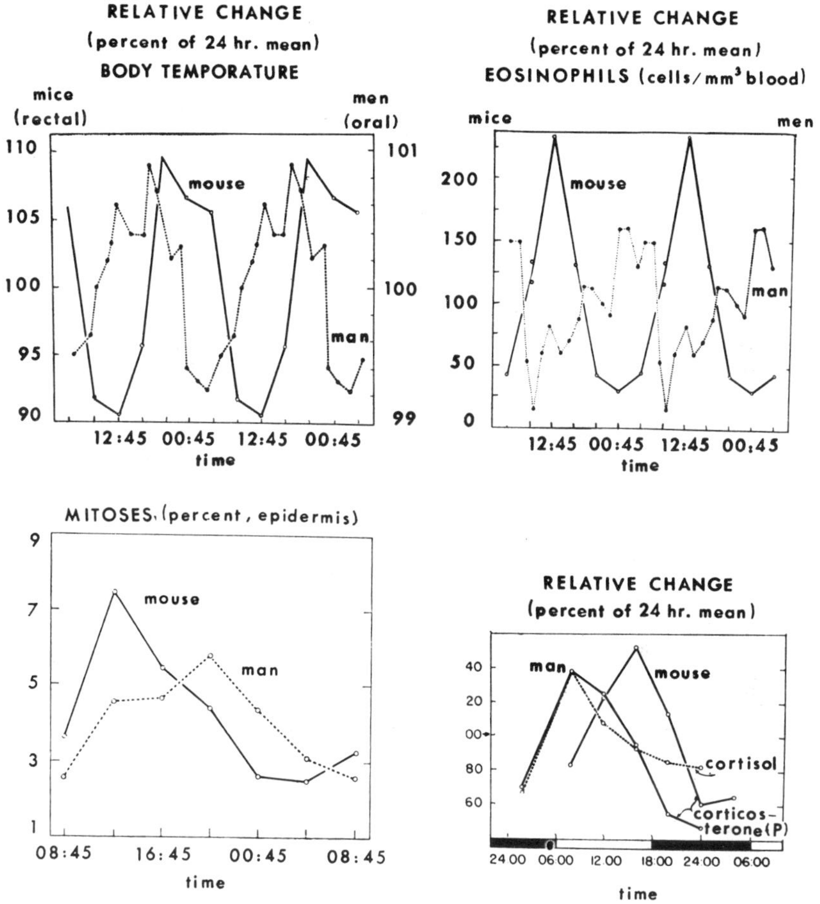

Figure 3. Species Differences in the Mode of Synchronization of Circadian Rhythms

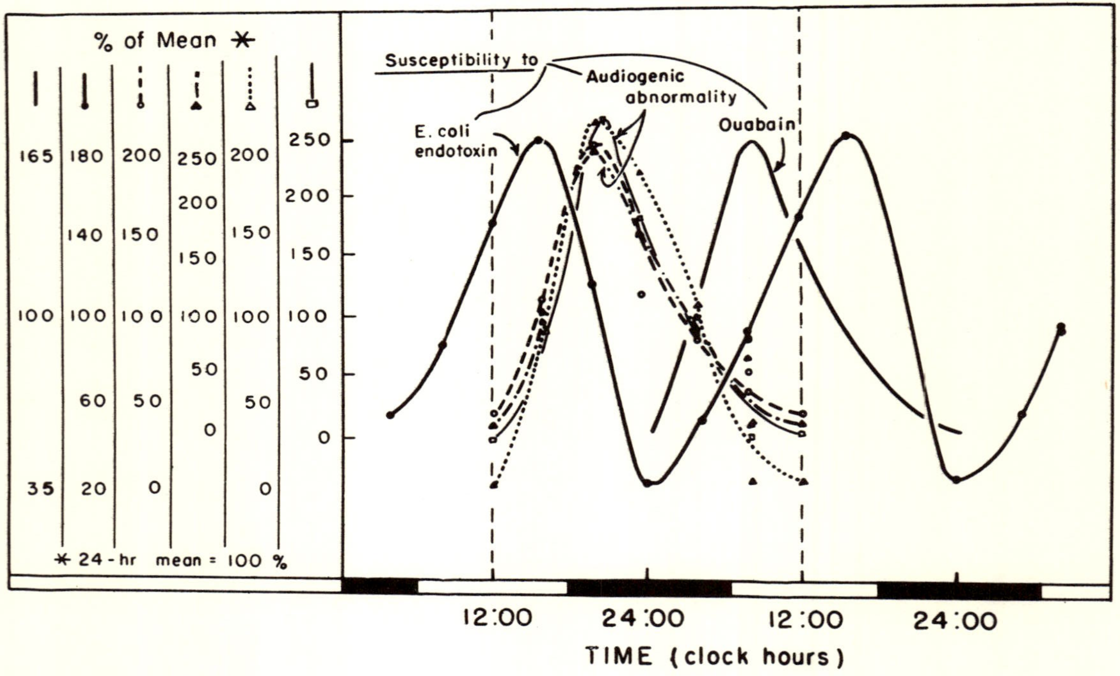

Figure 4. Hours of Changing Resistance

different susceptibility rhythms can be synchronized, yet only with certain differences in phase.

Such experiments require, of course, control of factors other than the periodicity under study. It is with provisions made to reduce genetic and anamnestic variations that one can reliably document the critical extent to which circadian changes underlie our ability to withstand damages. If the agent under study is called a "stressor," one might say that the stressor was kept constant, while the physiologic state was allowed to vary, as it does whether or not that is the variable under study. With such a procedure, periodicity can be shown to tip the balance toward death or survival of the organism exposed to trauma, as is readily apparent in Figure 4.

MECHANISMS

At the two ends of their scale, comparative physiologists are dealing with unicellullar forms of life, devoid of conventional nerves and hormones, and with certain Strategic Air Command aviators, not subject to habitual daily schedules. Including these extremes, a variety of organisms show circadian synchronization of their functional changes. Different numbers and types of intermediate steps are likely to be involved in the mechanisms of different rhythms and/or species. Models of rhythms, therefore, will vary in complexity among different forms of life, as sketched in Figure 5.

In unicellulars and mammals, the common denominator of periodicity is probably a cellular cycle. A cell, just as the organism as a whole, does have a division of labor in time; neither do all of its processes peak at the same time, nor do they change in rate haphazardly. The bottom row of Figure 2, for instance, visualizes three metabolic stages of cell activity by the leads and lags in phase of various hepatic functions. Stage A starts with a mitotic peak; we begin a cellular cycle at the time when most new daughter cells enter the population. This stage ends with peaks in relative specific activity (RSA) of microsomal phospholipid and RNA. Stage A, which began with an event involving largely the nucleus, ended with metabolic peaks more characteristic of the cytoplasm. Stage B, following A, lasts until the peak time in RSA of DNA, while Stage C extends from the DNA peak to that in cell division (8,15).

In simpler forms of life the cellular cycles are more autonomous

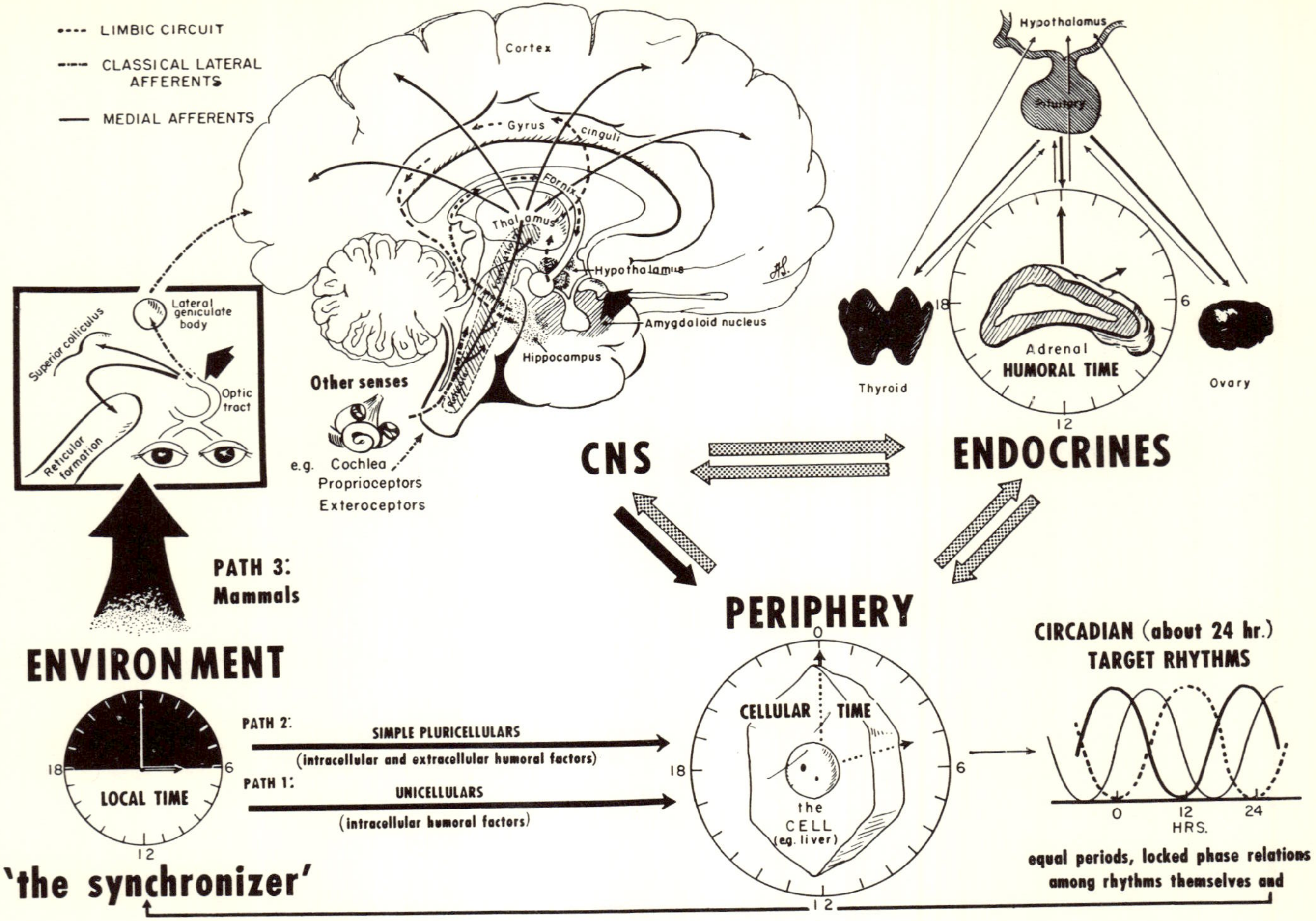

LIMBIC CIRCUIT
CLASSICAL LATERAL AFFERENTS
MEDIAL AFFERENTS
Cortex
Gyrus
cinguli
Fornix
Thalamus
Hypothalamus
Amygdaloid nucleus
Hippocampus
Lateral geniculate body
Superior colliculus
Optic tract
Reticular formation
Other senses
e.g. Cochlea
Proprioceptors
Exteroceptors
Hypothalamus
Pituitary
Thyroid
Adrenal
HUMORAL TIME
Ovary
18
6
12
CNS
ENDOCRINES
PATH 3:
Mammals
PERIPHERY
ENVIRONMENT
LOCAL TIME
'the synchronizer'
PATH 2:
SIMPLE PLURICELLULARS
(intracellular and extracellular humoral factors)
PATH 1:
UNICELLULARS
(intracellular humoral factors)
CELLULAR TIME
the CELL (eg. liver)
0
CIRCADIAN (about 24 hr.)
TARGET RHYTHMS
0
12
24
HRS.
equal periods, locked phase relations
among rhythms themselves and

than in the mammal, where they are under multiple controls originating from adjacent cells and from other hormonal and neural mechanisms (Figure 5). Some cellular rhythms in the mammal, but not all of them, are dependent, in particular, upon the adrenal glands since they are obliterated following adrenalectomy (9). The adrenal cycle, in turn, interacts not only with the periphery but also with the central nervous system. It seems particularly interesting that the corticosterone rise does not lag behind the daily onset of gross motor activity: the former is not a simple reaction to the latter; instead, the adrenal cycle leads in phase cerebral cortical activation as well as some peripheral rhythms (9, 16; Figure 1, top).

The temporal functions of the nervous system and the adrenals are sketched in Figure 5 with particular reference to the way in which lighting schedules influence the phase of circadian rhythms. Stimuli such as light (or sound) are received by transducers such as the eye (or ear). From the sense organ, potentials are transmitted corticipitally by conductors (a) via classical lateral pathways to the special sensory areas such as the striate area and (b) via medial pathways to the reticular formation and hypothalamus. A multitude of impulses reaching the brain must now be mixed, weighted and combined, after "biologic noise removal," perhaps in the reticular formation. The anatomy and the physiological characteristics of this general area of the brain have been highlighted at this symposium by Dr. Magoun (17).

Somewhere in the brain, and somehow, a "comparison" must be made between the composite phase information from within the body and that from without, COPI and CEPI, respectively. The composite *organismic* phase information (COPI) may be yielded by the mixing, weighting, and combining of information from various feedbacks, psychogenic, neurogenic, hormonal, and metabolic. The composite *environmental* phase information (CEPI), in turn, may schematically be subdivided into the potentials evoked by stimuli originating in the physico-chemical environment (EPIp; light and food, for instance), and into those evoked by other signals, arbitrarily designated as "socio-ecological" (EPIs; 1, 4).

Most likely EPIs, our social schedule (and our emotional response to it), is more critical in determining the phase of bodily rhythms in urbanized human beings, while EPIp seems more pertinent for men in settings such as an isolated farm. But to analyze interactions of EPIp and EPIs, a major undertaking when human subjects are studied, is more readily feasible in certain experimental animals, even though in the latter EPIs also has dramatic and often unexpected effects.

The electroencephalographic changes occurring, for instance, in the unanesthetized rabbit when it is confronted with the investigator, probably involve the equivalent of "emotional" components and these alerting responses are actually more striking than the corresponding changes evoked by physical stimuli (18). Moreover, "emotional" responses to EPIs, interfering with EPIp, involve not only brain waves, with their short periods, but also the rhythm in body temperature and even the periodic sequence of cellular metabolic events and mitoses (1). Unless we anticipate these varied effects, their contribution via EPIs to CEPI will remain uncontrolled.

In studying the effect of a change in EPIp (e.g., in the lighting schedule or in our routine) we must evaluate for experimental animals, as well as for human beings, possible concomitant changes in EPIs. Ambiguous results obtained in studies of effects of EPIp can quite easily be brought about by our failure to evaluate inadvertent yet critical changes in EPIs (1, 8).

At any rate, changes either in EPIp or in EPIs (or in both) can alter CEPI. Accordingly, a physiologic mechanism (a neural phase comparator) is now confronted with a new CEPI and an old COPI; it will compare the two and if the phase relations of COPI and CEPI are found to be altered, an appropriate message will be sent to various bodily rhythms to speed up or to slow down, as need be. Moreover, the phase comparator will continue to send messages until the rhythms are again in step with the environment, i.e., until the abnormal relations between CEPI and COPI have been corrected.

From the ill-defined physiologic equivalents of a neural "phase comparator" and, perhaps, from an as yet hypothetical neural "oscillator" (8), information is channeled neurally to the periphery (Figure 5); but, in addition, some of it also travels from the hypothalamus to the pituitary. In the pituitary, messages from above might be again "compared" with hormonal feedbacks from target glands; at any rate, if the phase relations of CEPI and COPI are altered, the pituitary will send appropriate messages to the "generators" of rhythms which appear to be (in part) the appropriate target glands (8, 9); the latter are stimulated by their tropins to speed up, or they are slowed down by throttling of tropin secretion until normal phase relations are reestablished.

The path from the central nervous system via the pituitary does not seem to be obligatory, however, for the transmission of phase information to the target glands, in all instances (8). Of interest in this connection is ample direct evidence as well as indirect evidence of continued aldosterone secretion by the adrenal cortex in the absence of pituitary function.

In the field of central nervous mechanisms of periodicity, promising work has already been begun (19–21) on problems that are important to the topic of this symposium. Is it useful to approach sensory isolation by periodicity analysis as a CEPI-deficiency at its extreme? Data on human rhythms in confinement with sensory deprivation will be of interest. CEPI-deficiency in the face of an intact COPI seems deleterious and periodicity analysis might reveal how such damage might come about and what may be needed to prevent or correct it.

PHASE-SHIFTING

The lighting regimen may be called a primary synchronizer of rhythms in the mouse (1, 4). Sociologic factors, according to which we adjust our watches, play the corresponding role in civilized human beings. Changes in daily routine of human beings may be instituted and maintained in order to shift the phase of their rhythms (Figure 1), so long as the schedules used are physiologically acceptable and certain other factors do not interfere critically.

One must recognize, of course, that frequency-synchronization between a rhythm and the lighting regimen, for instance, does not imply that rhythms are not responsive to factors other than lighting; times of feeding, of exposure to aggressors, actually any changes in sensory inflow, exert effects upon phase and/or form of rhythms (1). These factors, among others, are potential (secondary) synchronizers; their effects on a given organism vary in degree, if not in kind, among different rhythms, particularly at various physiologic organization levels. But if such effects are not exerted day after day at a fixed time, they will be modulating rather than synchronizing; these effects (interacting with the primary synchronizer) bring about phase changes only if they are exerted with "acceptable" periodicity.

Such interaction among synchronizers (Aschoff's competition of time-givers) occurs in time as well as in intensity of effect. Synchronizer-interaction is positive if the difference in time of their application and/or in their effects approaches zero; e.g., if effects of a primary synchronizer (such as the lighting regimen for fully fed mice) coincide with another effect (such as that of the feeding time); feeding then merely reinforces lighting. Interaction is negative when the primary and secondary synchronizers act with significantly different effects or at different times. Some oversimplified rules apply to the environmental phase control of several mammalian rhythms (1, 4–6, 8, 22).

1. There is the superficial equivalent to a refractory period: even if the shift of synchronizer is sudden, extensive phase-shifts are gradual. A transient refractoriness of rhythms to extensive changes in timing of synchronizer(s) seems equal in adaptive value to a certain degree of modifiability (see above). At least for a while, the exigencies of the temporal integration of diverse functions within the organism may override claims of new schedules, particularly at the cellular and hormonal levels (23, 24; Figure 6). It is only with a lag that the organism will ultimately be able to supply and transport the "old compounds," in the "old amounts," to the "old places"—at "new times"! For this purpose, essential steps in a sequence of periodically integrated metabolic events may be shortened or lengthened, rather than eliminated or reversed in order.

2. The shift-time increases with the degree of shift in timing of synchronizer, inversion time (180° shift of rhythm) being the longest.

3. The shift-time usually increases with the complexity of the species, other things being comparable (for a given variable, synchronizer, and degree of shift).

4. Shift-time also is a function of the synchronizer(s) involved. Shifts are fastest under control of the primary synchronizer, slower if controlled by secondary synchronizers.

5. Shifts depend further upon factors other than the synchronizer being dominant at a given time; shift-time may be several weeks longer following an inversion of the feeding-time of mice severely

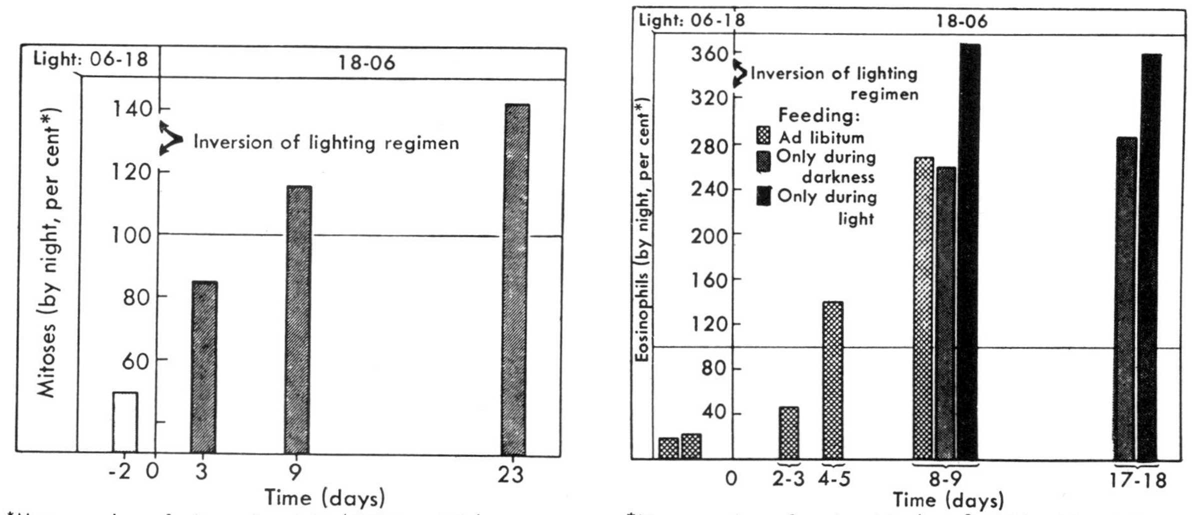

*Mean number of mitoses by night / 3000 nuclei / mouse—as per cent of the corresponding day value (=100%)

*Mean number of eosinophils / mm.^{3} of blood by night—as per cent of the corresponding day value (=100%)

Figure 6. Gradual Shift of Rhythms in Pinnal Mitoses and Blood Eosinophils in the Mouse Following Abrupt Inversion of Lighting Regimen

Note difference in synchronization time, suggestive of transient desynchronization.

restricted in calories, as compared to the shift-time in response of fully-fed mice to shifts in lighting (23). In this instance, the secondary synchronizer had to override the effect of lighting persisting on the old schedule. Thus, if other environmental interaction with a given shifted schedule is positive, it will reinforce the shift and shorten shift-time; if it is negative, it will delay the shift (or prevent it). In exploring the effects of new schedules one must, therefore, examine the number and the nature of those factors possibly persisting with the old timing.

6. The shift-time further depends upon the plasticity of the organism's particular rhythm; in the same species and individual, shift-times may differ from one rhythm to another. In the mouse, inversion times (by lighting reversal) differ for rhythms in blood eosinophils and tissue mitoses (25). The same may apply for the same species and synchronizer with respect to the same function in different tissues. Thus, inversion of mitotic rhythm in liver parenchyma was detected at eight days after initiation of lighting reversal (8); at that time after inversion of lighting (in the same animals) the mitotic rhythm in pinnal epidermis was not (yet) reversed.

7. If different rhythmic functions of the same organism shift with different speed, optimal time relations among such functions might be disturbed at some time during the shift. Shifts may therefore involve a transient (reversible) desynchronization. Such acute desynchronization, per se, may have no obvious ill effects under usual conditions.

Susceptibility to trauma, however, might change during shifts. Little information, mostly on experimental animals, is available on this topic. Thus, at nine days following inversion of the lighting regimen, peak-susceptibility to audiogenic convulsions occurred at the time of trough in mice on the opposite schedule and vice versa; the within-day difference in convulsions was statistically significant, whether or not the mice had been subjected to a change in schedule. Irrespective of circadian periodicity, however, over-all susceptibility to convulsions and deaths from convulsions had increased by shifting (26). A decrease in resistance to certain types of trauma (during transient frequency-desynchronization of rhythms) may be an unspecific aspect of shifts. There may be an equally unspecific subsequent increase in resistance, which overshoots the initial levels, once all shifts are completed (during optimal resynchronization).

Studies of rhythms during phase shifting of men are of great practical importance to aviation and space medicine (27). We shall have to define the exact shift times of various functions and we shall have to explore the possibility of shortening them by medication. If astronauts are assigned to staggered schedules of activity and rest, it will be necessary, of course, to shift them to their respective regimen and to allow for an appropriate synchronization-time on the new schedule before take-off.

FREE-RUNNING OF RHYTHM FROM ENVIRONMENTAL SCHEDULE

During the past decade, we have studied rather extensively the desynchronization of temperature rhythm in mice and human beings (1; cf. 4, 5, 22). Figure 7 shows rectal temperatures measured at 4 hour intervals after blinding or sham-operation on several groups each composed of over 20 singly housed animals. The mice were kept at 24.5 + 1° C., in light from 06:00 to 18:00 (alternating with 12 hours of darkness).

In blinded mice a lead in phase of temperature rhythm was hardly detectable during the first few days post-operation. Figure 7 shows that with the 4-hourly sampling interval used our data did not suffice for the detection of free-running circadian periods during the first few days following blinding. Thereafter, a lead in phase of rhythm in blinded mice became more apparent with each day; by day 22, the rhythms had passed through temporary antiphase; temperatures were higher in blinded mice at the time of the low in sham-operated mice and vice versa.

By day 33, in turn, the rhythms in blinded and sham-operated animals were roughly back in phase again. Thereafter, the curve for mean temperatures in blinded mice was affected by the desynchronization of individual rhythms from each other. Finally, a resynchronization among individual rhythms, on one hand, and their environment on the other, became apparent at late time points post-operation (1).

Spot checks suggest further that free-running circadian periods characterize the rhythms in blood eosinophils, tissue mitoses, and body activity of blinded mice as well as their temperature rhythm (8). The changes brought about by blinding are statistically significant in all of these variables.

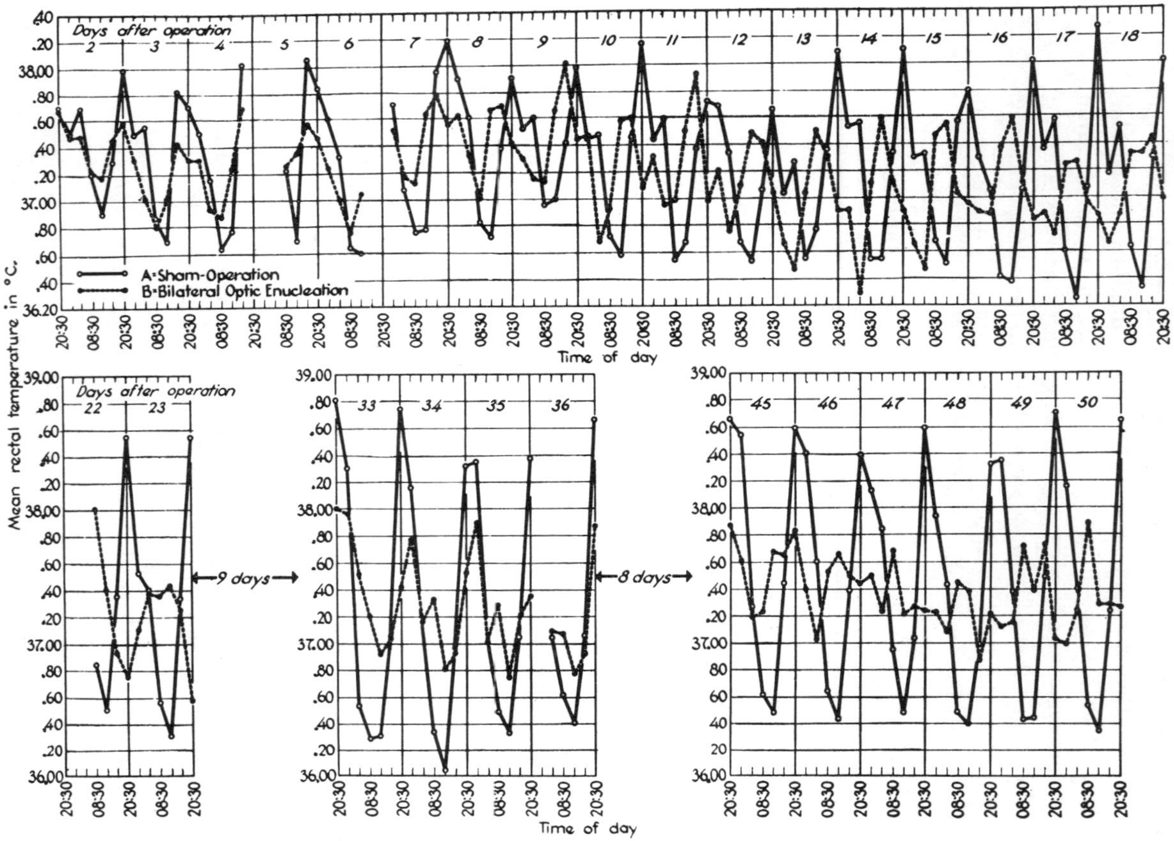

Figure 7. Mean Rectal Temperature Behavior during 50 Days Following Blinding

The temperature rhythm of blinded mice, free-running from the 24-hour schedule, leads in phase that of sham-operated mice.

Circadian periods that are free-running from the local time scale have been most frequently recorded for activity rhythms studied under conditions of environmental constancy and their significance and ubiquity were demonstrated by the studies of Dr. Aschoff (4) and Dr. Pittendrigh (22). Dr. Tribukait, in Aschoff's laboratory (4), has shown that there are limits beyond which the activity rhythm

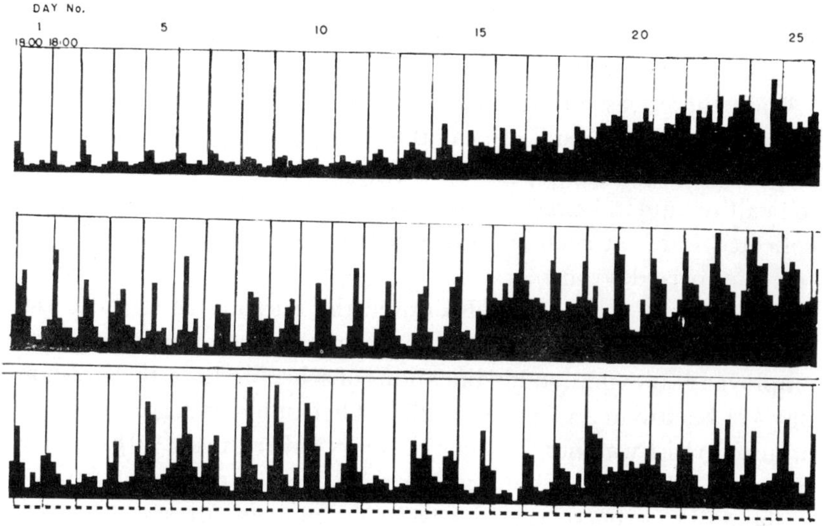

Figure 8. Activity Rhythm of Three Mice Kept in Light for Four Hours Alternating with Four Hours of Darkness

Activity in arbitrary units. Note circadian periodicity free-running from the 24-hour clock (24 hours shown by the vertical lines).

of the mouse can no longer be frequency synchronized by unusual lighting regimens. In Tribukait's experiments, rhythms that were free running from the 24-hour clock were recorded whenever the mouse was exposed to schedules deviating by more than a few hours from a "24-hour day." Figure 8 shows unpublished data from our laboratory, obtained in cooperation with E. Bakken and Y. Anderson, on locomotor activity of mice, free-running on an "8-hour day."

PERIOD OF RHYTHMS IN HUMAN BEINGS ON UNUSUAL SCHEDULES

Kleitman and Jackson have studied, among other schedules, a routine providing for the uninterrupted succession of four hours of duty and eight hours of leisure (28). Nine navy recruits, seventeen to twenty-five years of age, followed this "4-on, 8-off" schedule for two test periods, each of two weeks' duration. Concerning the results of a schedule with hours of duty 0 to 4 and 10 to 16, the authors state that the shape of the diurnal temperature curve did not reveal any bimodality, such as was previously found in the diurnal curves of submarine crews operating on a "4-on, 8-off" watch schedule (29). With respect to the second experience with the "4-on, 8-off" schedule (but hours of duty 8 to 12 and 20–24) they state: "Again there was no bimodality in the group diurnal temperature curve." Thus, it would appear that "4-on, 8-off" schedules, in the study cited, were not predominating in the temperature rhythms of healthy human beings. It would be interesting to examine suitably collected data on such schedules for possible free running periods (e.g., by periodograms).

Lewis and Lobban (30) also raised the question as to the period of rhythms in human beings living on unusual schedules. They employed less extensive modifications of schedule than the "12-hour day" of Kleitman and Jackson (28). Their subjects carried specially adjusted wrist watches showing 12 hours either during $10\frac{1}{2}$ ordinary hours or $13\frac{1}{2}$ ordinary hours; thus they lived on a 21-hour day or a 27-hour day. These routines were maintained for several weeks, while the subjects lived in two isolated communities in Spitzbergen under unusual conditions of environmental constancy. Moreover, this study is of methodologic importance, since data were examined by a modified form of Fourier analysis. Estimates of the variance of their periods are of interest.

In Lewis and Lobban's subjects, initial adaptation of certain excretory rhythms to a 21-hour routine or to a 27-hour routine was uncommon. Such adaptation progressively improved, however, with time. It was seldom complete, even after six weeks on the new environmental routine.

The authors point out that watches were worn to facilitate strict adherence to experimental routine, even when the subjects were away from base. This aim had been achieved. The question arises, however, as to how easy it was for the subjects to compute from one look at the clock (giving experimental time) the corresponding "control" time (24-hour time, BST). If the new time schedule according to which activities were scheduled may have been "compared," occasionally, with time on a 24-hour day basis, the degree to which one or the other excretory rhythm had adapted to the new routines could have depended upon the dominance over phase control of one or the other time schedule.

The same investigation by Lewis and Lobban has a bearing upon a most important point, namely, the dissociation among different circadian rhythms on a given unusual routine. Thus the temperature rhythm adapted almost immediately to the experimental routines in most subjects, while for excretory rhythms the reverse held true. Moreover, rhythms in the excretion of water, chloride, and potassium also revealed dissociations, that in potassium excretion usually being out of phase with those in water and chloride (31).

Such dissociation among different rhythms in a given individual may occur on 24-hour routines as well. The rhythms in blood eosinophils and serum iron may desynchronize in healthy human beings (25). This was noticed in changing from a 3-meals-a-day routine to the consumption of 4 isocaloric meals at 6-hour intervals (while continuing to live in the usual environment), and by changing then again to the 4-meal routine in a constant temperature room (with its additional effects of "confinement" and "detachment").

Dr. Welch has already reported at this symposium on men adapting to an "8-hour day," studied by Hauty *et al.* at the U.S. Air Force School of Aviation Medicine. Different physiologic and psychologic functions adjusted to a varying extent to this unusual schedule (32). Moreover, the extent of adaptations differed among subjects, as it had in earlier related work (30, 31). Figure 9 shows autocorrelograms done on Dr. Hauty's data with the help of Mr. James Smith of the IBM Research Center in Minneapolis, Minnesota.

We are now dealing with trained individuals, singly confined in a sealed 50-cubic foot chamber (P_B and PI_{O_2} at 380 mm and 150 mm Hg, respectively; PI_{CO_2} from 4.25 to 27.5 mm Hg). Temperature and humidity varied, but not 24-hour periodically; the level of illumination was constantly high and there was no visual contact with outside. Constant internal noise, $\approx$85 db, effectively masked external sounds. For 7 days, a given subject was committed to alternate 4-hour periods of rest and work (provided by a complex operator system). The subjects had wrist watches set to local time but "thought mostly" in terms of 4-on/4-off.

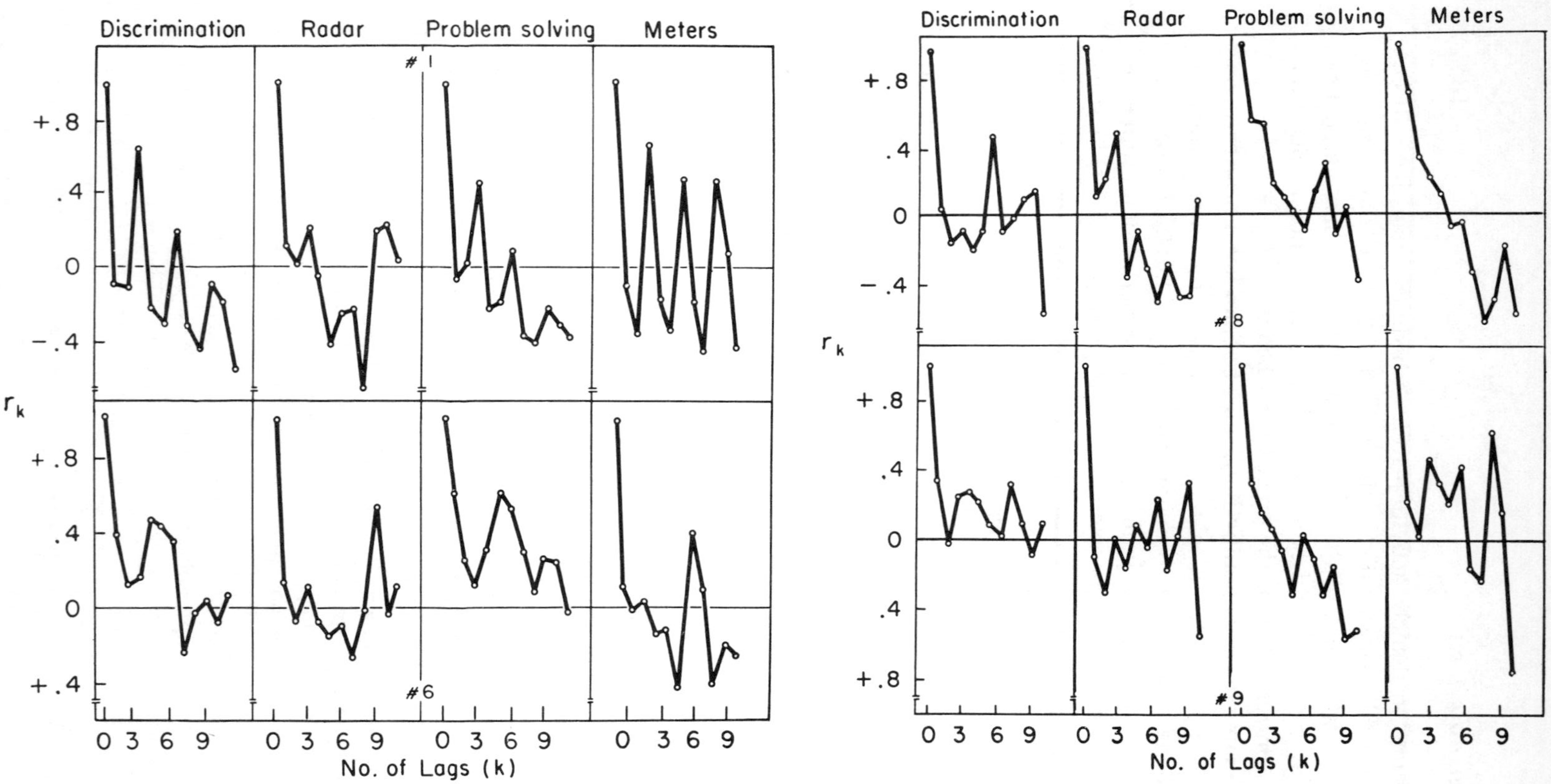

Figures 9a and 9b. Autocorrelograms on Performance Data Available at 8-Hour Intervals from 7-Day Flights (32)

Note that circadian component is most prominent in data from flight 1, from the subject with the poorest behavioral adaptation to the flight. Note further differences in circadian component of variation among functions and subjects.

These autocorrelograms of Figure 9 uncover circadian periodicity for several types of performance evaluated on an "8-hour day." Additional autocorrelograms carried out by E. L. Bell at the U.S. Air Force School of Aviation Medicine, as well as in Minnesota, show in addition circadian components of variation in heart rate and respiration rate of these subjects. It seems established that at least for a week, and probably for much longer, significant circadian components characterize several functions of human beings living on artificial routines that are drastically different from a 24-hour schedule. Analysis of the same data obtained by Hauty *et al.* further suggests that the circadian components of physiologic variations in performance were more significant in subjects whose over-all adaptation to an "8-hour day" was behaviorally more difficult (Figure 9). These suggestions are tentative, since the data are limited; more work along similar lines is indicated.

DESYNCHRONIZATION AMONG RHYTHMS

In mice kept for five days in constant darkness, the rhythm in susceptibility to ethanol persists as shown in Figure 10. Similar findings have been made, among others, on the activity rhythms of various species kept in constant darkness (4, 5, 22). The mean circadian period of animals kept under constant conditions of darkness or light is only rarely 24 hours long. More often, the mean period of functions studied in constant darkness differs slightly, although consistently, from exactly 24 hours. It also is established that rhythms that are free-running from the environmental 24-hour clock involve circadian periods that differ from one animal to the next (1). But the added and equally important question arises whether under conditions of environmental constancy different rhythms may also free-run from each other, i.e., can we find differences in the circadian periods of different functions in the same organism.

Evidence suggesting such internal circadian desynchronization among physiologic rhythms under conditions of constant darkness is scarce. Recently, the writer kept 34 singly housed male D_8 mice, approximately one month of age, in constant darkness for four days. Half of these animals were then killed at noon, the other half at midnight and their livers and ears removed for mitotic counts on pinnal epidermis and hepatic parenchyma. The average number of hepatic mitoses (per 100 oil immersion fields) at noon and at midnight was 6.5 ± 1 and 2.7 ± .5 respectively. The corresponding difference in mitotic count of ear epidermis was not statistically significant (P > .55).

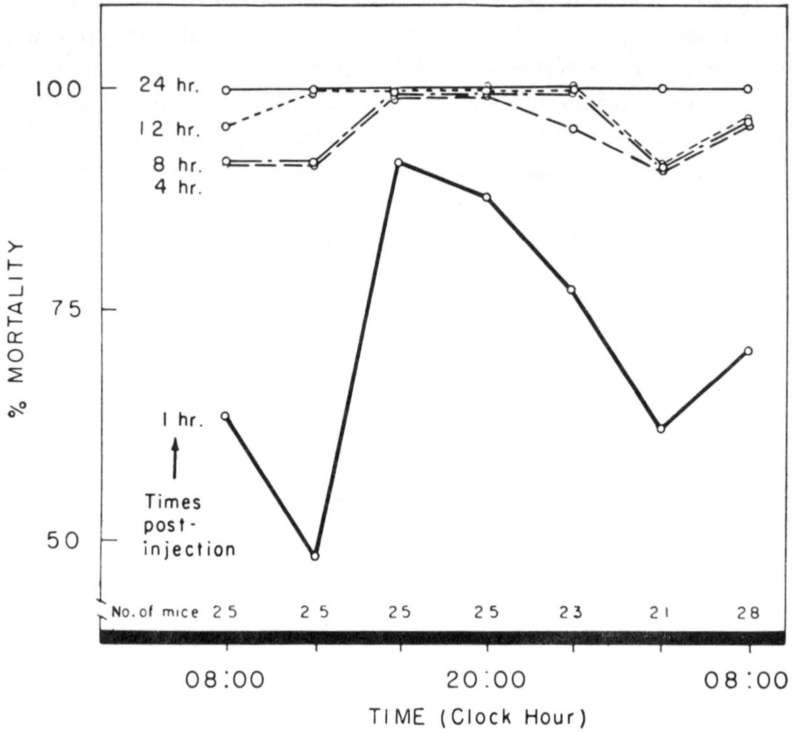

Figure 10. Susceptibility Rhythm to Ethanol in C Mice, 5 Weeks of Age (fifth day in constant darkness)

Prior to exposure to continuous darkness, the mice had been kept for several weeks in light from 6:00 A.M. to 6:00 P.M., alternating with 12 hours of darkness. The middle row of Figure 2 shows that under such conditions the noon and midnight sampling should have revealed significant differences in mitotic activity of pinnal epidermis as well as in that of liver parenchyma (cf. also 1). After several days in continuous darkness, however, the spot check revealed significant differences only for liver parenchyma.

This finding may be accounted for by the free-running of rhythm in pinnal mitosis from that in liver parenchyma. This view is supported by an earlier demonstration from our laboratory of the persistence of the rhythm in pinnal epidermis after blinding (33), among other considerations (8). With the limited data at hand, the possibility remains that the pinnal mitotic rhythm is rapidly

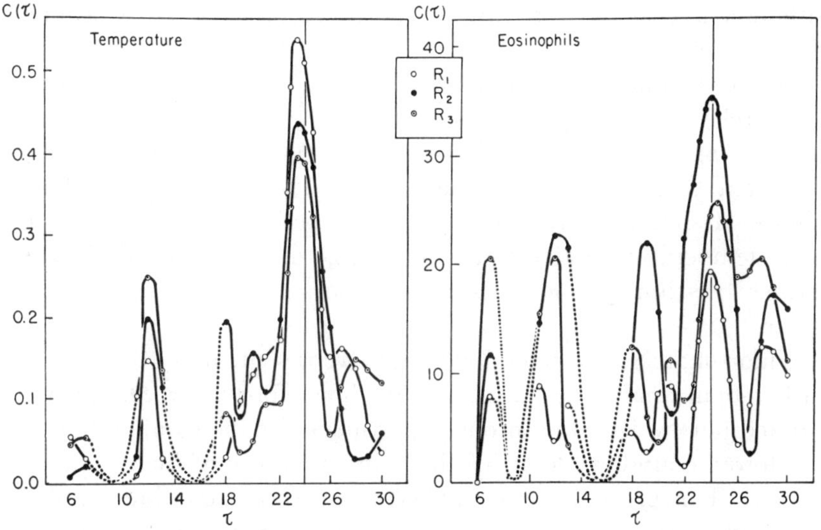

Figure 11. Mean Circadian Period for Three Human Subjects Subjected to 12-Hourly Regressive Electroshock Schedule (34)

Note that mean period of temperature rhythm appears to be shorter than that of eosinophil rhythm.

obliterated in constant darkness (while the mitotic rhythm of liver parenchyma persists). But even if this remote possibility be true, it can be concluded that the normal time relations of the two mitotic rhythms are altered in continuous darkness.

Free-running of circadian physiologic rhythms from each other also is suggested (but not proved) by studies on patients subjected to two electro-shocks every 12 hours for a week or two (34) until they are regressed. In three cases investigated, the rhythms in blood eosinophils and body temperature were only initially and feebly "driven" by the 12-hour shock schedule. Figure 11 reveals that both rhythms showed predominating circadian periods rather than a 12-hour period. The interpretation of these data must be qualified since we are dealing with psychotic patients rather than with normal subjects. For these subjects, however, it seems established that some of the most drastic stimuli applicable with non-circadian schedules to man (regressive electric shock) fail to erase the circadian periods. The body's circadian temporal structure for functional integration, although it is plastic, cannot be shortened or lengthened beyond certain limits.

At least equally interesting, however, is another aspect of the same data, relevant to the question whether the mean period for the rhythms in temperature and eosinophils was the same in a person subjected to the obviously unacceptable 12-hour shock schedule. Figure 11 shows differences in the mean period of the rhythms in body temperature and blood eosinophils, the mean period for the former rhythm being consistently shorter than that for the latter.

Unfortunately these periodograms represent only descriptive rather than analytical statistics (35). Therefore, a procedure was worked out by Dr. Rao in our department, for the computation of the lower bound, at least, of the standard error of the estimated period. This procedure was applied to the shock data but it failed to ascertain the significance of the deviation in mean temperature period from exactly twenty-four hours. Yet each of the three cases studied showed differences in the mean period of the rhythms in body temperature and blood eosinophils and in each the difference was in the same direction. It is suggested (not proved) that desynchronization among circadian rhythms is likely to occur in subjects exposed to trauma on drastic non-circadian schedules.

RESISTANCE TO TRAUMA ON UNUSUAL SCHEDULES

Work by Dr. E. Haus, F. Pass, and the writer now in progress deals with the relation of resistance to injury to the environmental routine. Results as yet are limited to one schedule ("8-hour day"), one agent (ethanol), one species (mouse), one sex (males); and they must be qualified further, since they involve only a relatively short-term exposure to unusual schedules. We cannot describe long-term adaptations. The experiments were designed to study the question whether the over-all level of susceptibility to a poison affecting the central nervous system will change in animals kept on drastically non-circadian routines.

For this purpose, three groups of mice were housed singly in three periodicity rooms kept for at least seven days in light from 6:00 A.M. to 6:00 P.M., alternating with 12 hours of darkness. Thereafter, one group was maintained on the same schedule while another group was subjected to the inversion of lighting regimen; a dark period was prolonged to 24 hours, with lights going on thereafter from 6:00 P.M. to 6:00 A.M., in alternation with darkness from 6:00 A.M. to 6:00 P.M. At the same time, a third group of mice was switched to a schedule providing for four hours of light alternating with four hours of darkness.

On the fifth day following the change in lighting, subgroups from each group were given .8 cc of a 25 percent solution of ethanol intraperitoneally, starting at 8:00 A.M. and continuing at 4-hour intervals until 4:00 A.M. the following morning. The mice continuing on the regular lighting schedule showed the previously described susceptibility rhythm to ethanol (14). As to the over-all level of susceptibility to ethanol (irrespective of the time chosen for injection), 27 out of 128 mice on the regular schedule died within 30 minutes post-injection. By comparison, 31 of 127 mice on the reversed schedule died at a comparable time point post-injection. Thus a difference in level of susceptibility was not ascertained ($X^2 = .38$; $P > .32$). A highly significant increase in over-all susceptibility to ethanol was seen, in turn, in the third group kept on the "8-hour day" (with light and darkness alternating every four hours). At 30 minutes post-injection, 51 out of 128 mice had died on the 4-on, 4-off light schedule, by comparison to only 27 out of the same total of mice kept on the regular schedule ($X^2 = 10.6$; $P = .002$). Moreover, an indication for the free-running of the susceptibility rhythm to ethanol in mice kept on the 8-hour day also was obtained.

It is premature to generalize beyond the scope of these available data. Differences in genetic background, age, sex, past history, among many other factors, will contribute to the ultimate physiologic preparedness of the body to withstand injury. Moreover, maximal physiologic preparedness to one agent will probably entail a deficit in the resistance to another (cf. Figure 4). Only with such qualifications can it be suggested that some schedules of activity are physiologically more acceptable than others and that efficient body functioning as well as resistance against various types of injury depends upon the routine of living.

The data on the significance of periodicity suffice, however, for suggesting that selection of astronauts should include studies of their circadian periodicity. Moreover, once a subject is selected, it seems likely that his efficiency and resistance to certain agents can be economically increased by the appropriate scheduling of rest and activity.

One can readily visualize situations when military and other sociologic factors gain precedence in determining work schedules. Even then physiologic considerations remain pertinent; whenever conditions arise that make optimal routines impractical so that physiologically less desirable ones are substituted, one should know of shortcomings in order to forestall deleterious effects. If, as seems to be the case, one cannot live most efficiently without physiologic considerations for scheduling rest and activity, one should adjust one's routine accordingly or make other provisions.

This paper will not conclude by suggesting certain schedules for astronauts, in preference to others. But methods are now available for studying this problem. At the present state of information it can only be said that the circadian temporal organization of body functions is a fact; that it was probably acquired through terrestrial evolution, and that this acquisition so useful adaptively on earth may not be readily lost in aerospace. Circadian components of some rhythms are now known to persist for a while on certain routines that are drastically different from 24-hour cycles. Life on such routines can entail reductions in the physiologic preparedness to withstand injury. Such deficits have been demonstrated experimentally on experimental animals kept on an "8-hour day," but much more extensive studies seem indicated.

One of the tasks at hand seems to be the application of periodicity analysis at different levels of physiologic organization to problems of human engineering for aerospace. It seems safe to predict that the longer the flights that we contemplate the more we shall have to be concerned with the possibility that circadian desynchronization may occur and that it may be detrimental.

REFERENCES

1. Halberg, F., Ztschr. f. Vitamin- Hormon- und Fermentforschung, 10:225, 1959.
2. Pittendrigh, C. S., V. G. Bruce, N. S. Rosensweig, and M. L. Rubin, Nature, 184:169, 1959.
3. Bruce, V. G., F. Weight, and C. S. Pittendrigh, Science, 131:728, 1960.
4. Aschoff, J., Ztschr. Tierpsych., 15:1, 1958.
5. Folk, G. E., Jr., and F. Sargent, Environmental Extremes and Mammalian Survival. Iowa City, Department of Publications, University of Iowa.
6. Bykow, K. M., Studien über Veränderungen physiologischer Funktionen des Organismus. Berlin, Akademi-Verlag, 1954.
7. Halberg, F., C. P. Barnum, R. H. Silber, and J. J. Bittner, Proc. Soc. Exp. Biol. and Med., 97:897, 1958.
8. Halberg, F., E. Halberg, C. P. Barnum, and J. J. Bittner, Physiologic 24-hour periodicity in human beings and mice, the lighting regimen and daily routine, in *Photoperiodism and Related Phenomena in Plants and Animals*, p. 803. R. B. Withrow, ed. Pub. 55, Amer. Assoc. Adv. Sci. Washington, D.C., 1959.
9. Halberg, F., The 24-hour scale: a time dimension of adaptive functional organization, Perspectives in Biology and Medicine, 3:491, 1960.
10. Halberg, F., Lighting regimen and experimental method: light-synchronized periodicity analysis, 12th Annual Conf. on Elect. Tech. in Med. and Biol. Digest of Technical Papers, 78, Nov., 1959.
11. Halberg, F., E. Johnson, W. Brown, and J. J. Bittner, Proc. Soc. Exp. Biol. and Med., 103:142, 1960.
12. Halberg, F., J. J. Bittner, R. J. Gully, P. Albrecht, and E. L. Brackney, Proc. Soc. Exp. Biol. and Med., 88:169, 1955.
13. Halberg, F., and A. N. Stephens, *Proceedings*, Minn. Acad. Sci. 27:139, 1960.
14. Haus, E., and F. Halberg, J. Appl. Physiol., 14:878, 1959.
15. Barnum, C. P., C. D. Jardetzky, and F. Halberg, Am. J. Physiol., 195:301, 1958.
16. Halberg, F., R. E. Peterson, and R. H. Silber, Endocrinology, 64:222, 1959.
17. Magoun, H. W., Proc. Assoc. Research Nerv. Mental Disease, 30:480, 1952.
18. Gangloff, H., and M. Monnier, Electroencephalog. Clin. Neurophysiol., 8:623, 1956.
19. Mason, J. W., in Reticular Formation of the Brain. Boston, Little, Brown & Co., 1958, p. 645.
20. Hume, D. M., and R. H. Egdahl, Annals of Surgery, 150:697, 1959.
21. Galicich, J. H., F. Halberg, and L. A. French, Corticosterone in mouse adrenal and serum following brain ablations with or without pituitary removal, in *Communications* of the First International Congress of Endocrinology, p. 55, 1960.
22. Pittendrigh, C. S., and V. G. Bruce, An oscillator model for biological clocks, in *Symposium, Society for the Study of Development and Growth.* Princeton, Princeton Univ. Press, 1957.
23. Halberg, F., M. B. Visscher, and J. J. Bittner, Am. J. Physiol., 174:313, 1953.
24. Flink, E. B., and R. P. Doe, Proc. Soc. Exper. Biol. & Med., 100, 1959.
25. Halberg, F., and R. B. Howard, Postgrad. Med., 24:349, 1958.
26. Halberg, F., E. Jacobsen, G. Wadsworth, and J. J. Bittner, Science, 128:657, 1958.
27. Strughold, H., J. Avn. Med., 23:464, 1952.
28. Kleitman, N., and D. P. Jackson, J. Appl. Physiol., 3:309, 1950.
29. Kleitman, N., in Human Factors in Submarine Warfare. Baltimore, Williams & Wilkins, 1949, p. 329.
30. Lewis, P. R., and M. C. Lobban, Quart. J. Exper. Physiol., 42:356, 1957.
31. *Ibid.*, Quart. J. Exper. Physiol., 42:371, 1957.

32. Hauty, G. T., G. R. Steinkamp, W. R. Hawkins, and F. Halberg, Fed. Proc., 19:54, 1960.
33. Chaudhry, A. P., Certain Physiologic and Pharmacologic Aspects of 24-hour Periodicity in Mitosis. Minneapolis, Minn., University of Minnesota Graduate School, 1956.
34. Fleeson, W., B. C. Glueck, and F. Halberg, Physiologist, 1:28, 1957.
35. Koehler, F., F. K. Okano, L. R. Elveback, F. Halberg, and J. J. Bittner, Exper. Med. & Surg., 14:5, 1956.

Physiological Data Acquisition

NEIL R. BURCH *and* HAROLD E. CHILDERS

I would like to simplify my consideration of physiological data acquisition to the following limited set of problems: What do you want to measure? How are you going to amplify and record? How are you going to transmit? How are you going to analyze? What is your interpretation going to be?

THE MEASURES

Table 1 presents three possible physiological profiles. Under

Table 1. Physiological Profiles

PROFILE A *Arousal*	PROFILE B *Basal Physiology*	PROFILE C *Cardiovascular*
1. EEG	1. Core temperature	1. EKG
2. GSR	2. Oximeter	2. Pulse wave
3. EKG	3. Endocrine assay	3. Blood pressure
4. Respiration	a. epinephrine	4. Ballistocardiogram
5. Skin temperature	b. norepinephrine	5. Heart sounds
6. EMG	c. 17-ketosteroids	6. Plethysmograph
7. Blood pressure	4. Blood pH	7. Leg plethysmograph
8. Plethysmograph	5. Blood count	8. Vital capacity
9. Eye movement	a. WBC	9. Mid position, thoracic volume
10. Movement (total)	b. Eosinophiles	
11. Salivation	6. Gut motility and pressure	
	7. Vital capacity	
	8. Tidal volume	

Dr. Burch is Associate Professor of Psychiatry, Baylor University College of Medicine, and Chief, Psychophysiology Laboratories, Houston State Psychiatric Institute, Houston, Texas. Mr. Childers is Research Associate in Biophysics, Baylor University College of Medicine. The research on which this paper is based was supported in part by the United States Air Force, through the Air Force Office of Scientific Research of the Air Research and Development Command and under Contract AF 41(657)-317 with the School of Aviation Medicine, USAF Aerospace Medical Center (ATC), Brooks Air Force Base, Texas.

profile A is an array of measures one would probably select for determination of state of consciousness or neurophysiological arousal. In terms of the stress response as outlined by Dr. Applezweig, this profile is primarily a measure of Selye's alarm reaction (9). This profile also reflects activity of the neurophysiological aspects of stress and the arousal system (7) described by Dr. Magoun. It is of interest to notice here that when one talks about measuring stress in man, and particularly in Air Force applications, you may not be interested in measuring what the physiologist considers to be the principal aspect of stress. You may be more interested in measuring the "alarm reaction" of the organism to the stressor in order to estimate deterioration in performance or perhaps to determine the state of consciousness.

Under profile B, the basal or core physiology, are some of the measures for relatively steady state changes in homeostasis. These measures would reflect stage II stress response or the stage of resistance. Some of these measures, such as oximetry or core temperature, may be a rather direct function of the ambient environment. Indeed, economy of instrumentation might recommend direct recording of the ambient environment itself rather than the physiological measures. Difficulty of remote measurement aside, endocrine assays and blood count show an unfortunate time lag in their changes to stressors that makes them impractical for relatively short term runs. Professor Kleitman might well shift core temperature into profile A and I would be in agreement with this, for it emphasizes the point that all of these measures shift back and forth from profile A to profile B to profile C depending on the particular interest of the investigator and on the particular systems under investigation.

Profile C would seem appropriate if one were interested in the stress response to some specific stressor, such as radial acceleration and its effect on the cardiovascular system. Under these circumstances of investigation the profile would be specifically designed to pick up physiological changes anticipated for the particular stress agent.

My proposition today is that we are primarily concerned with state of consciousness, and I have selected four measures from profile A for best economy of measurement and analysis. Economy of measurement and analysis of man in space subsumes such factors as the reliability of the total recording system, the cost of the system in weight and space occupied, the amount of "consciousness" information carried by the system, the number of telemetering channels required for transmission, the feasibility of analysis in real time, and, finally, the level of confidence associated with interpretation.

Table 2 outlines our suggested "state of consciousness" profile.

Table 2. State of Consciousness Profile

Measure	*Parameters*	*Interpretation*
1. EEG		
Left parietal-occipital	Frequency range 1–100	Major period
Right parietal-occipital	Period frequency	Minor period
	Wave shape	
	Amplitude	
2. GSR	Frequency range .02–2	Rate
	Count	Active GSR time
	Peak amplitude time	(sigma)
	Amplitude	
3. EKG	Frequency range .5–50	Rate
	Rate	Q-R-S time
	P-R interval	
	Q-R-S interval	
	S-T segment	
	Amplitude	
	Wave shape	

Two independent electroencephalographic combinations have been included to deliberately yield redundant information. This redundancy is directed by the EEG as a relatively sensitive measure covering a wide spectrum of consciousness but easily contaminated by the artifacts inherent in field situations. The galvanic skin response (GSR) presents a much simpler recording problem than the EEG but reflects state of consciousness information over a more restricted portion of the spectrum and is particularly insensitive to the fractional depressions which may be important to man in space. The GSR is not suited to the resolution of drowsiness versus moderate sleep, versus coma, etc. While the EKG is easily recorded and has the advantage of reflecting the cardiovascular state, it has the disadvantage of ambiguous interpretation in terms of arousal; in combination with the other measures it would seem to fulfill the requirement of reasonable economy.

THE INSTRUMENT

How do you amplify and record? The EEG should be taken with a pre-amplifier placed directly on the head. This pre-amplifier should be situated in a silicone rubber "frog" secured by plastic electrode rings cemented to the head; for long-term application dental acrylic proves to be quite satisfactory. Unfortunately,

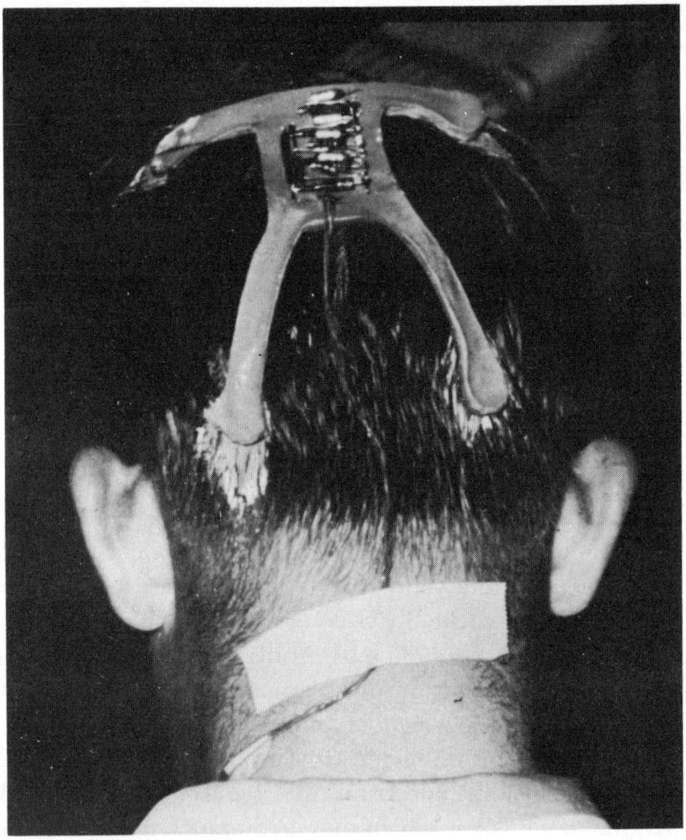

Figure 1. Pre-Amplifier in Place

The silicon rubber "frog" is secured by bentonite to subject's head in a left parieto-occipital, right parieto-occipital placement. The exposed transistor pre-amplifier is "potted" in ordinary application.

dental acrylic is very difficult to remove and we have to cut off some of the hair with the electrode, so it is not a good technique for standard daily laboratory application; here we substitute collodion or even bentonite (Figure 1). From this pre-amplifier system weighing less than an ounce, leads should go to a post-amplifier system contained in a special vest worn by the subject. The post-amplifier system, as designed and utilized in our laboratories, is a three-stage transistorized amplifier with a push-pull input of fifty thousand ohms impedance and a single ended output with a gain of approximately ten thousand. (Dimensions: $6'' \times 1\frac{1}{2}'' \times 1\frac{1}{2}''$.) This total system weighs less than twelve ounces with fifty-hour batteries included, and it amplifies the microvolt potentials of the EEG to a level of ten to twenty volts, adequate for transmission by available telemetry, adequate for both recording and analysis within the vehicle itself.

Band pass or selective filtering is extremely important for the recording of the EEG under field conditions. There should be a fairly sharp roll-off in the band pass which cuts off at 2 cycles per second at the low end, and some 40 cycles per second at the high end. I think that most of the state of consciousness information is retained with this band pass, and the artifacts are considerably decreased.

The galvanic skin response is one of the best peripheral measures of state of consciousness (2). We have worked with the GSR as a measure of neurophysiological arousal (1) for a number of years, and I must warn you that I am quite prejudiced in favor of its use. Our GSR amplifier has not been transistorized, although this could be done without appreciable difficulty and the package would probably be considerably smaller than the EEG system.

For EKG the band pass characteristics of the EEG post-amplifier are easily changed to the .5–50 cycle per second range. This post-amplifier alone, without preamplification, serves as an excellent EKG system.

THE ANALYSIS

How do you analyze? I suggest that a process we have developed called period analysis (8) should be applied to the EEG, the GSR, and the EKG. Figure 2 illustrates the process of period analysis. The top trace in this figure is a synthetic function generated by two

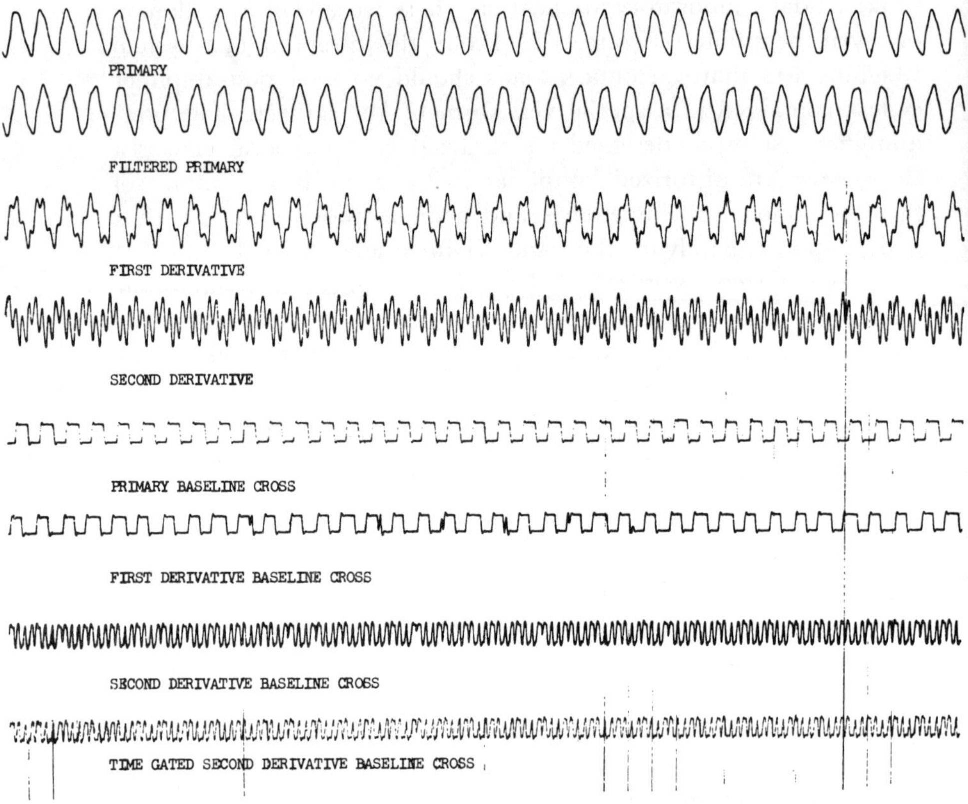

Figure 2. Pulse Width Conversion: Synthetic Function

Two oscillator signals, one at 9½ cycles per second and a much lower amplitude 36 cycles per second are mixed to produce a distorted "primary" sinusoid function. The analytical process of period analysis is illustrated in the three square wave trains of trace five, six, and seven. Paper speed 60 millimeters per second.

oscillators, one at a dominant frequency of some 9½ cycles per second, with the second frequency of 36 cycles per second having much smaller amplitude. It will be noticed that the amplitude of the superimposed frequency is so low in relation to the dominant frequency that the resultant is more a distortion in wave shape than a "mixture"; the superimposed frequency is not in itself clearly apparent. The second trace is the same function after a selective filtering system. In the process of period analysis we employ the primary trace; the first derivative of this trace and the second derivative. In the third line of Figure 2, the first derivative accentuates the almost hidden superimposed frequency of 36 cycles per second; the second derivative accentuates the "low voltage fast" activity to a degree that it becomes the major component of the wave. We then take the baseline cross of each of these three functions. A square wave is generated at the base line cross points of each function so that we produce our primary square wave, our first derivative square wave and our second derivative square wave. Again you see in the primary train of square waves (major period) that the dominant frequency is faithfully represented. In the first derivative there are a few little spikes which are repetitive over time and show the beat that is occurring between these two frequencies. The second derivative base line cross (minor period) clearly shows the previously hidden 36 cycle per second component. My proposal is that we utilize this method in the analysis of all three of our selected measures: the EEG, the GSR, and the EKG. We have applied this process to the EEG for a number of years (4). We are now using this method with the GSR; we have just recently started an attempt to process the EKG in this way.

Figure 3 shows the recorded EEG in the top trace. The second trace, the filtered EEG. This band pass, because it is a laboratory situation, is from 1 cycle per second to 100 cycles per second. The first derivative and the second derivative functions are shown as they are generated by R-L-C networks. The respective baseline cross square waves are indicated. It can be shown that if we recombine these three square wave trains in a particular way (integration-mixing-integration) we can essentially reconstitute the original function. This indicates that the majority of data is carried through the processing and that the analytical process approximates a

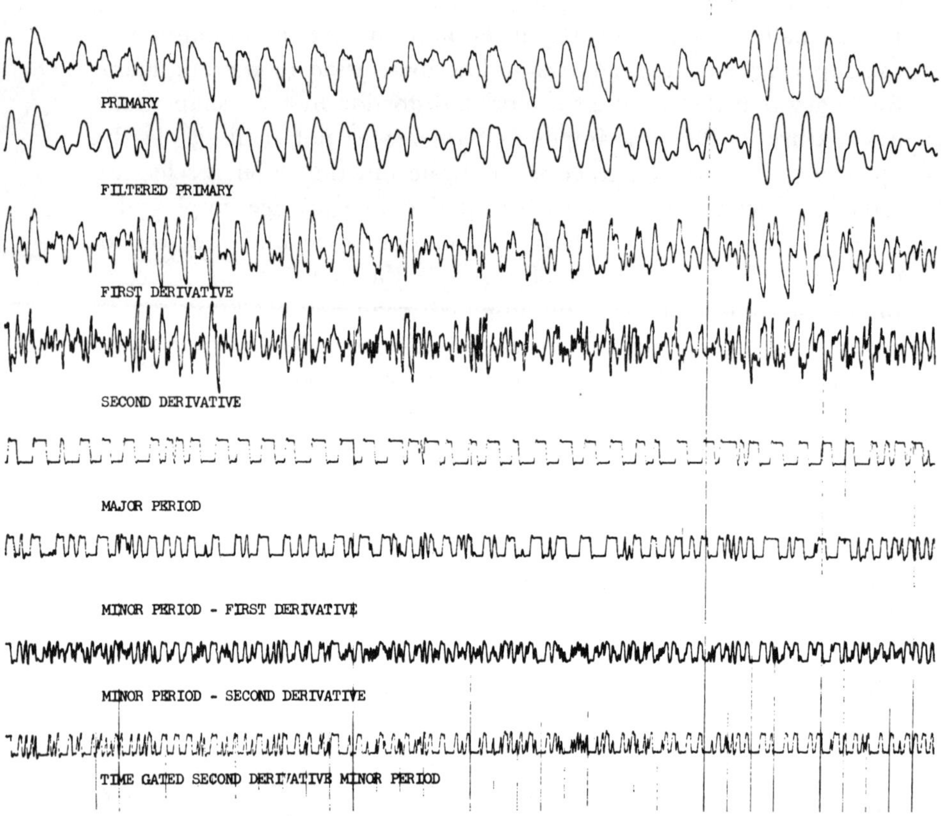

Figure 3. Pulse Width Conversion: EEG

The process of period analysis applied to the left parieto-occipital electroencephalogram. The 60 cycle per second artifact superimposed on the original primary trace is markedly reduced by the rejection notch of the selective frequency amplifier, as seen in the filtered primary. The "fragmented" appearance of the second derivative minor period results from the high inertia pen system which cannot follow a true square wave at these frequencies. Paper speed 60 millimeters per second.

reversible transform. The last trace of Figure 3 designated "time gated second derivative minor period" is the second derivative minor period gated through a special purpose digital computer which rejects all square waves with a time duration corresponding to frequencies higher than 100 cycles per second.

Figure 4 is an example of period analysis applied to the GSR. The top trace is the primary GSR as it is recorded through an amplifier with an 8-second time constant. The bottom trace is the first derivative as generated by an operational amplifier; the heavy black line running through the bottom trace is an artificial baseline which was drawn in after the record was taken to emphasize the relation between the continuous first derivative and the baseline cross square waves shown in the middle of the figure. This "baseline" was "seen" only by the circuits at the time of ongoing analysis.

The important parameters to be measured in the analysis of the GSR are both contained in the square waves of the first derivative baseline cross. These parameters are the number of square waves per unit time or GSR frequency and the duration of the square waves per unit time which we have called sigma in Figure 2 and designated as "active GSR time." Here we assume that the "active" GSR time is the duration of membrane depolarization (5), or the time from the onset of the GSR to the point of peak amplitude.

Figure 5 indicates the potential application of period analysis to the EKG. You must be aware that this record is processed with an analytical system designed for the EEG and not for the frequency range of the EKG. It can be seen that the primary square wave train yields a square wave for the P wave, the Q-R-S complex and the T wave; the square wave for the P seems to be somewhat too long, the square wave for T may also be a bit prolonged although within normal limits (the expected median values for the P and T waves are .085 and .15 seconds respectively (6), compared to the major period durations in Figure 5 of 0.2+ and .15 seconds, respectively). This artifact in the P wave major period may be due to a shifting baseline that is designed for the positive-negative area symmetry of the EEG wave; the assumption of such area symmetry is not directly applicable to the wave form of the EKG and probably should be compensated for by a fixed baseline system more similar

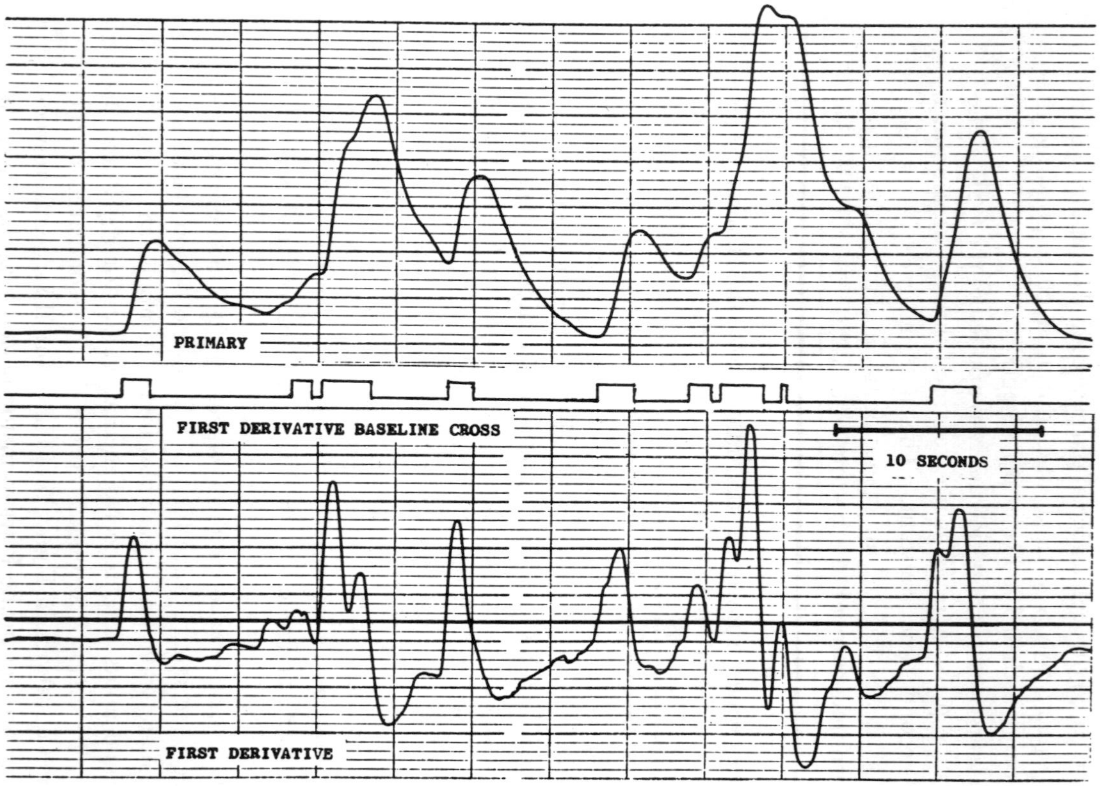

Figure 4. Period Analysis of GSR

Recorded through an 8-second time constant. The heavy black line hand drawn through the first derivative trace establishes the approximate base line "seen" by the circuits during ongoing analysis. The square wave duration is generally a linear function of primary amplitude.

to our GSR analysis. Of course we intend to pursue this study and optimize the system by modifying it for the wave shape, amplitude distributions and the band pass frequency of the EKG. The

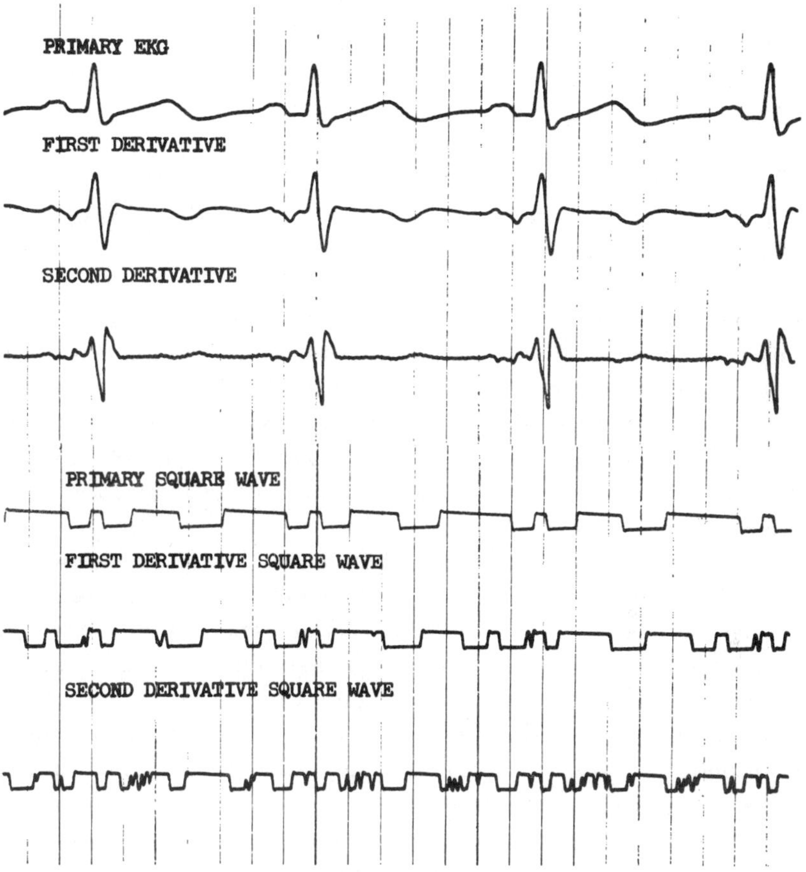

Figure 5. Period Analysis of EKG

Record shows the utilization of circuits designed for EEG signal parameters; the discrepancies from expected results are noted in the text. Paper speed 60 millimeters per second.

derivatives in Figure 5 yield baseline cross square waves proportional to the T wave shape in the primary and if we were interested in rather exact measurements of the T wave shape, or any other parameters of the clinical EKG, we might well use a small special purpose digital computer coded by various combinations of the square waves from the primary and derivative trains. The "notch" in the T wave is seen to be emphasized in the continuous first derivative (second trace) and even further emphasized in the continuous second derivative (third trace).

I have suggested that we might record, amplify, and analyze in a particular way. We shall next approach the problems of interpretation and long-term recordings.

THE INTERPRETATION

If our psychophysiological interpretation of the physiological measures allows smoothing in time, such as sampling or total measurement over an epoch, we are assured of one economy factor: we may transmit all of our physiological data over a single telemetering channel. A 10-second epoch is as short a sampling interval as is necessary for the proposed recordings. It follows that we could sequence multiplex some ten pieces of information of amplitude "spikes" on our single channel. In addition to this aspect of measurement economy the single spike per epoch makes for more convenient reading and interpretation.

Figure 6 is a case in point in which each black vertical line is a "spike" of amplitude proportional to the number of periods occurring in a 10-second epoch. The major period reflects the "dominant frequency" of the clinical electroencephalographer and is the number of major periods or baseline cross square waves of the primary trace that have occurred in the 10-second epoch. The minor period count of second derivative baseline crosses in a given 10-second epoch is a reflection of EEG desychrony and superimposed fast activity; as might be expected the minor period is far more sensitive to minimal changes in the EEG than the major period.

All of the figures designated as I.V. epinephrine are the several different measures, automatically analyzed and "smoothed" in time from the same psychophysiological experiment. In this particular experiment the subject was placed on a comfortable bed in a shielded, sound resistant, lightproof room. A continuous I.V. drip was fed from the outside of the room into the subject. At a time unknown to the subject the various drugs were injected into the tubing and the "arrival time" estimated from the rate of drip. This particular subject was a sophisticated physiologist who often dispatched his animals with massive doses of I.V. air. During the beginning of the run, where the record is marked "anxiety," the subject was quite sure that he heard large bubbles gurgling down the I.V. tube. The results of this spontaneous anxiety can be seen mirrored to a greater or lesser extent in Figures 6, 7, and 8, but they were particularly noticeable in the minor period analysis of the EEG. In Figure 6 it would seem that the early spontaneous anxiety not only resembles the epinephrine effect, but may be synergistic in action with the 5 gamma epinephrine dosage; that is, the 5 gamma per minute I.V. epinephrine immediately after anxiety produced more minor period activation in the EEG than subsequent 10 gamma per minute epinephrine in a later period of no background anxiety. The minimal change in the major period throughout the total run indicates that the electroencephalographer would see no appreciable change in the clinical record. The record would be seen as a slight change in synchrony, somewhat poorer organization, or a suggestion of increased superimposed fast activity that accompanies moderate arousal.

Figure 7 is an example of the GSR automatically analyzed and automatically plotted with time. We have an hour's worth of GSR analysis in these four 15-minute sections. The 5 gamma epinephrine increases the number of GSRs as shown in the top portion of the slide; anxiety also increased the GSR rate. The 10 gamma epinephrine shows more activation of the GSR than it did in the EEG. The lower portion of Figure 7 is another way of measuring degree of GSR activity by taking the percentage of the active GSR time from duration of baseline cross square waves. In our interpretation of the GSR we feel that the number of these square waves increase as a monotonic function of the state of arousal. As one pours more Metrazol or epinephrine into an individual, GSR rate increases. The amplitude of the GSR and the related measure of "active GSR time" is not a monotonic function, but will increase only to a point of alertness; if you push the individual further toward panic, the amplitude of response will decrease (3). Toward the other end of the arousal spectrum, depression induced by I.V. Pentothal, as in the third and fourth records of Figure 7, decreases both the number of GSRs and the total active GSR time. The initial dose of 50

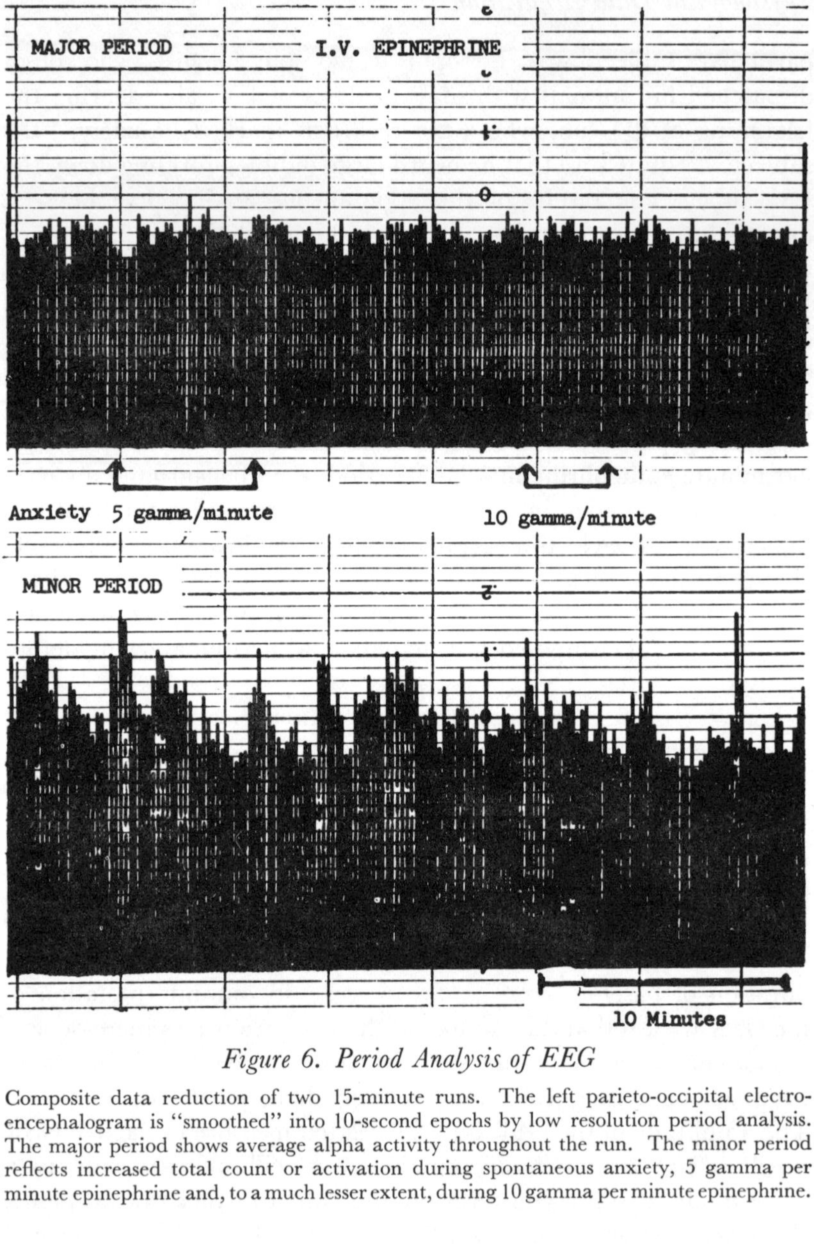

Figure 6. Period Analysis of EEG

Composite data reduction of two 15-minute runs. The left parieto-occipital electroencephalogram is "smoothed" into 10-second epochs by low resolution period analysis. The major period shows average alpha activity throughout the run. The minor period reflects increased total count or activation during spontaneous anxiety, 5 gamma per minute epinephrine and, to a much lesser extent, during 10 gamma per minute epinephrine.

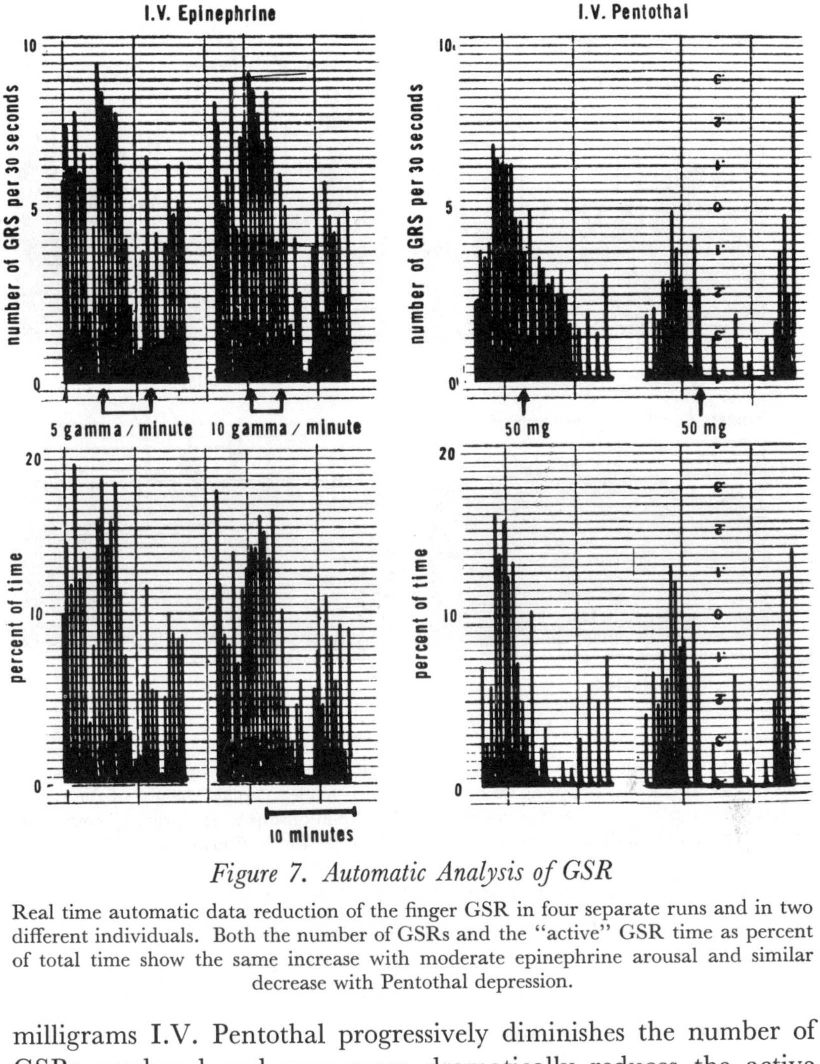

Figure 7. Automatic Analysis of GSR

Real time automatic data reduction of the finger GSR in four separate runs and in two different individuals. Both the number of GSRs and the "active" GSR time as percent of total time show the same increase with moderate epinephrine arousal and similar decrease with Pentothal depression.

milligrams I.V. Pentothal progressively diminishes the number of GSRs produced and even more dramatically reduces the active GSR time. After a 30-minute rest period, indicated by the separation between record three and four, there was still some residual relaxation as compared to the first part of the Pentothal run. The second dose of I.V. Pentothal practically abolishes the GSR activity until the onset of increased arousal in the termination effect; an effect often seen when the subject is aware that the experiment is about to end.

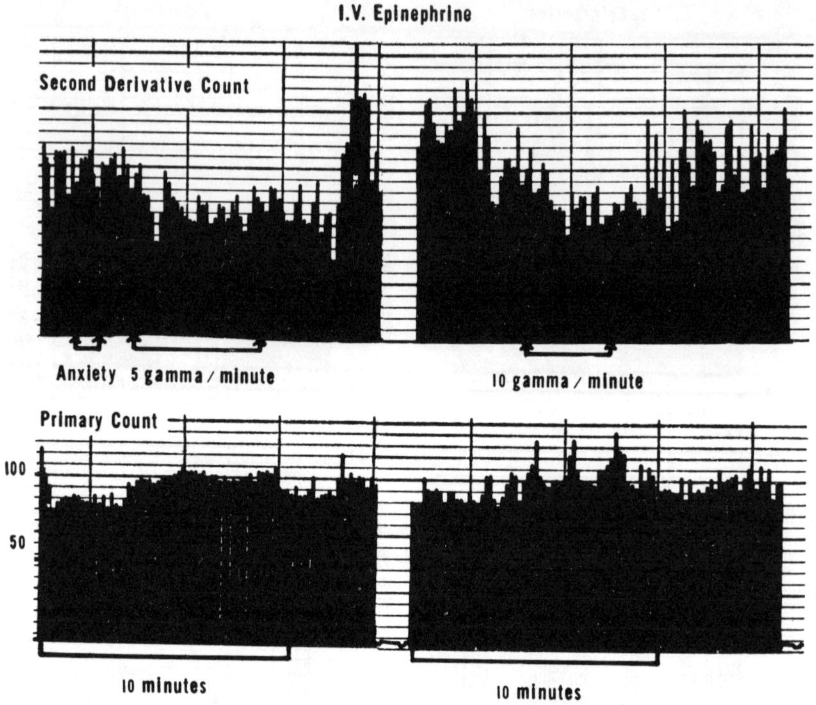

Figure 8. Total EKG Count

Automatic data reduction of the EKG with period analysis shows the expected increase in rate per 10-second epoch as illustrated by the increase "spike" height of the bottom trace. The top trace shows a peculiar reciprocal relationship to the primary count rate; the interpretation of the second derivative count is open to question as suggested in the text.

Finally, Figure 8 is a writeout of the EKG automatically analyzed in 10-second epochs. The bottom record is the primary count, each spike representing a 10-second total. The 10-gamma per minute I.V. epinephrine increases heart rate considerably more than the 5 gamma per minute dose, but in a cyclic pattern—as if the subject "breaks through" the epinephrine effect to drop back to a heart rate of some 100 beats per minute, only to once again activate to the 120–130 beats per minute level. The top records of Figure 8, identified as second derivative count, do not carry an ordinate because, with the hybrid system we were using, I have no interpretation for this measure. Theoretically, an increased total count of the second derivative reflects an increased complexity of the wave shape; perhaps as the heart rate increases, or under an epinephrine effect, the wave shape complexity of the EKG is reduced. There may be alternate explanations for this apparent simplification of EKG wave form, and the problem requires extended investigation.

SUMMARY

I have suggested that physiological data acquisition is really a problem of what you want to measure and what you can measure with reasonable economy in a particular situation. I have suggested that for the man in space we have the equipment, we have the method of processing, we are able to automatically analyze and record over long periods of time. The recording and analyzing instrumentation could be completely transistorized and reduced in size and weight to allow complete data reduction within the vehicle. This would offer direct and immediate feedback of state of consciousness information to the astronaut as well as the economy of time sequence multiplexing for all physiological data telemetered to the ground station at the expense of only one channel. In brief, we are very nearly ready to measure the psychophysiology of man in space.

For future physiological data acquisition I think that it is quite important to pursue three parallel research efforts. Not only should we concentrate on instrumenting the man in space for state of consciousness, but we should also carry the same measures into the clinical psychophysiology laboratories for normative studies and, lastly, we should continue to conduct theoretical work on the analytical process itself.

REFERENCES

1. Burch, N. R., and T. H. Greiner, Response of human galvanic skin reflex to drugs that influence reticular formation of brain stem, Fed. Proc., 14:1, 1955.
2. Burch, N. R., and T. H. Greiner, Drugs and human fatigue: GSR parameters, J. Psychol., 45:3–10, 1958.
3. Burch, N. R., and T. H. Greiner, A bioelectric scale of human alertness: Concurrent recordings of the EEG and GSR, Psy. Res. Reports 12, pp. 183–193, Jan. 1960.
4. Burch, N. R., H. E. Childers, and W. A. Spoor, Period analysis of the electroencephalogram. Paper presented before the Southwestern IRE Conf., Houston, Texas, 1960.
5. Edelberg, R., T. H. Greiner, and N. R. Burch, Some membrane properties of the effector organ in the galvanic skin response, J. Appl. Physiol., 15:691–696, July, 1960.
6. Katz, L. N., Electrocardiography. Philadelphia, Pa,. Lee and Febiger, 1946.
7. Magoun, H. W., The Waking Brain. Springfield, Ill., Charles C. Thomas, 1958.
8. Saltzberg, B., and N. R. Burch, A rapidly convergent orthogonal representation for EEG time series and related methods of automatic analysis, in *IRE Wescon Convention Record*, Part 8, 1959.
9. Selye, H., The Stress of Life. New York, McGraw-Hill, 1956.

PART 3

Problems of Human Reliability

Sensory Overloading

JAMES G. MILLER

It is possible that critical situations in space flight may overload a man in space with the necessity of responding simultaneously to information from multiple dial readings, auditory signals, and other sensory input. As a result of this overload he might be unable to process information adequately, and a serious breakdown in performance might result. It is therefore important to know what are the maximum and optimum channel capacities of individuals, what processes of adjustment do they use to compensate for information input overload, and if possible, what are the respective costs to a person of forced performance at various rates of information input, as well as the cost of the respective adjustment processes to overload.

GENERAL BEHAVIOR SYSTEMS THEORY

I intend to describe here a research program just being completed at the Mental Health Research Institute of the University of Michigan. Before I give a general description of our findings, I want to present a brief survey of our general orientation to an integrative study of the biological and social aspects of behavior. We refer to our approach as general behavior systems theory (1), and it is based on the assumption that there are in the universe a hierarchy of concrete systems which exist in space-time, including the particle, nucleus, atom, molecule, and crystal. About at the level of the crystal a structure known as the tobacco mosaic virus, which crystallizes, emerges as a primitive form of life. From there on up there are a series of levels of behaving systems, including the cell (like the neuron), which is a component of the organ (like the liver or brain), which are components of the individual, who is a component of small face-to-face groups (like the family), which are components of social

Dr. Miller, Professor of Psychiatry and Psychology, is Director, Mental Health Research Institute, University of Michigan, Ann Arbor, Michigan.

institutions and societies. Larger than these living systems are other combined living and nonliving systems such as the planet, the solar system, the galaxy, and so forth. The approach of general systems theory is to look for formal models which can represent identities in some characteristics across these various levels of systems. Whether or not in the very smallest nonliving systems and the very largest systems there are any such formal identities is beyond my competence to say. General behavior systems theory limits itself to the special subset of living systems, and attempts to find certain regularities or formal identities in them.

It is not too implausible that such analogies could be found. After all we have found similarities among individuals while studying individual differences in psychology or physiology, and we have found similarities across species in sciences like comparative anatomy, comparative physiology, or comparative psychology. Why should there not also be a third level of generality in which, while explicitly recognizing interindividual variance and interspecies variance, we also look for cross-level similarities from cell to society?

All of these living systems at whatever level are faced with comparable problems. They exist in an environment based fundamentally upon the chemistry of water, in a relatively restricted range of pressures, temperatures, radiations, and hydrations. They are all composed of protoplasm which is primarily constituted of proteins composed of a handful of amino acids. They all share fundamentally the same genetic inheritance going back to the original forms of life. Therefore it would not be too surprising if we should find certain formal identities among them.

What do these organisms, or organizations, or living systems share in common? In the past, various general systems theorists like Lotka (2) and Volterra (3) have emphasized that certain types of functions, growth characteristics, and interactions with the environment are common. Bertalanffy (4), a modern general systems theorist, has emphasized the fact that these are open systems with throughputs of energy and information maintaining equilibria in an environment and apparently carrying on purposive activities which can be explained by a mechanism he has called equifinality. Wright (5) and Gerard (6), among others, have recognized many specific characteristics of these systems which are similar. Gerard pictures the different levels of these living systems as having three common aspects—being or structure, behaving or function, and becoming or history. The difference between behaving and becoming in this equilibrium theory of these systems, which are maintaining stabilities within their boundaries by negative feedback or cybernetic mechanisms, is that behaving or alterations of function around an equilibrium point are reversible and can return to that point. On the other hand, becoming, or changes from maturation, decay, or trauma in a system, includes processes in which the equilibrium point of the system is transmuted to a new one, so that its structure is fundamentally altered to a new structure. So we conceive of a Chinese box-like hierarchy of systems composed of subsystems composed of subsubsystems, which are components of suprasystems which are in supra-suprasystems, and so forth. Each of these systems has inputs and outputs of energy and/or matter, as well as inputs and outputs of information.

Since these systems must maintain life, they must fight the entropic tendencies described by the second law of thermodynamics (7). They do this by taking in foods or fuels of high negative entropy, required to maintain their stability. So living systems cannot be entirely walled off, and there must be a minimal rate of input of a series of necessary forms of energy or matter for life to go on. Whenever inputs are less than adequate or extremely high, they constitute stresses. So one can have a stress of anoxia or inadequate rate of input of oxygen or one can have oxygen poisoning, too high a rate of input of oxygen. The same can be true of water and other essential materials.

We ask whether there must also be a minimal rate of information input to maintain life in the organism, and whether there can be lack and excess stresses of information upon these living systems—underloads or overloads of information. The evidence accumulating indicates that both are possible.

INFORMATION INPUT UNDERLOAD STRESS

Recently there has been much talk and several somewhat confusing research reports about one type of informational stress, what we would call information input underload, a lack stress. The most common name for this is sensory deprivation.

Heron, Doane, and Scott, working with Hebb at McGill (8), greatly diminished the inputs through several sensory modalities to their subjects, and after a few hours they had hallucinatory experiences which were in many ways like psychotic states. Lilly (9), working at Bethesda, suspended himself and another subject naked in a tank below the water level, wearing a blacked-out headmask for breathing which also kept out light. The water temperature was constant, and somatic sensation was minimized by the immersion. After a short time both subjects experienced psychotic-like manifestations.

This evidence suggests that there must be a certain minimal rate of input of information into the organism for it to function normally. Other sorts of evidence confirm this. For example, Riesen (10) found that if you raise a chimpanzee in darkness for the first three months of its life and then bring it out into the light, it will never see adequately again. The lack of informational input into the visual nervous system causes permanent structural damage. On the other hand, if the chimpanzee is raised in light for the first three months and then in darkness for as long as six months, when coming back to the light it temporarily has trouble seeing but rapidly regains perfect vision. In other words, as Freud pointed out in a very different context, early informational experiences may have more significance than later ones, after development has gone farther.

Recent investigations indicate that cutting the amount of energy coming through the sense organs does not produce sensory deprivation (11). Rather, it is the amount of patterning, of sensory message, of information in the input which is significant. Whenever this information falls below a minimum, these phenomena appear. So you may put white noise into the ear at a loud intensity, and the subject can still suffer from sensory deprivation, because he hears noise only, without any informational patterning of sound. The same is true for visual presentation.

We are therefore thinking of doing experiments in which we can control the amount of information coming to the individual by any sensory pathway, using an apparatus which systematically increases the patterning seen or heard by the subject. We will then correlate the time of onset of sensory deprivation phenomena with the previous amount of input information. This might be done, for example, by having the patient wear earphones and peer into a screen (both of these usually present noise to him), and from time to time increase the amounts of patterned signals on top of the noise. The amount of this patterning would be correlated with the rate of onset of the sensory deprivation situation.

INFORMATION INPUT OVERLOAD STRESS

Just as there can be lack stresses of information input, or sensory deprivation, so there can also be excess stresses. We have studied the effect of such excess stresses, or information input overload, upon behaving systems at five levels—cell, organ, individual, group, and social institution (12). We found that there was a similarity in the relations between rate of information input and rate of information output at all these levels. For each system, if the rate of information input in bits per second is increased, the rate of output follows it exactly as a linear function for a period of time. Then it begins to level off until it reaches the channel capacity or maximum rate of output possible for the system. Then it maintains this channel capacity, even though the input rate increases. Finally, as the input rate speeds up even faster, the output falls drastically, sometimes to zero. The system is overloaded and can no longer transmit information. We are not certain yet from our data whether this overload phenomenon of catastrophic collapse occurs in the larger systems, or whether they have built-in mechanisms which permit them to keep to their maximum channel capacities regardless of the input rate.

Even though the curves were similar for all the levels of behaving systems, we found an interesting systematic difference among the levels. We discovered that a single neural fiber of the sciatic nerve of the frog, when dissected and stimulated electronically, has a channel capacity of about 4,000 bits a second, assuming optimal pulse-interval coding. This is a remarkably rapid rate indicating high efficiency for such a small biological system. The total visual nervous system of a rat, between the electrically stimulated optic nerve and a single cell in the optic cortex, can transmit information at a channel capacity of about 50 bits per second, assuming the same sort of optimal coding. In experiments which we carried out with our IOTA apparatus (Information Overload Testing Aid), the maximum channel capacity of individual subjects was about

6 bits a second. A four-man group with the IOTA apparatus had a maximum channel capacity of about 3 bits a second, and a simulator of the United States Air Raid Warning System composed of three groups transmitting information concerning symbols for planes arriving randomly in time and space, was of the order of about 3 or 4 bits per second per channel maximum. There were about the same number of components in each channel in this simulator as in the group.

Apparently the more components there are in an information processing system, the lower is its channel capacity. There are several reasons for this. Two of the most obvious are that at the border between each component and the next a recoding of information is necessary, and such recoding always results in loss of a certain amount of information. Moreover, if there are *n* components in any system, one must have a lower channel capacity than the others, and the statistical probability of there being such a slow component is always greater as *n* increases. This sluggish component constitutes a bottleneck, since no channel is faster than its slowest component. So much for the performance characteristics of systems with different rates of information input. It is apparent that they can be overloaded, and that breakdown in information processing capacity can occur.

It seems that such overload can lead to psychopathology, just as information underload can. Since we first reported these data, various clinicians and others dealing with situations in real life have called to our attention such overload phenomena. It appears that when executives must make decisions in a brief period of time their information processing capacity may break down. Collapse of the "ability to cope" with situations may be another example. I have received from a personnel psychologist reports of individuals who have asked to be transferred from important positions or refused to take responsibility because they said they could not handle the rate at which information processing had to go on in their jobs, even though they recognized that other people could do so.

PROCESSES OF ADJUSTMENT TO RATES OF INFORMATION CHANGE

A mounting body of evidence suggests that the reticular system has an important role in responding to the quantity of information coming into the nervous system. The usual picture of the sensory modalities is that they transmit patterns of information in the fields of audition, vision, somesthesis, taste, and so forth, and that behavior consists largely of learned responses to these patterns. Now the development of information theory mathematics enables us to quantify the total amount of information being processed through a sensory channel or through a central channel in the nervous system, independent of the particular patterning of it. It now appears that perhaps the role of the reticular system is to react to this total quantity of information coming in through all sensory pathways, rather than to the patterning. For example, when we close our eyes, darken the room, and relax our muscles in a standard temperature in bed, alertness—a function of the reticular system—drops. Here we have intentionally created a partial sensory deprivation situation, as Jacobson's relaxation theory (13) implied many years ago. The alertness of the nervous system decreases under the control of the reticular system, and we sleep.

On the other end of the scale, when the nervous system is bombarded with high rates of information input over a number of sensory modalities such that the channel capacities of the central decision-making mechanisms of the nervous system are exceeded, the reticular system appears also to have a role in limiting this total amount by selectively filtering out inputs exceeding what can be handled. In the past this has traditionally been viewed as a central mechanism, called attention. Recent research by Hernández-Peón and others (14), however, has indicated that this process occurs more peripherally than previously suspected. A chronic electrode placed in the cochlear nucleus of a cat ordinarily would record a transmitted impulse every time a click occurred in its ear. However, as Hernández-Peón and his co-workers showed, if a glass bottle containing mice is placed in front of the cat, he gives preferential attention to the mass of fascinating visual information coming to him, and possibly under the control of the reticular system, the click is not transmitted to higher nervous centers. A fish smell or a painful shock produces the same effect as the sight of the mice. This is very possibly a preventive measure to keep the central nervous system from being overwhelmed by information input overload.

In our studies we discovered that the following processes of adjustment, or mechanisms of defense, are used by living systems against the stresses of information input overload. Not all living systems have all of these mechanisms (indeed, systems can be classified in terms of whether they do or do not have them). The smaller systems, like the neuron, appear to have fewer than the larger systems, like the society, which not only have all of them but also have complicated variations of them. These appear to be the fundamental mechanisms:

omission, which is simply not processing information whenever there is an extreme of overload;

error, which is processing incorrectly and then not making the necessary adjustment;

queuing, which is delaying responses during peak load periods and then catching up during lulls;

filtering, which is systematic omission of certain categories of information, according to some sort of priority scheme;

approximation, which is an output mechanism whereby a less precise or accurate response is given because there is no time to be precise;

multiple channels, parallel transmission subsystems that can do comparable tasks at the same time and consequently handle altogether more information than a single channel can transmit alone;

decentralization is a special case of this; and, finally, there is

escape, which is leaving a situation entirely or taking any other steps that effectively cut off the flow of information.

In our researches with the IOTA apparatus we found that both individuals and groups, once they had learned about all the adjustment processes, tended to try to use various ones. At slow rates of information input this was not necessary. At medium rates, all of them were attempted wherever possible. However, at high rates, with the IOTA apparatus at least, filtering and particularly omissions were the primary processes used. At the very rapid rates it got so that perhaps as much as 98 percent of all information transmitted into the system was omitted, rather than being transmitted out. By this process the individual was able to keep operating, even though little of the total input information was transmitted.

It is apparent that there is also an economic problem involved in information input overload. There is a certain rate of information transmission at which the system is most efficient. Intuitively we would think that at very high rates, when confusion tends to develop and many symbols are being omitted, or errors made, or queuing or other mechanisms of adjustment are being employed, the costs in terms of some value of the system undoubtedly are increased. We hope to be able to carry out investigations on this. Also we are concerned with the costs of the various processes of adjustment. Some are clearly more expensive in given situations than others. For example, a priority system whereby unimportant information is filtered out and only critical information transmitted may be useful in some circumstances, but when one is not certain which information is potentially important and which is not, filtering is an expensive or dangerous mechanism. Similarly, in some situations a few errors may not be important, but in other situations where a single mistake may mean death or destruction of a system, errors may be inadmissible. Also, it is obvious that at times a process of adjustment of random omission may be adequate, but at other times it will not be. Specific man-machine systems must be investigated, then, in terms of the optimal strategy for utilizing these processes of adjustment, since the fundamental channel capacity of an individual in space flight or in any other man-machine situation apparently cannot be importantly altered.

I say "apparently" because we have conducted researches recently which have demonstrated that Dexedrine (dextroamphetamine sulphate) definitely increases an individual's information-processing capacity and delays the point of overload. Dexedrine may produce side effects which are undesirable, but this research does suggest that new drugs might significantly alter information processing capacity of the nervous system. Also, it might be possible to develop new compounds which do not have side-effects. All this, however, is at the moment in the realm of speculation, because no definite clues to the nature of such compounds exist.

I shall conclude by reemphasizing that in a multi-person system there is clearly a limitation of channel capacity, resulting from the limitations of the individuals and of their subsystems. There are definite points of overload, and this must always be considered in designing the equipment and communication facilities for space flight. However, processes of adjustment of different costs are available, and part of space-vehicle design in the future should consist in determining quantitatively the optimal strategies for utilizing these different adjustment processes in the given situation.

REFERENCES

1. Miller, J. G., Toward a general theory for the behavioral sciences, Am. Psychol., 10:513–531, 1955.
2. Lotka, A. J., Elements of Physical Biology. Baltimore, Md., Williams and Wilkins, 1925.
3. Volterra, V., Leçons sur la théorie mathématique de la lutte pour la vie. Paris, Gauthier-Villars et Cie, 1931.
4. Bertalanffy, L. v., The theory of open systems in physics and biology, Science, 111:23–28, 1950.
5. Wright, S., Gene and organism, Am. Nat., 87:5–18, 1953.
6. Gerard, R. W., ed., Concepts of Biology, Behavioral Science, 2:92–215, 1958.
7. Schrödinger, E., What is Life? Cambridge, The University Press, 1955.
8. Heron, W., B. K. Doane, and T. H. Scott, Visual disturbances after prolonged perceptual isolation, Canad. J. Psychol., 10:13–18, 1956.
9. Lilly, J., in *Illustrative Strategies for Research on Psychopathology in Mental Health*, pp. 13–20. Group for the Advancement of Psychiatry, Symposium No. 2, June, 1956.
10. Riesen, A. H., Arrested vision, Scientific American, 183:16–19, 1950.
11. Wheaton, J. L., Fact and fancy in sensory deprivation studies, Aeromed. Rev., No. 559, Air Univ. School of Aviation Medicine. USAF, Brooks Air Force Base, Texas, 1959.
12. Miller, J. G., Input overload and psychopathology, Am. J. Psychiat., 116:8:695–704, 1960.
13. Jacobson, E., Progressive Relaxation. Chicago, University of Chicago Press, 1938.
14. Hernández-Peón, R., H. Scherrer, and M. Jouvet, Modification of electric activity in cochlear nucleus during "attention" in unanesthetized cats, Science, 123:331–332, 1956.

Sensory Deprivation: Effects upon the Functioning Human in Space Systems

D. EWEN CAMERON, LEONARD LEVY, THOMAS BAN, *and* LEONARD RUBENSTEIN

There has been a rapid development of interest in the phenomena which may be produced in the human being by a reduction in sensory input. It would appear that the work in this field was first started in the early 1950s with animals and was concerned primarily with the effects of reduction of sensory input upon the development of the animal. As in the opening up of any new field, there were precursory lines of investigation which eventually led to this area.

One of the earliest of such investigative lines was inaugurated by work done by Hebb (1) in contrasting the development of rats blinded in infancy with normal rats. The two groups were tested subsequently by a rat intelligence test. A far greater degree of intelligence was observed in maturity in the controlled rats than in the blinded animals.

A study which began to approach more closely the field of reduced sensory input was one carried out at the same time by Hebb on rats reared in small cages as contrasted with those brought up in a much wider environment.

A few years later, Hymovitch (2) studied rats reared in a setting in which demands on them for decisions and problem solving were lessened and pain was greatly reduced. He contrasted them then with controlled rats brought up where there were many problems in food seeking and in conflicts with other rats. He showed that the rats brought up in the protected environment with reduced demands revealed in adult life a lasting inferiority in problem solving.

Dr. Cameron is Professor of Psychiatry and Chairman, Department of Psychiatry, McGill University, Montreal; Psychiatrist-in-Chief, Royal Victoria Hospital; and Director of the Allan Memorial Institute. Doctors Levy and Ban, and Mr. Rubenstein, are on the staff of the Allan Memorial Institute.

Even earlier than this, important studies were carried out by Mackworth (3), who was requested by the Royal Air Force towards the end of 1943 to determine the optimum length of watch in connection with radar operation in anti-submarine control. Lapses in attention had been observed in those engaged in such monotonous activities. Apparently, even before this, work had been carried out in the Middle East where the optimum duration of such watches had been recommended as one hour. The Mackworth studies served to clarify the observation that where close and prolonged attention must be given to some part of the environment in which little change is occurring, or where it is occurring at very regular intervals, there tend to occur lapses of attention despite possible serious consequences. This constituted one of the first hints of the possible effects of decreased sensory input and tied in with similar work being carried on by Sharpless and Jasper (4). They reviewed and reported that where stimulation fails to change rapidly, it loses its power to evoke response.

Still another investigation leading to the present field of decreased sensory input was instituted by myself at the Albany Medical School in 1938 (5). This was concerned with nocturnal delirium in the aged. We were interested in the number of aged individuals with marked restriction in the memory span who, during the night, passed into a confused, delirious, excited stage from which they emerged during the daylight hours. After considerable experimentation, it was found that if these individuals were placed in a quiet room during the daytime with their eyes bandaged, they would not only pass into an identical confused and extremely anxious state, but they would show some very interesting phenomena, such as a tendency (while still bandaged and asked to describe their image of the room) to state, for example, that there were four windows instead of one, three beds instead of one, four dressers instead of one. Apparently, there was a breakdown in the synthesis of the various sense impressions of the objects in the room which they had gained at the time of entry. On removal of the bandages they rapidly recovered from their delusions.

From this it was concluded at the time that, in order to maintain a time and space image, we ordinarily rely upon two major factors: (a) our continued sensory input, and (b) our memory. In these individuals the memory span was so limited that it was impossible to retain a space-time image over the period of one hour during which they were blindfolded and kept in a quiet room, as the quietness of the room and the bandaging of the eyes cut off their only other means of maintaining their space-time image.

Considerable anxiety was provoked in these persons as their space-time image became disturbed. This is a phenomenon which—as will be reported later—quite frequently appears in states of reduced sensory input.

These were the early lines of investigation which ultimately brought us to the present field. The essential development of the concept of sensory isolation, however, took place in the psychology laboratories of Professor D. O. Hebb of McGill University. A report on the effects of decreased variation in the sensory environment in the adult human subject was published by Bexton, Heron, and Scott in 1954 (6). They reported on the effects of decreased input of stimulation on 22 male college students. These students wore translucent goggles, gloves, and cardboard cuffs and remained in a partially soundproof cubicle with a U-shaped foam rubber pillow for reclining the head. It was difficult to keep some of the subjects in the test area for more than 2 or 3 days. Since most of the categories of phenomena subsequently reported as occurring in consequence of decreased sensory input were described in this report, they will be listed here.

They are essentially an early somnolence followed in the later days by restlessness, unusual emotional lability, reduction in the capacity to concentrate on a topic for any length of time during the test, together with "blank" periods. Subjects also showed considerable decrease in ability to make words out of jumbled letters, and visual hallucinations—and occasionally auditory and somatesthetic—were noted. Reference was also made to disturbance in the body image. One subject reported that he felt as if his head were detached from the body; another reporting that his mind seemed to be a ball of cotton wool floating above his body. It was noted that subjects coming out of the area of reduced sensory input seemed at first to be dazed. There was some disturbance in vision—usually lasting not more than a minute or two and consisting in difficulty in focusing and objects appearing fuzzy—and the environment seemed to be two-dimensional, with the colors more saturated than usual. Confusion, headaches, and a mild nausea and fatigue were also reported, but these conditions lasted no longer than 24 hours.

Hebb himself gave further structure to the concept of sensory isolation in his article published in 1955, "The Mammal and His Environment" (7), in which he points to the connection between these observations and studies carried out on brain stimulation and, particularly, the concept of cortical arousal.

Lilly in 1956 reported on a somewhat different approach (8). Part of his report consisted in a description of two human subjects suspended with all but the top of the head immersed in a tank containing slowly flowing water at 34.5° C. The subjects wore a blacked-out mask for breathing. In so far that this study was based on an extremely short period of exposure to reduction in sensory input and is characteristic of certain others which have appeared, we will report it in some degree of detail.

Lilly stated that for the first three-quarters of an hour, the ongoing thinking of the day persisted, then relaxation occurred, with feelings of being isolated in space. During the next hour there was growing tension, and hidden methods of self-stimulation developed, such as slow swimming movements. The tension rose to the point where the subject might have to leave the tank. While in the tank, the subject's thinking was directed towards fantasies of a highly personal and emotionally charged nature. Finally, there might occur a stage where there was projection of visual imagery. He also reported another approach, namely, a study of autobiographical records of individuals who suffered long periods of partial isolation, such as in shipwrecks and in the polar winter. A considerable diversity of findings were reported, such as increased passivity, an increased vividness of the inner life and a gradual loss of visual acuity. Visual hallucinations were also noted.

Since then, a considerable range of contributions has been made. The field was reviewed by Wexler *et al.* in 1958 (9), and a symposium on the subject was held in Boston in that year. Vosburg *et al.* (10) reported, in a study of 12 adult college students, that in experimental sensory deprivation there is first a stage of adaptation characterized by repeated excursions into memories, then a breakdown in adaptive behavior, and, finally, either panic or flight. These results were obtained over a three-hour period in an anechoic chamber. Rosenzweig (11) has compared sensory deprivation and schizophrenia and states that he feels that perceptual interference produces the primary symptoms of schizophrenia more closely than does mescaline or LSD 25.

The more recent publications indicate a growing sophistication of approach. Gruenbaum *et al.* (12) suggested that the task of the investigator is to study the following three major variables: (1) experimental variables dictated by the nature of the experiment, namely, the types of interference with sensation and, in particular, whether there is a reduction in the total amount of sensation, or essentially, an interference with the pattern of sensory input; (2) variables arising from the subject's personality, his motivation, and other characteristics; and (3) variables arising from the relationship between the experimenter and the subject. They were not able to find any relationship between clinical ratings of what they termed "ego integrity" and the production of disturbances in perception. They considered that since sensory deprivation did not serve to explain the psychodynamics of personality, save in terms of reactions to loneliness, it did give an opportunity to study the interrelations of the various components of the perceptual apparatus.

Davis *et al.* (13) approached the matter from the point of view that it is not the absence of sensory stimulation which reduces the effects, but the absence of meaningful stimulation. They found that random visual stimulation was not sufficient to prevent the occurrence of aberrations and concluded that meaningful contact with the outside world is essential for normal functioning rather than the quantity of or change in sensory input.

From the survey of the literature, it is clear that we are now moving from an earlier conception of the importance of the reduction of the total quantity of sensory input to a conception that, in addition, the quality of input is also significant.

We would also like to draw attention to something which we believe to be important, namely, the concept of the individual himself concerning the duration of reduction of sensory input. In certain circumstances the duration may be entirely in his hands, hence he may structure it as he will. Secondly, it may be structured by the investigator, and the investigator may impart this to the subject: e.g., it may be said to the subject that he must remain for three days. And, thirdly, there may be no structuring whatsoever, hence the subject may feel that there is no definite limitation to the extent of his stay in the area of reduced sensory input.

Before proceeding to a review of the findings from our Institute, may I state that the field has now reached sufficient complexity that we may recognize six major areas of study and investigation. The first is with respect to reduction of sensory input during the developmental years in animals; the second refers to reduction in sensory input in fully developed animals and human beings; the third relates to reduction in sensory input incidental upon monotonous occupations; the fourth has reference to historical and anecdotal reports of individuals who have been shipwrecked, who have remained throughout the winter in lonely Arctic regions, and in other situations in which there was marked reduction in sensory input; the fifth consists in the effects of reduction in sensory input by blockage of conduction within the body of sensory stimuli; and the sixth is concerned with the effects of reduction in the responsiveness of the individual to stimulation.

At the Allan Memorial Institute, the effects of reduced sensory input upon human behavior have been studied in three different ways: (1) by reduction in the amount of stimulus coming from the environment and received by the individual through his eyes and ears, and an attempted reduction of some of the tactile stimuli by limitation of the use of his hands; (2) by reduction of input achieved through interference with the conduction of stimuli from the external receptors to the central nervous system; and (3) by reduction of the responsiveness of the individual to stimulation.

During the last several years, by far the greater amount of work at the Institute has been done with respect to the reduction of stimuli from the environment. The earliest published reports from the Institute are by Azima and Cramer-Azima (14). In their experiments, sensory isolation was achieved by covering the eyes with goggles, keeping the arms in cardboard cylinders, and reducing verbal communication to twice a day for the purposes of interviewing. The psychoneurotic and schizophrenic subjects were maintained in a darkened room and told they could terminate the study any time they wished. They remained in the room for periods ranging from one to seven days. Feelings of depersonalization appeared in 8 of the 15 patients. It was felt by the workers that repression and aggression turned against the self led to the depersonalization syndrome. In addition, hallucinations occurred in 4 patients. There were moderate to marked changes in the body scheme of 8 patients.

Our later investigations in reduction of stimuli have depended upon a more rigorous and sustained reduction in sensory input. The patients were in a darkened room with goggles, and their ears were covered with rubber eardrums into which was led white sound. White sound was also led into the room. The arms were covered with cardboard cylinders. The patients were fed and toiletted in the rooms. The nurses had instructions to reduce all communication to a minimum, and the timing and composition of the subjects' meals were changed unpredictably; e.g., soup might be given for breakfast. The duration of stay in such sensory isolation was increased to a maximum of 16 days. We also carried out a brief duration (5 to 7 hours) exposure to reduction in sensory input using occlusion of the eyes and enclosure of the arms in cardboard cylinders. The patients were located in the soundproof room of our Sound Laboratory. (In this laboratory sound can be reduced from the low circumambient level by 50 to 60 decibels.) It can be stated categorically that an increase in the rigorousness of sensory isolation did not result in a proportionate increase in the disturbance of behavior.

We observed that subjects vary considerably in the degree to which they show changes attributable to reduction in sensory input, but it is not yet defined with precision what factors determine the extent to which individuals will be affected by sensory input. As a working hypothesis, however, we consider that it is probable that individuals who customarily are self-contained and self-dependent, rather than highly sociable and dependent upon others, are capable of withstanding the effects of reduction in sensory input for more prolonged periods of time.

A second general observation which may be made is that individuals tend to take active measures to protect themselves against the disturbing effects in the reduction of sensory input. Four of these steps may be recorded: A number of individuals develop such intense anxiety in the situation that it is necessary to remove them from the conditions of reduced sensory input. It is also generally reported that individuals so exposed resort increasingly to reminiscence—in this way, as it were, maintaining their sensory input by drawing upon their inner world for the necessary input rather than upon the outer world. Other subjects endeavour to maintain their sensory input by purposeless movements, such as hand play or head movements—or by questioning the staff on any occasion when they are aware of the staff. The third step is apparently an increased sensory perceptiveness. For instance, one subject was able to maintain her space-time image by noting the very faint rumble which penetrated the white sound and the occluding earmuffs and which came from a plane passing overhead on its way to New York at 9 o'clock in the morning and 1 o'clock in the afternoon. It may be said that the staff was quite oblivious both of the plane passing overhead and of the fact that it did pass at these times. Other patients structured their space-time image by noting the composition of the meals, their number and intervals. By varying these intervals and by changing the menu from the expected time we were able to break up this structuring.

Moreover, once the effects of reduced sensory input were clearly observable in our subjects, we initiated another experiment based on an attempt to change the personality characteristics of the individual by running in a series of verbal signals designed to produce change. We noted that the subjects at once became dependent on these signals and would call the staff at once with considerable distress if the apparatus broke down. In addition, this dependence upon this form of sensory input persisted—although in lesser form—for days and weeks after the patient was removed from the conditions of reduced sensory input.

When we turn from consideration of these steps taken by the subject to maintain his space-time image to other effects produced by reduction in sensory input, we may note increased passivity, relaxation, and dependence, which appear within the first few days. There is increased introspection and fantasy production, sometimes with increased physical concern about the body. Auditory and visual hallucinations we found to be quite rare, even though the subject was on one occasion kept under such conditions for as long as 16 days.

When reduced sensory input was ended, there was in a few cases a degree of what was apparently a reactive euphoria, lasting in one or two instances for several days. There was some tendency to see objects as being rather flat and two-dimensional; this lasted, however, for only a few hours. We also noted what has been recorded by others: some measure of inability to speak with normal volume and some feelings of inadequacy. These findings were, however, not striking.

We now pass over to the second category of experiments, namely, the attempt to reduce sensory conduction within the body.[1]

It should be noted that we are on much surer ground in assessing the reduction of sensory input in the first category of experiments, where we directly reduce the amount of stimulus from the environment. When we attempt to reduce sensory conduction within the body, we are faced with the problem of the side effects of the agents which we use. And when we attempt to understand the effects of reduced sensory input by reducing the responsiveness of the individual to stimulation, we are faced with the still more complex problem of the considerable disturbance which we produce in thinking by the agents which we use for this purpose.

Sernyl appears to exert its action by the release of adrenaline and noradrenaline in association with the depression of the availability of serotonin in the brain (15). This is consistent with Brodie's hypothesis (16) that serotonin and noradrenaline are antagonistic chemical mediators regulating the central nervous system. Because of the importance of the kinesthetic input and the preservation of the body image, it was felt that Sernyl might throw valuable information upon the problem of the effects of the reduction in sensory input.

With our psychoneurotic subjects Sernyl produced apathy, then anxiety, followed by disturbance of body image, feelings of unreality and depersonalization. There were also thought disorder and disorganization of intellectual processes and difficulty in comprehension.

One patient experienced auditory hallucinations; two patients

[1] In this second category of experiments we used preparations furnished by Parke, Davis & Co. Ltd.: Cl 395 (Sernyl) and Cl 400. These substances were developed for their possible anaesthetic properties.

became hostile and paranoid. The body image disturbances which occurred in all patients were well recalled after the effects of Sernyl had disappeared. Feelings of floating in outer space were frequently described. There was a tendency for patients to maintain catatonic limb postures. This was not present under administration of Cl 400.

Our third set of experiments consisted in an attempt to reduce the activity of the individual. These studies, which also were carried out on psychoneurotic and schizophrenic subjects, involved the use of massive electroshock to a point where marked degrees of confusion occur. One finding which may be reported with some confidence, in that it is present in the other two sets of experiments where we studied the effects of reduction in sensory input, is that at the point where electroshock is beginning to interfere with the maintenance of the space-time image there occurs marked anxiety, and often hostility. The deeper levels of disorganization which occur as electroshock is continued are so greatly affected by disturbances in the whole process of thinking that very little information concerning interference with sensory input can be learned. In these deep states of confusion, which we term states of "complete depatterning," the individual's span of awareness is usually limited to the immediate present. He is concerned only with whether he is hot or cold or hungry. He communicates in very simple terms—quite unaffected by memories or by anticipations.

DISCUSSION

In opening the discussion on this review of the effects of markedly reduced sensory input upon performance, effectiveness, and general integrity of the functioning human being, it is necessary to state a fundamental working hypothesis: that a basic activity of all human beings is to maintain and extend control over their internal and external environments. Where this control is interfered with, as, for instance, in loss of control over body equilibrium, in disorientation, in amnesia, in organic brain disease, or where the individual is forced to operate in a dangerous situation without adequate means of control, anxiety constantly appears.

Control over the environment requires the integrity of an interlocking series of images. It is necessary, for successful interaction with the environment (both internal and external), that there should be, intact, a self image. States where this is interfered with, and which we commonly call states of "depersonalization," are almost always associated with a great sense of insecurity and anxiety on the part of the individual.

Interlocking with this image of the self, there is a body image. And, here again, disturbances in the body image are of serious consequence, as where, subsequent to temporal lobe damage, there is difficulty in locating the position of a given arm or leg. And then again there is the space-time image; and interference here, as in certain toxic and organic states, creates much apprehension and anxiety for the individual, leading, as it quite clearly does, to considerable frustration in his attempts to control his world.

These images are customarily maintained by our memorial processes. When our memorial processes are intact we can, for instance, awaken in a darkened room and immediately grasp the disposition of ourselves in time and space. Where the memorial processes are intact, the amount of sensory input necessary to maintain these images at their full effectiveness is quite limited.

Hence, for this reason, I should be inclined to raise the question whether the disturbances reported as resulting from very short periods of reduction in sensory input—namely, a few hours—are really valid manifestations; or whether it might be more accurate to say they are manifestations of (a) increased introspection, which commonly arises in solitude; (b) a decrease in sensory threshold resulting from such introspection; and (c) anticipation—a placebo effect, as it were.

It would appear that we are now at the end of the period of preliminary exploration of the phenomena brought about by reduction of sensory input and from here onwards progress is likely to be made only by the most closely controlled experiments. Variables to be studied are: (1) the degree of reduction of sensory input; (2) the pattern of reduction (cf. Davis *et al.* [13] and their comments concerning disturbance in the meaning of sensory input as contrasted with the amount); (3) anticipations of the subject with regard to what is to happen; (4) the effects of simple drowsiness upon thinking and upon experiencing in general; (5) the effects of the recumbent position maintained over many days; and (6) different ways of strengthening the duration of stay for the patient in a situation of reduced sensory input.

Thus far we are on soundest ground in demonstrating the effects of reduction of sensory input where we report on studies of reduced sensory input upon the development of animals, and where we carry out the reduction over prolonged periods of time.

The many analogous but not planned situations which occur may give leads but these cannot give definitive answers. Among these are anecdotal reports of deprivation of human relationship, solitary confinement in jail, religious retreats, experiences in an iron lung, the break-off phenomena in high flying, and kayak sickness.

CONCLUSIONS

Behavioral changes can be produced in adult human subjects by exposure to reduction of sensory input.

There is some reason to consider that changes may also be produced in such subjects by exposure to marked changes in the meaning of the sensory input.

Reduction in input can be achieved by: (a) interference with reception of environmental stimuli; (b) less certainly, by blocking of conduction within the body; and (c) still less certainly, by interference with reception by the brain.

There is variation from person to person in susceptibility to reduction in input. The factors controlling the variability are as yet unknown.

There is no definite evidence that extending the duration of exposure to reduction in sensory input or increasing the reduction in input beyond a given level increases the extent or range of change.

Periods of exposure of less than one day probably do not produce changes properly attributable to reduction in input. Such changes as do occur after a few hours may well be due to (a) changes in behavior which normally occur when people are by themselves—i.e., there is an increased amount of reminiscence and introspection; (b) lowering of the sensory threshold; this lowering being part of the means which the individual adopts to protect himself against the effects of sensory deprivation; and (c) anticipation—i.e., a placebo-like effect.

These possibilities can only be tested effectively where controls are used.

All changes in the intact person are of a low order of intensity relative to those commonly produced by the application of drugs, physical agents or by potent physiological factors.

In brain-damaged persons, the changes are likely to be considerably more severe.

Changes tend to disappear within about a day after removal from the area of reduced input.

Persistent and extensive changes are reported in animals exposed during their developmental period to prolonged reduction in sensory input.

REFERENCES

1. Hebb, D. O., The effects of early experience on problem solving at maturity, Am. Psychol., 2:306–307, 1947.
2. Hymovitch, B., The effects of experimental variation on problem solving in the rat, J. Comp. Physiol. & Psychol., 45:313–321, 1952.
3. Mackworth, N. H., Researches in the Measurement of Human Performance. Med. Res. Council, Spec. Report Series, London, No. 268, 1943.
4. Sharpless, S., and H. Jasper, Habituation of the arousal reaction, Brain, 79:655–680, 1956.
5. Cameron, D. E., Studies in senile nocturnal delirium, Psychiat. Quart., pp. 1–7, Jan., 1941.
6. Bexton, W. H., W. Heron, and T. H. Scott, Effects of decreased variation in the sensory environment, Canad. J. Psychol., 8:70–76, 1954.
7. Hebb, D. O., The mammal and his environment, Am. J. Psychiat., 111:826–831, 1955.
8. Lilly, J. C., Mental effects of reduction of ordinary levels of physical stimuli on intact, healthy persons, Psychiat. Res. Rep., 5, March, 1956.
9. Wexler, Donald, Jack Mendelson, Herbert Leiderman, and Philip Solomon, Sensory deprivation, Arch. Neurol. & Psychiat., 79:225–233, 1958.
10. Vosburg, Robert, Norman Fraser, and John Guehl, Imagery sequence in sensory deprivation, Arch. Gen. Psychiat., 2:356–357, 1960.
11. Rosenzweig, Norman, Sensory deprivation and schizophrenia: some clinical and theoretical similarities, Am. J. Psychiat., 116:326–329, 1959.
12. Gruenbaum, Henry U., Sanford J. Friedman, and Milton Greenblatt, Sensory Deprivation and Personality, Am. J. Psychiat., 116:878–882, 1960.
13. Davis, John, Wm. F. McCourt, and Philip Solomon, Effect of visual stimulation on hallucinations and other mental experiences during sensory deprivation, Am. J. Psychiat., 116:889–892, 1960.
14. Azima, H., and F. J. Cramer-Azima, Studies in Perceptual Isolation, Dist. Nerv. System (Monograph Supplement), 18:1–6, 1957.
15. Levy, Leonard, D. E. Cameron, and R. C. B. Aitken, Observation on two psychotomimetic drugs of piperidine derivation—Cl 395 (Sernyl) and Cl 400, Am. J. Psychiat., 116:843–844, 1960.
16. Brodie, B. B., Serotonin and norepinephrine as antagonistic chemical mediators regulating the central autonomic nervous system, in *Neuropharmacology.* 3d Conf. Josiah Macy Jr. Found. pp. 323–340, 1956.

Experiments in Solitude, in Maximum Achievable Physical Isolation with Water Suspension, of Intact Healthy Persons

JOHN C. LILLY *and* JAY T. SHURLEY

Originally, one of the aims of this investigation was to test the neurophysiological hypothesis that, in the drastic attenuation of physical stimuli below the usual level, the activity of the brain and its contained mind would be that of sleep. Findings in our experiments (1, 2) and in those of other groups (3, 4) in this field demonstrate that sleep is not necessarily the outcome over a short time period. A parallel, though not identical, aim was to observe what, if any, effect such experimental conditions might have in altering ego function both in the present moment and over the longer time period; i.e., ego choices and ego structure. A more specific aim has been to establish methods of self-observation by finding, defining, and setting limits for the subject's psychological sets for these experiments and by seeking those sets which would give the maximum of information from the subjective sphere. The collection of data has been mainly by notes and recordings by the subject alone.

At the outset two conditions seemed essential, and these have been maintained throughout. All observers first prepare themselves by participating as subjects; those who participate in this experimentation first do so in the role of subject, then in the role of "safety man" (observer), and, finally, in the role of self-observer in solitude. The second crucial condition is that of the restrained and minimal participation of the "safety man"; his role is to stay out of and not interfere with the phenomena which occur in the self-observer.

Dr. Lilly was Chief, Section of Cortical Integration, Neurophysiological Laboratory, Research Branch, National Institute of Mental Health, Bethesda, Md. He is now Director of the Communication Research Institute, St. Thomas, U.S. Virgin Islands. Dr. Shurley is on the staff of the Veterans Administration Hospital, Oklahoma City, Oklahoma.

TECHNIQUE

A systematic consideration of the technique illustrates how these aims are carried out in this particular set of experiments.

The Physical-Physiological Level

1. The simultaneous attenuation of all known external physical stimuli to the lowest possible level (including light, sound, odor, taste, light pressure, deep pressure, and other gravity-opposition forces, vibration, heat, cold, etc.). These characteristics of the experimental environment were achieved with relative success by use of a water immersion tank in a soundproofed chamber.

2. The maximum simultaneous attenuation of intra-integumentary sources of stimuli which, in the order of importance in our experiments, have included low-level pain and discomfort because of an unsatisfactory position in the tank; muscle stretch; slow motions of limbs moving through the water; internal sources such as hunger; full bladder; full rectum; gas in the GI tract; unusually active cardiovascular system; local pressure ischemia leading to pain; irregular changes in respiratory rhythm, rate, or depth; accumulating carbon dioxide; reduction in oxygen.

3. The maintenance of a constrained and restrained situation voluntarily: Obviously in a system such as the human body, efferent activity leads to afferent activity in a continuous and circular fashion; therefore in suspension in a liquid the subject is instructed to voluntarily inhibit movement, including vocalizations, to his maximum possible ability.

4. Special case of skin temperature: We have found that thermal differences over the skin of the body are intensely stimulating when the other sources of stimuli have been attenuated. The use of water suspension (in which the water is slowly flowing by the body) allows an isothermicity of the unclothed skin surface which is difficult to achieve by other methods. At 34.5° C. (94.1° F.) the water seems to disappear in the thermal sense; i.e., the subject feels neither hot nor cold, and this temperature allows a steady state of heat exchange at a constant normal body temperature at the reduced level of metabolism that can be achieved under these conditions. In addition, the slowly flowing water allows continuous removal of waste products of the body.

5. The position and suspension of the body in water: Because the body parts are not of uniform density it is necessary to add weight to certain parts and to add buoyancy or support to certain other parts. These additions are done in such a way as to avoid chronic low-level discomfort and pain caused by unusual degrees of angulation of spinal or other joints and that caused by pressure ischemia.

We found that the position of the body of each subject must be very carefully worked out in order to avoid low-level discomfort and pain. Unless this is done we found that we were studying the effects of a chronic low-level pain on our subjects in a relative absence of other sources of stimulation. If a given subject is exposed to too much pain for too long a period, the experiment becomes extremely distasteful to him. We do not feel that we have found the ideal method of buoyancy adjustment, and that a good deal more work could be done on this phase of the experiments, possibly by using liquids of two densities, one for the limbs and one for the chest and head, or, possibly, by using a liquid of greater density than the fresh water which we have been using. In summary, water suspension allows most of the gravity-opposing forces to be distributed evenly over the whole surface of the body; thus the unit pressure is greatly decreased over any one area. Because fresh water of the proper temperature was available, we used this liquid.

6. The mask: Since the subject is suspended in the liquid, breathing requires a mask with certain characteristics; (a) minimum inward pressures over the surfaces of the skin, (b) maximum sealing without undue local pressure, (c) minimum flow resistance, (d) minimum dead space, (e) minimum back- or fore-pressure during the respiratory cycle, and (f) as great a degree of equalization of the pressure in the mask with that over the chest as can be achieved. An approximation to the last requirement can be reached if the subject is suspended just below the surface of the liquid with his chest parallel to that surface so as to minimize pressure difference across the thoracic and abdominal walls while breathing air at one atmosphere from the room. Such an apparatus has the virtue of extreme simplicity and maximum control by the subject. We have employed a through-and-through breathing system with an inspiratory valve and an expiratory valve with two different tubes (Figure 4) leading to the small space (approximately 100 cc) in the mask immediately

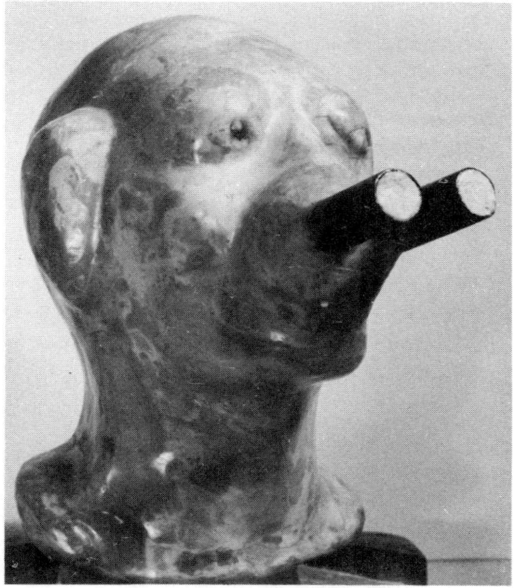

Figure 1. Underwater Mask Manufacture I

Positive plaster cast of one subject's head and neck (J.S.), with spaces over eyes, nose and mouth, and ears filled in, and (bakelite) tubing in place. Note smooth surface from which later casts in plaster or latex may easily be separated.

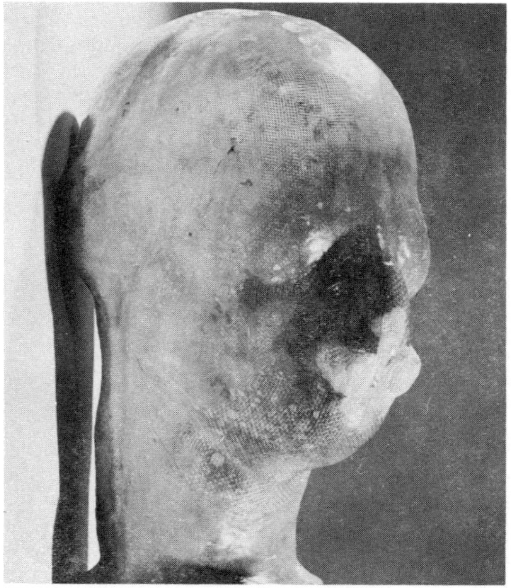

Figure 2. Underwater Mask Manufacture II

Dipping form for one subject (J.L.). A plaster bandage cast (negative) is made from the modified reproduction of the head and neck casting (Figure 1) with a separating agent. Inside this negative mold, fiberglas cloth and resin is inserted to construct the positive reproduction shown in this figure. The two white areas between nose and chin are the bumps for positioning the two tubes shown in Figure 3. The two halves of the fiberglas reproduction are assembled and fastened together with fiberglas tape and resin, and finally sanded. A base with a socket for a 75-watt heating lamp is inserted in this model.

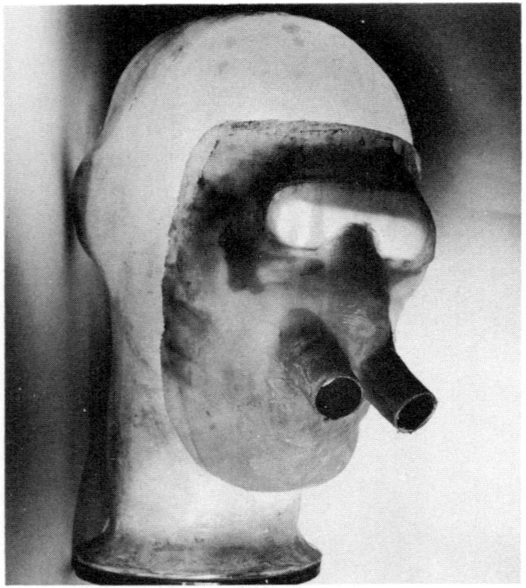

Figure 3. Underwater Mask Manufacture III

The dipping form: mask insert in place on the face. (Heating lamp is lighted.) The mask insert is built of Fiberglas on the dipping form with latex as the separating agent. The inspiratory and expiratory tubes (stainless steel) and the window (Lucite) are inserted and embedded in the Fiberglas at the proper stages; three layers are built up. This form is separately dipped into latex, put on the head-form, and the assembly dipped to generate the

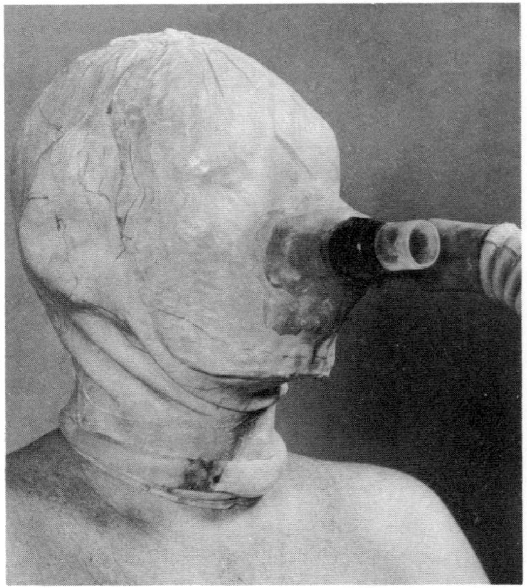

Figure 4. Underwater Mask Manufacture IV

This is a finished mask formed by dipping cast shown in Figure 1, which does not contain a Lucite window before the eyes—note breathing tube connected on one side. Note also the loose folds of latex at the neck which seal out liquid without undue constriction of subject's neck. Mask is donned simply by pulling down over head, much as a stocking would be. In place, it fits face and head closely, is smooth and is completely comfort-in front of the nose and the mouth, breathing air at one atmosphere from the room. This system can be easily repaired by the subject and does not require as much maintenance as a more complicated, continuously flowing gas system at a higher pressure. However, again, we do not consider this ideal, and would prefer a very simple system operating at a higher pressure so that the subject could be less constrained as to depth of immersion.

Environmental Control at the Social and Community Level

1. The maintenance of physical-physiological isolation and solitude in the midst of a community implies barriers to intrusion by persons or sources of physical stimuli; i.e., such isolation implies that eventually one is in solitude (of course solitude per se does not necessarily imply physical isolation). Such consideration requires a building which houses the tank and constructed in such a way as to bar any continuous traffic through its structure and which permits no invasion by people or animals or other objects which may be sensed by the subject; a lock on the door is required but not sufficient. The safety man is instructed to act as a buffer agent for the subject, both before, during, and after the experiments and to maintain privacy. The safety man also must check the in-flowing water temperature, lights, telephone, etc.

2. The issue of privacy seems to us to be so important that we give it separate consideration here. Relevant privacy includes present and future communications including all of those between the subject and the safety man. For optimal conditions privacy requires the firm assurance to the subject of his control of the secrecy of his individual data indefinitely into the future. Maximum ego freedom and voluntariness of the subject in these experiments can be achieved through such kinds of privacy. It also implies that the subject chooses his own times for beginning, ending, and the total duration of exposure as well as the control of whatever restraints, voluntary inhibitions, and supports are needed. Privacy also implies trust and respect for the ego of the subject on the part of the safety man; i.e., the elimination (or at least attenuation) of any observer encroachment, exploitation, or invasion of each experience and of its data indefinitely (even to the extent of avoiding invited, available, encroachment by the subject).

When the safety man and the subject both consider it is safe for the subject to become a self-observer free of the safety man, i.e., to enter solitude, these matters must be considered with great intensity and care. It is at this point in our experience that the subject is likely to use disguised methods of appealing for help from the safety man, or from others, in one form or another. After the first few experiences it may help him as a self-observer to function as a safety man for another subject. The introduction of any new factors into the experiment, (especially variables important to survival, such as changes in the respiratory apparatus) require a self-observer to return to "subject status" temporarily and bring a safety man back into the situation.

Of course, privacy also implies that the abstraction of, and the distribution of, the results of the experiments are also under his control. In this regard one must consider all media of communication including gossip (professional and otherwise), newspaper accounts, scientific journal accounts, and scientific meetings. One keeps in mind possible future uses of the material by persons other than the subject; the revealed material is carefully scrutinized by the subject in order to contain only those observations and shorthand descriptions which contribute directly to the generalizations which are found. Minimal disguise of data allows maximum transmission of the true pictures of what occurs but are carefully balanced against what Freud called, in his communications of his self-analysis, "the point at which one owes discretion to oneself."

The future research plans are also maintained in privacy and are set up by those who have reached self-observer and safety man status. In functioning as safety man the necessity for certain specific plans and organization becomes apparent and obvious.

3. The process of selection of subjects: Normal, healthy volunteers of equal social and professional status to the previous subject-observers have been the source of our subjects. Neither much younger nor much older, higher or lower, persons are chosen in order to give maximum freedom to the particular person involved. This condition is required for the attenuation to our maximum ability of any factors which might resemble a draft, a persuasion, or coercing of the subject in his or our view. In addition, this process implies that not only each experiment or exposure but each series of

exposures requires that social isolation be maintained. The fact that experiments may be going on is protected in the local community. This technique has been worked out as a result of provocative and disturbing experiences during the course of our experiments.

SCIENTIFIC METHOD AND THE SELF-OBSERVER

Objections can be raised that under these rules an ego observing itself generates only circular data; i.e., that it experiences only what it wishes and allows itself to experience, and that the use of an outside observer can avoid such difficulties. We have found that these objections have a limited validity and for our purposes an outside observer inordinately complicates the situation and the data in which we are interested. Within certain limits yet to be determined experimentally, it seems to us that the mind is the only province of science in which what one believes to be true is, or becomes, true (5). Our experimental task in these studies is to determine what these limits are. However, it is felt that it is important to remember that one must give subjects the permission to experience what *can* be experienced and not make suggestions as to what may or *will* be experienced.

It is our conviction that the range of phenomena available to the normal human mind is much greater than "society" will apparently permit or accept (1, 2, 5); consequently, the safety man becomes the intercessor between the individual and the community. As such, he grants the subject permission to experience whatever he can experience; i.e., the right to exercise any function, strictly leaving open the content of what is experienced. If you will, the individual is "indoctrinated" in the principle of freedom for his own ego with the internal experiential sphere. As is mentioned below, the results of such experiences in a given subject generally turn out to be surprising to that subject; i.e., so far as the subject is consciously aware, new data occur quite spontaneously.

CONCLUSIONS

Detailed results are to be reported in a later paper. However, some general conclusions of these studies may be of interest.

When given freedom from external exchanges and transactions, the isolated-constrained ego (or self or personality) has sources of *new information* from within. Such sources can be experienced as if they are outside with greater or lesser degrees of awareness as to where or what these sources are (projected imagery, projected sounds, doubling of body parts, emotional states of euphoria or anxiety, etc.)

Any other person, observer, or safety man can be made to appear as if he is a "source" to which is attributed the origin of the new information.

Transference-related drives may become extremely intense. In a given exposure, such needs increase in intensity with time and may ultimately demand direct release; i.e., such as leaving the tank and participating in one's active life with other persons (2, 5). Multiple exposures lead to better control and increase awareness of these effects.

The relationship of any residual stimulus to these needs is carefully evaluated. "Negative and positive" transference problems arise from extremely small and unlikely kinds of stimuli under these conditions; i.e., a "wrong" word, too many suggestions, implied judgements of accuracy or performance, or their "positive" opposites. The safety man must be, as it were, an ideal and keenly aware diplomat when faced with such problems. It has been found that having once experienced the lowest possible level of stimulation oneself makes it very much easier to function as a "diplomatic," tolerant, and considerate safety man. Hurt feelings, overenthusiastic reactions, and replication of experience reported by others are examples of the kinds of phenomena to be found and dealt with.

The positive, enjoyable results were achieved only at those times when the inner and the outer disturbing stimuli were minimizable. Any residual discomfort made it impossible to achieve the euphoric state; any anxiety induced by faulty apparatus or technique blocked the possibility of enjoying or profiting from the experience. Until we were able to attenuate physical discomfort and fear by better techniques, multiple exposures, and careful training, we saw mostly "negative" phenomona. As the levels of stimuli were lowered closer to zero, the positive, more blissful, enjoyable states and the positive transference phenomona appeared. No addiction to these states has occurred: the internal satisfactions of needs achieved in the tank are limited in the same sense that, say, day-dreaming is limited. Basic satisfactions of needs felt in the tank require later exchanges with other persons and with physical reality.

As has been published (1, 2), it is felt that such experiences are not necessarily psychotic, or even mentally aberrant, and after training can be constructive and invigorating. Eventually, after many exposures, each subject can learn enough to enjoy and not fear or dislike his own experiences.

REFERENCES

1. Lilly, J. C., Effects of physical restraint and of reduction of ordinary levels of physical stimuli on intact, healthy persons, in *Illustrative Strategies for Research on Psychopathology in Mental Health*, Symposium No. 2, Group for the Advancement of Psychiatry, New York, 1956.
2. Lilly, J. C., Mental Effects of Reduction of Ordinary Levels of Physical Stimuli on Intact, Healthy Persons, Psychiatric Research Reports 5, American Psychiatric Assoc., Washington, D.C. 1–28, June, 1956.
3. Heron, Woodburn, The pathology of boredom, Scientific American, 196:52–56, 1957.
4. Bennett, A. M. H., Personal communication.
5. Lilly, J. C., Some considerations regarding basic mechanisms of positive and negative types of motivations, Am. J. Psychiat., December, 1958.

Assessment of Individual Resistance to Sensory Alteration

ROBERT R. HOLT *and* LEO GOLDBERGER

When one reviews the literature on isolation and sensory alteration (1, 2), two facts are especially striking. First, there are certain abnormal mental phenomena, changes in cognitive and affective states, which have attracted a great deal of attention. But just as remarkable is the second fact: that individual differences in reaction to any such altered environment have been very marked. Some men break down easily when removed from the support of their usual surroundings and companions; others withstand remarkable hardships, deprivations, or both. Clearly, any program that involves exposing people to highly unusual environments and situational stresses, such as a program for the exploration of space, must take careful account of these differences and must seek to learn the qualities of a man that fit him for such unusual missions.

Even the briefest space flights will involve separating men from the support of perceiving their usual environments, especially the loss of bodily sensations of gravity, and prolonged flights in which there will be little for the astronauts to do will expose them to the stresses of monotony and confinement as well as the lack of familiar earthly sights, sounds and other sensations. For these reasons, there may be something to learn about selection for space flight from a study of reactions to experimental confinement, isolation and perceptual monotony, and attempts to find aspects of personality that predict such reactions. Any such study will have to settle on operational definitions for three critical sets of terms: (1) terms

Dr. Holt is Professor of Psychology and Director of the Research Center for Mental Health, New York University. Dr. Goldberger is on the staff of the Research Center. The work on which this paper is based was done with the support of the Aerospace Medical Laboratory, Wright Air Development Division, Wright-Patterson Air Force Base, under Contract No. AF33(616)-6103.

describing the exact situation of sensory alterations used—perhaps different types of persons will do well under different types of experimental conditions; (2) variables measuring the subjects' reactions to the situation, or measures of its effects—such measures may vary from objective tests of intellectual or motor performance to subjective evaluations of spontaneous productions; (3) variables of personality that can be measured and correlated with individual differences in experimental effects—we measured such variables by means of objective tests of personality.

We shall describe two experiments in which we have found aspects of personality that may predict reaction to our experimental sensory alteration, achieved by techniques similar to those of the McGill experimenters (see diagram). Subjects spent eight hours in a lighted room, lying on a comfortable bed, with the auditory and visual senses occluded. Halved ping-pong balls were attached with rubber cement to the eye-sockets, so that only diffuse white light was visible to the subject. He wore a light leather Air Force helmet containing padded earphones, through which a steady white noise (a mixture of random frequencies) was fed into his ears. The two experiments differed in minor respects, but principally in the fact that, for the first sample, there was occasional slight contact between experimenter (E) and subject (S) when luncheon was brought in and when S indicated that he needed to go to the toilet. In the second experiment, subjects had a chemical toilet in the room with them and took sandwiches in for lunch.

In both studies, the instructions to S were to lie quietly and from time to time to report whatever was going through his mind. All verbalizations were tape-recorded, as was an interview that was held with S at the end of the eight hours, in which he was questioned closely on his experience. In addition, a number of tests were given before and after the isolation experience, but the results of these will not be reported here.

So much for the situation to which subjects were exposed. As just noted, we did not find it profitable to use test findings as measures of effect. The measures we found useful stem from the theoretical basis of our interest in these experiments. Our investigations have been conceptualized in terms of the psychoanalytic theory of thinking, in which a leading role is played by the concepts of primary and

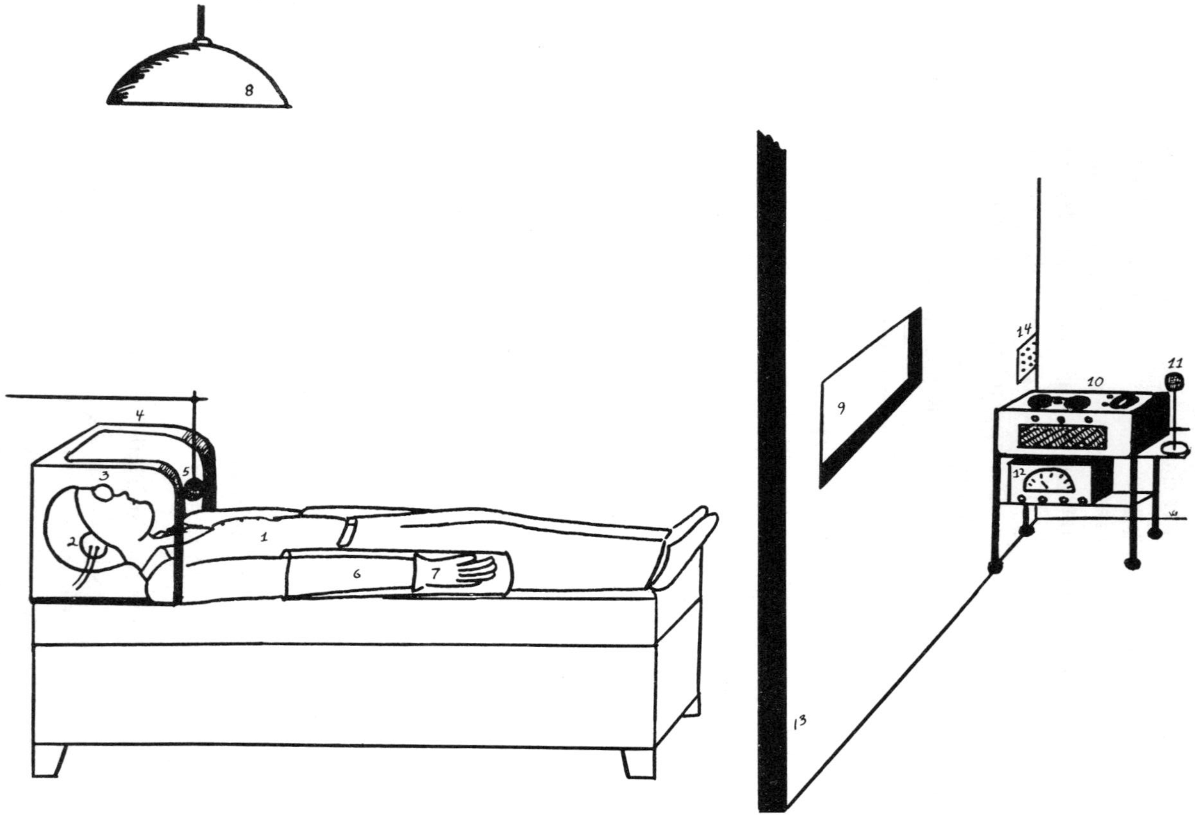

1. Subject
2. Helmet with earphones
3. Eye cups
4. Foam rubber head enclosure
5. Microphone
6. Cardboard arm cuff
7. Gloves
8. Light
9. One-way mirror
10. Tape recorder
11. Microphone
12. Random noise generator
13. Wall
14. Electric binding post

secondary process. The primary process is a hypothetical extreme of disordered, dream-like, hallucinatory, unrealistic and fantastic thought operations, most closely approximated in acute schizophrenia. The secondary process, by contrast, refers to an ideal of logical, orderly, realistic, and adaptive thinking processes.

In the psychoanalytic theory it is assumed that the drives are almost always active and ready to take over thinking and force it towards the primary process extreme if contact with ordinary, well-structured reality is removed. At the same time, according to Rapaport's (3) theory of ego autonomy, a person who is in touch with his drives and has a well-compensated, highly differentiated set of ego structures is able to maintain secondary process thinking despite a severance of contact with reality, and is also able to allow primary process into his conscious waking thought without being disturbed or overwhelmed by it. In any event, we relied on this theoretical framework, in selecting variables in terms of which to study the effects of sensory alteration.

ANALYSIS OF DATA

After the protocols of the subjects' spontaneous verbalizations and the interviews had been typed up, they were read and rated by two independent judges,[1] each of whom rank-ordered the subjects according to the following variables: imagery; controlled primary process thinking; poorly controlled primary process thinking; unimpaired secondary process thinking; impaired secondary process thinking;[2] stimulus-bound thinking; pleasant affect; unpleasant affect; immobility; self-stimulation and exploration; quitting; sleep; and verbal output. In the first study, the reliabilities of rating range from .80 to .99; in the second study, from .25 to .885. Except for two variables (controlled primary process: .25; and immobility: .27) the reliability of judgments was satisfactory in the second study, the next lower Rho being .68 (regressed secondary

[1] In the first study (4, 5, 6), the authors; in the second, one of the authors, Leo Goldberger, and Dr. Gokce Cansever, to whom we wish to express our thanks for her skilled help. The ratings by Leo Goldberger were used in all further analyses.

[2] Actually, this variable underwent a change. In the first study, it consisted largely of complaints of inability to think consecutively and productively; in the second, there were few such complaints, and instead the raters fell back on rating the presence of regressed secondary process in the form of disjointed, free-associative sorts of remarks.

process). The poorer agreement between judges in the second study is partly a function of reduced range of variation in the sample, and the fact that in the second study, there was no one-way vision mirror in the soundproof room in which S stayed for the experiment, so that immobility had to be inferred rather indirectly.

For each sample, these variables were intercorrelated, and in both instances, they fell into two syndromes (7). New rank orders were then made up for the two syndromes, and they were correlated with rank orders on a variety of tests of personality, cognitive style, and intellectual functioning. All subjects had been given a sizable battery of tests as part of a personality assessment.

RESULTS

In both samples there emerged a similar pattern of intercorrelated reactions to isolation, which we call the *adaptive syndrome* (see Tables 1 and 2). In both samples, this included unimpaired secondary process thinking, controlled and accepted primary process, imagery, self-stimulation and exploration. In the first sample, pleasant affect and verbal output also formed part of this syndrome; in the second sample, regressed secondary process was part of the syndrome, plus sleep, which correlated negatively with all the other variables. In the first sample, the median intercorrelation was .67; in the second sample, .66.

The second cluster of intercorrelating variables, most of which were unrelated to the components of the first syndrome, was called the *maladaptive* reaction to isolation. In both studies, this included unpleasant affect and quitting (that is, preoccupation with terminating the experiment). With the first sample, the maladaptive syndrome included also poorly controlled primary process thinking,[3] complaints of impaired secondary process thinking, and general disturbance on a questionnaire. In the second sample, it included two variables both of which correlated negatively with unpleasant affect and quitting: pleasant affect, and immobility. (Note that these were both part of the adaptive syndrome in the first sample; both had a few correlations with components of the adaptive syndrome in the second sample, but fit best into the maladaptive one.)

[3] In the second sample there was not enough variance on poorly controlled primary process even to rank-order this variable.

Table 1. Rank-Order Correlations (Rho) between Measures of Isolation Effect, Study 1
(N = 14 except as noted)

	1	2	3	4	5	6	7	8	9	10	11	12
1. Pleasant affect												
2. Controlled primary process[a]	.84[d]											
3. Free secondary process	.67[d]	.67[c]										
4. Self-stimulation	.45	.71[d]	.37									
5. Imagery[a]	.68[c]	.88[d]	.77[d]	.60[c]								
6. Immobility	.36	.60[c]	.32	—.15	.68[c]							
7. Verbal output	.72[d]	.70[d]	.95[d]	.29	.87[d]	.41						
8. Sleep	.18	.22	—.05	.28	.05	.00	—.13					
9. Unpleasant affect	—.67[d]	—.43	—.52	—.53[c]	—.56	—.16	—.56[c]	—.28				
10. Poorly controlled primary process	—.09	.33	.13	—.02	.30	.02	.19	—.10	.37			
11. Impaired secondary process[b]	—.58[c]	—.16	—.44	—.44	—.22	—.10	—.42	—.01	.53	.75[d]		
12. General disturbance[a]	—.46	—.14	—.29	—.40	—.19	—.01	—.34	—.22	.52	.58[c]	.64[c]	
13. Quitting	—.61[c]	—.26	—.17	—.18	—.05	—.26	—.15	—.40	.58[c]	.37	.25	.37

[a] N = 12 [b] N = 13 [c] .05 level [d] .01 level (two-tailed test)

Table 2. Rank-Order Correlations (Rho) between Measures of Isolation Effect, Study 2
(N = 16)

	1	2	3	4	5	6	7	8	9	10	11
1. Controlled primary process											
2. Free secondary process	.91[b]										
3. Self-stimulation	.71[b]	.61[a]									
4. Imagery	.64[b]	.47	.58[a]								
5. Regressed secondary process	.61[a]	.76[b]	.52[a]	.40							
6. Sleep	—.73[b]	—.67[b]	—.68[b]	—.66[b]	—.66[b]						
7. Unpleasant affect	—.02	—.14	.32	.19	—.23	—.24					
8. Quitting	—.11	—.24	.14	.06	—.45	—.02	.81[b]				
9. Pleasant affect	.42	.54[a]	.02	.40	.64[b]	.30	—.65[b]	—.76[b]			
10. Immobility	—.19	—.04	—.60[a]	—.41	.11	.15	—.36	—.52[a]	.40		
11. Verbal output	.00	.00	—.23	—.28	—.11	.27	.22	.20	.08	.35	
12. Stimulus-bound thought	.12	.12	—.09	.32	.07	—.22	—.36	.10	.02	.27	.21

Note: The questionnaire that gave rise to the variable of "general disturbance" was not used in Study 2. An attempt was made to measure *Poorly controlled primary process*, but there was too little variance in it to make possible a rank-ordering.

[a] .05 level [b] .01 level (two-tailed test)

In the first sample, the median intercorrelation was between .52 and .53; in the second sample, it was between .58 and .59.

In both samples, the two syndromes did not show any significant degree of correlation, much as they may appear at first glance to be logical opposites of each other. In the first sample, the maladaptive and adaptive syndromes correlated —.33; in the second sample, the corresponding correlation was —.07. Thus, the maladaptive reaction is not just a lack of adaptive manifestations; it is characterized by active complaining (statements of discomfort, threats of walking out, and the like).

Before the correlations between the reactions to isolation and the measures of personality can be properly understood, a word has to be said about the two samples of subjects who were tested. The first sample was composed of undergraduate freshmen in the New York University School of Education. Their ages ranged from 17 to 29. They were preselected so that all scored at the 40th percentile (or better) of college students on the Ohio State Psychological Examination (a group test of intelligence). They were further screened by means of the Minnesota Multiphasic Personality Inventory, a screening interview, and a Rorschach test. Subjects with insufficient motivation or time for the experiment, and others whose adjustment seemed to be too fragile or pre-psychotic were eliminated in this way. An important further specification about this sample is that it included a variety of vocational interests, despite the fact that all were attending the same teachers' college. Some were studying physical education, with the intent of becoming athletic coaches; others were studying manual training (shop work). At the other extreme, there were students of art education and would-be teachers of social science, English literature, and other college subjects.

The sample in the replication study was quite different in many respects. Subjects were all unemployed actors, recruited from Actors Equity in New York, and paid at the same rate as the undergraduate students. They were screened much the way the earlier subjects were, except that no restriction was made on intelligence; one of them had a Wechsler-Bellevue IQ of 105, the upper extreme was an IQ of 143. Ages of the actors ranged from 21 to 42; 12 of the 16 were under 30. They too were screened by means of the MMPI, an interview, and the Rorschach; not quite one out of every six applicants who took the MMPI was finally accepted as a subject after being put over these successive hurdles. Because of the high incidence of overt homosexuality in this population, we did not consider that a sufficient basis on which to exclude a subject if in other respects his adjustment seemed reasonably sound. As a consequence, among the 16 subjects used in the second study there were at least 5 who had a predominantly homosexual orientation.

When we turn to Tables 3 and 4, which present the personological correlates of the two syndromes of reactions to isolation in the two studies, it is at once apparent that the findings of the first study were not replicated by the second one. Only two measures correlated similarly with the adaptive syndrome in the two studies: the MMPI measures of hypochondriasis and of ego-strength.

Table 3. Correlates of Syndrome I: Adaptive Reaction to Isolation

	STUDY 1		STUDY 2	
	Rho	*N*	*Rho*	*N*
A. *Acceptance of one's passive, feminine side/masculinity*				
Barron-Welsh Art Scale (14)	.75[b]	11	−.28	11
Esthetic value (A-V-L)	.66[a]	12	.36	15
Ranking of Path 3 (Nurturant love of others)	.64[a]	10	−.84[b]	13
DPI Early Oral Scale (or Oral Dependence) (15)	.62[a]	11	−.30	13
Ranking of Path 12 (active somatotonic mastery)	−.62[a]	10	.28	13
DPI Feminine identification scale	.55	11	−.22	13
DPI Masculine identification scale	−.11	11	.75[b]	13
Jenkins Transexual identification (16)			−.70[b]	14
Economic value (A-V-L)	−.42	12	−.66[b]	15
Political value (A-V-L)	−.49	12	.59[a]	15
B. *Intellectual flexibility*				
Brick uses: flexibility (17)	.65[a]	11	.30	16
C. *Emotional freedom vs. emotional disturbance, constriction or ungenuineness*				
Rating of Path 10 (Stern Spartan self-control)	−.79[b]	11	−.28	15
Ranking of Path 10 (Stern Spartan self-control)	−.64[a]	11	−.03	13
MMPI: Psychasthenia	−.64[a]	12	−.43	14
MMPI: Hypochondriasis	−.55	12	−.62[a]	15
MMPI: Barron Ego-Strength			.73[b]	15

[a] .05 level [b] .01 level (two-tailed test)

We are not, however, dealing with the usual melancholy situation of regression to the mean. Although many variables that correlated significantly in the first study show no relation to the behavioral measure in the second, there are three that correlated significantly in both samples, but with the signs reversed! Supporting the hypothesis that the results are nonrandom is the fact that though the pattern of correlates in Study 2 is quite different from that in Study 1, it is still internally consistent and meaningful.

The headings in Tables 3 and 4 were made up in an attempt to characterize groups of correlates that seemed meaningfully related to each other in Study 1. Though these headings are not appropriate for Study 2, they still may be used to guide our approach to these results.

In the first study, there are many measures that seem related to a general personality picture of passivity and feminine interests (including esthetic interests and tastes). Two of the direct reversals occur in this cluster, and there are a couple of other nearly significant correlations in Study 2 that are more or less opposite in meaning to the general purport of the correlations in Study 1. In general, the change may be summarized by saying that in the sample of actors, it was the more masculine, less orally passive subjects who reacted adaptively to the isolation situation; thus, one test measure of cross-sex identification correlates negatively and another test measure of masculine identification positively with the adaptive pattern in the second study. Going along with that meaningfully are a positive correlation with the political value and a negative value for an ideal of service to others.

The key to this change in the pattern of correlations may be found in the ego-strength scale for the MMPI. The high positive correlation of the Barron ego-strength scale (14) with the adaptive reaction in the second study suggests that, in this group of actors for whom passivity was generally quite congenial, and among whom homosexuality was such a problem, those who are more masculine tend to have the stronger egos. Among the students of education (where the same correlation approached significance), the ones with high scores on masculine identification presented a picture of hypermasculinity in which manliness was identified with violent muscular activity. For such young men, to lie quietly and passively was too great a threat; in this group, the presence of feminine interests was highly correlated with a set of values and interests that connoted a rich inner life and congeniality for a situation of lying around and thinking. Among the actors, on the other hand, those who were at the masculine extreme of the distribution were in many respects not far from the subjects who reacted adaptively in the first sample; in them, a reasonably balanced mixture of masculine and feminine interests did not preclude the existence of ego-syntonic passivity and an adequate inner life, but was a sign of generally more effective personality organization. At the low end of masculinity in the group of actors were a couple of compulsively promiscuous homosexuals with rather disorganized ego structures.

Another way to look at the results in the second study is to note that the adaptive syndrome there includes sleep, unlike the first study. Moreover, this most passive of reactions to the situation of isolation is negatively correlated with the group of positive, adaptive reactions. Also, in this population, motor passivity (as measured by immobility, which was part of the adaptive syndrome in the first study and not in the second) now is part of the maladaptive syndrome. Thus, although we have been using the same term for the similar clusters of reactions to isolation in the two studies, there are several differences between them, one of which seems to be focused on the issue of passivity. Therefore, it should not be surprising that the pattern of personality correlates differs.

In this picture of change, there are three variables that show much the same pattern of relationship to adaptive reaction to isolation in the two samples. The MMPI measure of hypochondriasis is a measure of diffuse bodily symptoms; it is not surprising that a person who admitted to many such symptoms on the MMPI would be low on the adaptive syndrome in both studies. Seemingly unrelated to this finding are the two other variables, both of them representing a situation of near-significant correlation in one sample and significant correlations in the middle .60's in the other. These borderline results say that, in both samples, the adaptive reactors tend to have esthetic values and to be low on economic values (both as measured by the Allport-Vernon-Lindzey scale; 9). In the first sample, these values fit together into the picture of the somewhat idealistic and esthetically inclined students of art education, future teachers of the social sciences, literature, and the like. It is a little less easy to see why this kind of pattern should be related to the adaptive reaction among the actors, all of whom tend to have relatively strong esthetic values and weak economic ones. Seemingly, someone who reversed this pattern would be a misfit in acting, hardly a lucrative and certainly an esthetic field!

When we turn to Table 4, to examine the correlates of the maladaptive syndrome in these two samples, the picture is a little less clear. Again we find a strong positive correlation in the first sample flip-flopping to a significant negative one in the second, with the

Table 4. Correlates of Syndrome II: Maladaptive Reaction to Isolation

	STUDY 1		STUDY 2	
	Rho	*N*	*Rho*	*N*
A′. *Masculine, "hard-headed" interests*				
Economic value (A-V-L)	.78[b]	12	−.11	15
DPI: Masculine identification scale	.55	11	.14	13
J′. *Dislike of dependence and "claustral" situation*				
DPI: Prenatal scale (womb fantasies)	−.73[b]	11	−.10	13
Rating of Path 13: Submissive dependence	−.62[a]	11	.15	15
B′. *Intellectual rigidity and poverty (lack of resources)*				
Brick uses: fluency	−.70[b]	11	.06	16
Rorschach: Adaptive regression (18)	−.46	12	.39	16
K. *Other-direction and field-dependence*				
Ranking of Path 5: Social extraversion, pure other-direction	.80[b]	10	−.61[a]	13

[a] .05 level [b] .01 level (two-tailed test)

ranking of the "path of life" (10) that expresses an ideal of social extraversion and pure other-direction. There is no obvious reason that this variable should correlate highly with a maladaptive reaction to isolation in either direction: one can argue that an other-directed person might be very sensitive to the wishes of the experimenter and thus compliant and uncomplaining in the situation (as may have happened in Study 2); on the other hand, one can just as easily argue that the other-directed person is so dependent on the continued presence of approving others and tends to be so field-dependent in Witkin's sense (11)—that is, physically unsteady and insecure without the orienting and reassuring framework of visual reality—that anyone strong on this variable would find our situation of isolation quite intolerable. When it is so easy to rationalize such opposite findings, perhaps the best course is not to belabor the point!

At any rate, the most significant correlations in the first study suggest that the maladaptive response to isolation, which was largely a complaining one, was characteristic of people who were actively opposed to passive, dependent, sheltering situations which they presumably perceived as infantilizing and threatening to their masculinity. These complainers also were notable for their lack of intellectual flexibility and for their economic interests. In the second sample, this whole pattern disappeared. But then, the similarities between the maladaptive syndromes in the two studies are even more tenuous in the case of this syndrome than in the case of the first one. The only two variables in common in the two studies are unpleasant affect and quitting; and even so, the variable of quitting has quite different significance in the two studies. In the first one, the three subjects who were highest on this variable actually walked out of the situation. In the second study, no subject walked out nor even came very close to doing so. In effect, then, we were sampling two different regions of the distribution of concern with or predisposition towards quitting in the two samples. In the first sample, the maladaptive syndrome included complaints of impaired secondary process thinking, and poorly controlled primary process thinking; there were no such variables pertaining to thinking in the maladaptive syndrome of the second study. Indeed, among the actors, evidences of regressive secondary process thinking correlated *positively* with the other aspects of the adaptive syndrome! It seems that, in this group who found the whole situation so much less threatening and unpleasant than the students did, those who reacted adaptively also tended to verbalize a good deal of a disjunctive, loosely organized kind of thoughts which still did not contain any obvious evidences of the primary process but had to be scored as regressed secondary process. In the first sample, there was less of this kind of thing, and what tend to be scored under the similarly named variable were *complaints* like the following: "My thoughts kept jumping around"; "I can't concentrate"; such complaints were rare in the actors' sample.

Complaining is the common element in the two maladaptive syndromes (as expressed by the verbalizations we measured as statements of unpleasant affect and concern with quitting), but in the second sample, such complaints were negatively correlated with positive statements of enjoyment and a perhaps relaxed acceptance of the suggestion to lie still. The maladaptive syndrome in the first sample did not include restlessness, and is complicated by the presence of a variable (questionnaire: general disturbance) that was not used in the second study.[4]

CONCLUSIONS

The two experiments reported here, with the failure to replicate a seemingly promising pattern of personality correlates of reactions to a situation of sensory alteration and isolation, point up two principal conclusions.

First, reactions to an altered sensory environment may be predictable from a knowledge of the specific nature of the situation and personality variables that are meaningfully relevant to such alterations. By this statement we mean to imply both a faith that there is order in our data and that personality is predictably related to behavior in the experimental situation, and also to stress the specificity of the cogwheeling of particular personality dispositions and particular situational specifications. To call the altered environment of our study and of, for example, the tank studies of Lilly (12) and Shurley (13) by the same name of "sensory deprivation" is to overlook many major differences in the actual predicament of the subject. There is every reason to think that such specifics will have a good deal to do with the personality correlates that come out of such different studies. For example, our situation called for complete passivity, in contrast to any likely condition of space flight. It might be quite erroneous, then, to take too seriously the correlation of the adaptive reaction with passivity, in any actual application.

Second, the exact pattern of correlations between personality and reactions to sensory alteration depends heavily on the nature of the sample of persons studied. When we changed from a sample of freshmen in a school of education to an older group of unemployed actors, we were aware that these were two very different breeds of men indeed, and were not surprised to find that the predictive variables in one group did not work with the other. Indeed, these variables of personality themselves were quite differently interrelated and patterned in the two groups.

[4] Since the present report was focused on looking for replicates of the personality correlates found in the first study, we have not as yet combed through all of our measures of personality to find and list all of those that correlated with the two syndromes.

From these two points it follows clearly that none of the substantive findings from either of our two studies can be directly applied to the problem of selecting space crews, nor to any other such practical application as the Air Force may be interested in. Our *method*, however, does seem to us to have worked well in both studies and to offer promise for such problems as the selection of space crew personnel. For research of this latter kind, it would be necessary, first, to simulate the particular pattern of sensory alteration to be expected in the criterion situation—including the duties of the subject—as closely as possible, without the introduction of specific conditions (such as prolonged bed rest) that will not be present in the target situation. And, second, it will be necessary to experiment in this work-sample situation with samples of men drawn from the population that will actually be screened for the mission in question. Granted these specifications, relevant reactions to the experimental situation might well be correlated with the same battery of personality tests that we used. Ideally, the resulting predictors should be cross-validated on another, similar sample of subjects before the findings are applied to the actual selection of astronauts. The more we can approximate relevant parameters in the situation and in the sample of subjects, the more confidence we will be able to have in the practical utility of the research findings.

REFERENCES

1. Solomon, P., P. H. Leiderman, J. Mendelson, and D. Wexler, Perceptual and sensory deprivation—a review, Am. J. Psychiat., 114:357–363, 1957.
2. Wheaton, J. L., Fact and fancy in sensory deprivation studies, USAF Sch. Avn. Med. Rev., No. 5–59, 1959.
3. Rapaport, D., The theory of ego autonomy: a generalization, Bull. Menninger Clin., 22:13–35, 1958.
4. Holt, R. R., and L. Goldberger, Personological Correlates of Reactions to Perceptual Isolation. USAF WADC Tech. Rep., No. 59–735, 1959. 46 pp.
5. Goldberger, L., and R. R. Holt, Experimental interference with reality contact (perceptual isolation): method and group results, J. Nerv. Ment. Dis., 127:99–112, 1958.
6. Goldberger, L., and R. R. Holt, Experimental interference with reality contact (perceptual isolation): individual differences, in P. Solomon, ed., *Sensory deprivation and social isolation.* Cambridge, Harvard University Press (in press).
7. Horn, D., A study of personality syndromes, Charact. & Pers., 12:257–274, 1944.
8. Barron, F., An ego-strength scale which predicts response to psychotherapy, J. Consult. Psychol., 17:327–333, 1953.
9. Allport, G. W., P. E. Vernon, and G. Lindzey, A Study of Values. Boston, Houghton, Mifflin, 1951. Rev. ed.

10. Morris, C., and L. V. Jones, Value scales and dimensions, J. Abnorm. Soc. Psychol., 51:523–525, 1955.
11. Witkin, H. A., *et al.*, Personality Through Perception: An Experimental and Clinical Study. New York, Harper & Brothers, 1954.
12. Lilly, J. C., Mental effects of physical restraints and of reduction of ordinary levels of physical stimuli on intact, healthy persons, Psychiat. Res. Rep., 5:1–9, 1956.
13. Shurley, J. T., Profound Experimental Sensory Isolation. Paper read at American Psychiatric meetings, Atlantic City, May, 1960.
14. Barron, F., Complexity-simplicity as a personality variable, J. Abnorm. Soc. Psychol., 48:163–172, 1953.
15. Grygier, T., The Dynamic Personality Inventory. Sutton, England, Banstead Hospital Management Committee, 1955.
16. Jenkins, T. N., The neutral theory of personality: new evidence and a revision of the argument, Trans. N.Y. Acad. Sci., 17:315–330, 1955.
17. Guilford, J. P., N. W. Kettner, and P. R. Christensen, A Factor-Analytic Study Across the Domains of Reasoning, Creativity, and Evaluation. Rep. Psychol. Lab., No. 11. Los Angeles, University of Southern California, 1954.
18. Holt, R. R., and Joan Havel, A method for assessing primary and secondary process in the Rorschach, in Maria A. Rickers-Ovsiankina, ed., *Rorschach Psychology*. New York, Wiley, 1960.

Interpersonal Relationships in Isolated Small Groups

JOHN H. ROHRER

There have been a variety of definitions given to the term "small groups," ranging from the two-person, dyadic groups as described by Sears (1) to the groups composed of 15 to 20 persons as studied by Lippitt and White (2). In this paper "small groups" will designate collections of people ranging in number from 5 to 24.

Isolation too, can have a variety of meanings. There is the absolute isolation for a period of time in which there is no escape possible and no possibility of receiving assistance from the external society (3, 4). There is the isolation to be found under conditions of sensory deprivation in which only one individual is involved, as described by Dr. Cameron. There is the isolation found in remote radar bases that has been described by McCann (5). All of the above conditions imply that the isolation is physical. There can be cultural isolation also, as in the internment camps of the Second World War and the Korean War.

There are three reasons why people enter isolation: (a) they volunteer; (b) they are captive; (c) they are victims of situational events.

The following motivations have been identified for those men who volunteer: (a) desire for prestige; (b) desire to escape from an unpleasant situation; (c) feelings of inadequacy that spur them to "prove themselves"; (d) desire to save money; (e) intellectual curiosity; (f) the challenge of the "unknown"—the "early explorer type."

The other two conditions which bring about isolation are forced upon the individual. First, there is the condition of isolation due to

Dr. Rohrer is in the Department of Psychiatry, Georgetown University, Washington, D.C.

captivity; e.g., (a) prisoners of war, or (b) internment as civilians—the concentration camp situation. The second condition of forced isolation is that brought about by situational events, such as shipwrecks, floods, disasters, and so forth.

When one considers the factor of time commitment to isolation, there are three conditions. One is a predetermined, definite time period for isolation, from which there is no escape possible and no possibility of receiving assistance from the external society during the period of isolation (4, 6). The second possibility is personal commitment to a definite period of isolation, but where, in emergencies, return to a larger society and assistance from it is possible. For example, this condition is met by some isolated stations in the Arctic (7). As will be seen later, the variable "degree of absolute isolation" is most important in determining the quality and nature of interpersonal relationships in isolated small groups. The last condition is where the people are in isolation for an indefinite period of time. The latter situation results largely from captive and situational events (8, 9).

The remaining discussion in this paper will be preoccupied with interpersonal relationships between individuals who have volunteered for duty in isolation for which there is a definite period of isolation, but until the end of that period, no return is possible and there is no possibility of receiving assistance from the external society. This eliminates many of the types of isolation described above. It also eliminates completely all of the research work that has been done on isolated large groups (50 or more people), since the social and psychological phenomena that occur in these large groups differ significantly from what is observed in the small groups (4).

Perhaps the best way to begin discussion of problems of interpersonal relations in isolated small groups is to indicate the phasic nature of those relationships during the period of isolation (4, 10).

The first period is marked by a considerably heightened anxiety on the part of all men. The degree to which the anxiety is heightened is a function of the degree of danger or threat that the given individual feels or perceives. For example, men entering into the Antarctic to be isolated for from 10 to 14 months, showed markedly heightened anxiety upon arrival, and it is at this point that those so predisposed have psychotic episodes. Of the eight men that had to be evacuated from the Antarctic because of psychiatric reasons, all of them had their psychotic episodes within a week after "getting on the ice" (4).

The heightened anxiety was explained in a variety of ways by the men: "not knowing what to expect," "a fear of the unknown," and similar statements. The major method used in the Antarctic to reduce this heightened anxiety was work. Work there has more meaning than just making preparations for the "wintering over" period. It is a frantic kind of work, with jerky bodily movements, and much half-running in order to get from the stock pile to a storage bin, and so forth. Literature on the submariners reports much the same kind of need for engaging in bodily activity under attack conditions. In one report (6) on a submarine which, during the Second World War, had been under bombing attack for 36 hours, the men stated that their anxieties were allayed most by "doing something with their hands." Walter Gibson (9), in describing his miraculous escape from a badly damaged coastal vessel in the Indian Ocean, characterized his compulsive washing of his teeth with sea water as one of the things that permitted him to come through without breaking down mentally.

The second phase of adjustment to isolation occupies the greatest period of time. It is the phase in which the group "settle down" and perform the routine duties to which they have been assigned. During this period their anxiety is lessened, but there is an increase in the amount of depression felt by the men. Depression is experienced by all members of the group, and it may increase periodically for some individuals. In discussing these periods of depression, with a highly observant person who had wintered over in the Antarctic, one man raised this question: "Sure I was depressed, but what is really wrong with being depressed? I got my work all done, and done properly." And he had a pertinent point! Anxiety levels during this long period of depression will vary; again, as a function of the perceived hazardous nature of the duty to be performed.

The third phase develops when individuals are about to leave isolation. It is characterized by increased affect expression, and differs from the other periods in that much anticipatory behavior occurs. Also, it is at this time that there is a great likelihood of the occurrence of aggressive behavior. This is a function of a lessening of the repressive processes that occur during the period of depression. The net result of the anticipatory responses is that the working habits are not as precise as before. A greater amount of error is evidenced, for example, in making scientific observations. Housekeeping and other daily routine chores tend to be neglected, and anxieties tend to rise somewhat.

I might remark that this same cyclic pattern of adjustment has been observed in individuals who entered into isolation for a three-day period. Here I am referring to some studies being carried out by the American Institute of Research, in Pittsburgh, on "fallout shelter habitability." During one weekend the same pattern did occur in a group of 28 people, ranging in age from 8 to 45, with mixed sex composition, and where all had volunteered for the three days of isolation. Apparently the cyclic adjustment pattern has considerable generality, and is not a function of a time factor per se.

Perhaps there is no place where one can observe more clearly the tremendous need man has for gratifying ego and affect-involved interpersonal relationships than in the small isolated group. Deprivation of such relationships by isolation from the group produces phenomena quite similar to some of the phenomena produced by sensory deprivation as described by Dr. Cameron. The behavioral syndrome produced by the exclusion from the isolated group I have labeled the "Long Eye" (4). I have at least ten documented cases where it occurred in the Antarctic. The syndrome can be produced by an attempt on the part of the group to use social censure as a control technique. This is the "silent treatment," where the rest of the men in the group decide that they will not talk or respond to a given member of the group. In from six to ten days the "Long Eye" phenomenon is produced. It consists of various combinations of sleeplessness, spontaneous bursts of crying, hallucinations, and a giving up of the usual habits of living, such as washing, eating, drinking coffee, and the like. Persons experiencing the "Long Eye" are apparently oblivious to external stimulation and are described variously as lying in their bunks, staring into space, or moving aimlessly about. A more vivid description of this "staring" was given to me by one person who said: "It's like a twelve-foot stare in a ten-foot room." Sometimes the phenomenon is accompanied by a repetitive, obsessive carrying out of rather simple acts, such as packing a box, unpacking it, repacking it. This "Long Eye" phenomenon, produced by social isolation from the small group, is temporary. As soon as the person is permitted to return to, and interact with the group, the symptoms disappear.

A universal phenomenon that occurs in isolated small groups in the Antarctic is that of sleeplessness (3, 4, 10). People will go at times for periods of from six to fifteen days sleeping only an hour or so per day. This is in contrast with submariners (11), among whom there tends to be a greater amount of sleeping than normally occurs in a more complex society. Sleeplessness in the Antarctic apparently is related to tenseness and to problems of anxiety. For example, a mechanic went through a period of five days of sleeplessness, while attempting to repair a piece of machinery. He was able to regain his older sleep habits when he finally admitted to himself that it was impossible to repair the equipment. A second person who had rather severe periods of sleeplessness told me that the only way he could overcome it was with tranquilizing drugs such as meprobromate. Seconal (a barbiturate) for example, did not aid him to regain his usual sleep habits.

With the rather intense repression of sex impulses that occurs in isolated small groups of the same sex, there is a corresponding increase in the importance of oral gratification. This is true aboard submarines (11) and in the Antarctic (3, 4, 10). In both cases, where the period of isolation is rather long, weight gains are reported by nearly all, and food preparation becomes of greater importance than it is in normal society. Correspondingly, the social status of the cook in these isolated small groups reaches heights unknown to a cook in our more complex society.

Leisure-time activities tend toward simpler, more fundamental types of activities such as reminiscing, telling "tall stories," and so forth. Both in submarines and in the Antarctic almost everyone, prior to becoming isolated, had made plans to use their leisure in a "constructive" manner, such as studying for rates, reading novels or technical books they have long wanted to read, studying languages, listening to technical and scientific lectures, and similar types of activities that are necessary steps for upward social mobility. Attempts at these types of upward mobility, "manufactured" leisure-time activities have been made by most all groups studied. Apparently aboard submarines (11) there was more success in achieving those goals (particularly in studying for advancement rates) than in the Antarctic. However, in both cases, with time these types of activities seem to disappear, being pushed out by the simpler, more fundamental, and perhaps more "earthy" types of activities. Correspondingly, there is much "status leveling" of group members in isolation.

I have said nothing about the adjustment of women to isolated groups, largely because there is such a paucity of information about their adjustment, and what exists is largely anecdotal. There have been at least three women who have wintered over in the Antarctic. Mrs. Ronnie and Mrs. Darlington (12) went along with their husbands on one expedition. A few years back there was one middle-aged Russian biologist who wintered over at the Antarctic Russian station at Murney. One woman survived with Gibson (9) after the ship had been torpedoed by the Japanese. But the conditions in all cases were so unusual that no generalizations can be drawn from them.

With this background of general adjustment patterns, we can proceed with a discussion of some of the underlying variables that influence interpersonal relationships in isolated small groups, for it would be a rather barren description that did not provide some explanatory conceptualizations as to why the observed behavior occurred.

In all of the literature that I have read on isolated small groups, the first time that the men get together as a group is when they are ready to enter isolation. Hence, they know very little about each other. This is true in the Antarctic groups, in the case of shipwrecks (a classic example here being Gibson's account), and it is true in the case of submariners on their first cruise.

These persons start out the period of isolation not as a group, but as a collection of people. True, the necessary skills for survival and performance of work duties are usually provided by the various members of the collection, but no functional group structure exists. However, informal group formation takes place quite rapidly in the small groups, even when there is a formal hierarchical structure. The formalized structure soon is replaced by a functional one, which may be isomorphic with the formal structure or may depart radically from that structure. Generally speaking, the initial "buddy" selections are of a temporary nature and shift after the period of initial anxiety is lowered. Apparently, during this first period friends and companions for leisure activities are chosen more in terms of their ability to lower anxiety for the selector than for any other reason. During this initial period too, any show of hostility is inhibited or displaced outside the group.

The closest relationships in the initial period are built up between men occupied with the same type of task. Where there are two different groups (e.g., civilian scientists and navy personnel), the original identifications that they brought into the group are determining factors in the original friendships that are formed. Under these conditions, one sees initially a considerable amount of over-identification with the pre-isolation in-group, and some show of hostility directed towards the pre-isolation out-group. During the second phase of adjustment these patterns change, although the work similarities of the various men tend to bring them together and into interaction more frequently and hence tend to build somewhat stronger emotional ties between them.

The depression produced during the second period of adjustment to isolation is due largely to repression, resulting in part from the fact that the social role of the individual has been greatly reduced as a function of his isolation. Under conditions of isolation, about the only social role that an individual has is that connected with his occupation. The temporary loss of such social roles as "husband," "brother," "father," "club member," and all of the other various roles that he occupies in normal society is a keenly felt deprivation. Because of these circumstances and the need for repressing thoughts about his latent roles, the work or occupational role becomes highly valued by the man, and he guards very jealously the work activities attendent to that role. This possessiveness extends from such roles as driving a snow weasel to the most complex of technical roles. As mentioned, the depressions apparently occur because of the reduction in the variety of roles available to be engaged in, plus the heightened anxiety resulting from the constant threat that the men experience.

The threat experienced may be due to at least three different reasons. First of all there is physical threat, brought about by a hostile environment. Second, there is the threat of isolation from the social group. Third, there is a threat that most everyone who has gone through isolation experiences at one time or another: the fear that the experience may result in their own personal psychic harm or destruction.

During this period of depression, hostility is greatly inhibited and is expressed most frequently as verbal hostile acts directed toward someone outside the group. One reason why this hostility is displaced is the mentioned fear of isolation from the social group. Going along with the increased repression that occurs in the second period of adjustment to isolation is an increased awareness of minute physical stimuli, stimuli that under less isolated conditions would not be attended to. This phenomenon has been described vividly by Giaever (13) and is apparently a function of the increased repression being used as a defense tactic.

The type of adjustment characterized by the third period or phase of isolation is one of lessened depression, probably due to the increased work activity that occurs. Accompanying the lessened depression is a greater show of hostility towards members in the group (indicating a lesser use of repression as a self-protective device), and an increased neglect of responsibilities to which the individuals had been assigned. During this period there is usually some aggressive behavior shown, inasmuch as the members of the group feel that they have accomplished their mission. They behave in a more adolescent manner with considerable "bragging"—which is a way of rewarding themselves for feeling that they have achieved a goal that was set. For the more restrained people during this third phase, there is an increase in frequency of psychosomatic problems, e.g. headaches (3). Real or imagined slights are verbalized more frequently that they were in the earlier phases of isolation.

In closing, perhaps justification should be made for eliminating the rather rich literature that exists on isolated small groups in radar bases and in the Arctic. The fact is that all the data reported in that literature indicate that the problems that exist there are completely different from the ones described in this paper. There is not the great degree of sexual repression that is noted in the completely isolated group. The factors that influence morale are quite different. Morale in the completely isolated group tends to center around freedom of social interaction, food, and the like. In the groups described in the literature on isolated radar and Arctic stations morale tends to center around the absence of good "liberty spots" and similar factors that influence morale in any of the smaller detached and somewhat isolated groups to be found in a complex society. Apparently the big problem here is one of acceptance of the commitment to complete isolation, for the people at both the radar and Arctic stations are not so committed. At any time they can break isolation if an emergency arises. Aboard submarines out for a three months' cruise, especially under wartime conditions, there is a "point of no return." The same is true for the small Antarctic groups. Total commitment to complete isolation for a definite time period, then, is a variable of prime importance in determining the quality and nature of the interpersonal relationships that will develop in isolated small groups.

REFERENCES

1. Sears, R. R., A theoretical framework for personality and social behavior, Am. Psychol., 6:476–483, 1951.
2. Lippitt, R., and R. K. White, An experimental study of leadership in group life, in G. E. Swanson, T. M. Newcomb, and E. L. Hartley, eds., *Readings in Social Psychology*. New York, Harper, 1952. 2d ed., pp. 340–355.
3. Mullin, C. S., Jr., and H. J. N. Connery, Psychological study at an Antarctic IGY station, Armed Forces Med. J., 10:451–462, 1959.
4. Rohrer, J. H., Some Impressions of Psychic Adjustment to Polar Isolation. Washington, D.C., Bureau of Medicine and Surgery, U.S. Navy, 1958. 52 pp.
5. McCann, G. C., Morale and Human Problems in A.C. and W.C. Sites. Technical Memorandum CRL-TM-56-5. Crew Research Laboratory Air Force Personnel and Research Center, Randolph AFB, Texas, 1956. 39 pp.
6. Duff, I. F., and C. W. Shilling, Psychiatric casualties in submarine warfare, Am. J. Psychiat., 53:603–613, 1947.
7. McCullum, E. L., Survey of Human Adjustment Problems in the Northern Latitude. Arctic Aero-medical Laboratory, Project 21-01-022, Program C, Part 1-A, Ladd AFB, Alaska, 1950.
8. Vaughan, Elizabeth H., Adjustment problems in a concentration camp, Sociol. and Soc. Res., 32:513–518, 1947–48.
9. Gibson, W., The Boat. New York, Houghton, Mifflin, 1953.
10. Law, P., The Sir Richard Stawell Oration. Personality problems in Antarctica. (Unpublished manuscript.) Antarctic Division, Department of External Affairs, Her Majesty's Government, London, 1959.
11. Kinsey, J. L., Psychologic aspects of the "Nautilus" transpolar cruise, Armed Forces Med. J., 10:451–462, 1959.
12. Darlington, Jennie, My Antarctic Honeymoon: A Year at the Bottom of the World. New York, Doubleday, 1956.
13. Giaever, J., The White Desert: The Official Account of the Norwegian-British-Swedish Antarctic Expedition. London, Chatto and Windus, 1954. Pp. 112-138.

Motivations and Emotional Reactions in Early Space Flights

PHILIP SOLOMON

In planning for space flights, perhaps the most difficult element to subject to scientific preparedness is that of the human equation. Pilot error is notoriously dependent on the precarious balance between strength and frailty of the human spirit, tied not only to the continuous efficiency of the intellect but also to the smooth operation of the underlying emotional forces which permit the mind to function. There is an old saying that you cannot teach a hungry child; you cannot teach an unhappy child either, or a worried one, and you cannot expect peak performance, or even rational behavior, from an adult who is bordering on panic or frenzy or despair. The motivations and emotional reactions of our early space travelers will be as important to the success or failure of their enterprise as the characteristics of their ship and the adequacy of their supplies.

Unfortunately, we know little of predictive value concerning the kind of behavior to be anticipated from particular individuals in moments of genuine crisis. Admittedly, we have whole batteries of tests for personality attributes, including measures of "emotional stability," "maturity," and "ego strength." Who can say how these would correlate with responses under conditions of actual life-or-death stress?

What I propose to do in this paper is to discuss, in frankly speculative terms, the role of motivation in the emotional reactions of a pioneer space traveler, and to analyze the more dangerous emotional reactions from the point of view of their unconscious derivations and their possible means of prophylaxis. In connection with the last of

Dr. Solomon is Physician-in-Chief for Psychiatry, Boston City Hospital, and Assistant Clinical Professor of Psychiatry, Harvard Medical School.

these, I shall draw upon our experiences at the Psychiatric Research Laboratory of the Boston City Hospital, where we have been conducting experiments in sensory deprivation over the past four years (1, 2, 3, 4, 5, 6).

Though space travel is now so new, the motivations of the astronaut with respect to it are probably not greatly different from those of the ship captain in the days of Columbus with respect to transoceanic travel. The unknowns and the dangers are different, but the challenges and rewards are basically the same.

The motivations may be divided into two types: aggressive and defensive. The aggressive motivations are those which are directed toward attaining some form of success, for example, furthering the aims and goals of mankind, science, one's country, one's military organization, or one's particular unit; also adventure, excitement, self-mastery, and self-fulfillment. Operationally, it may be expected that there will be no problem in choosing personnel in whom this form of motivation is very high; nor should it be anticipated that there will be any great difficulty in keeping it high throughout the course of the journey. Healthy human beings love nothing so dearly as they do success.

The defensive motivations are those that are directed toward avoiding any kind of failure, such as pain, injury, illness, invalidism, or discomfort generally; also, of course, danger and death. It is here that the chief problems with personnel may be expected.

Psychological reactions to danger involve both the intellect and the emotions. The former attempts to diagnose the situation and initiate appropriate action, the latter simply respond with some measure of fear and anxiety, and perhaps other emotions. The intellect may succeed in diminishing or eliminating the danger, or may at least set up proper preparations to meet it when it arrives; the emotions stir up changes within the body, such as increased heart rate, respiration and blood pressure, which are of value in fighting, running away, or doing whatever else is necessary in the emergency. Usually there is a mixture of intellectual and emotional reactions, but there may be a preponderence of one or the other. Words indicating such mixtures may be arranged in a kind of spectrum, with those signifying greater intellectual participation at one end, for example, "concern," "presentiment," "misgiving," "apprehension," "foreboding," and "disquiet"; those denoting greater emotional participation at the other end, for example, "fright," "dismay," "consternation," "horror," "terror," and "panic"; while those that are more evenly divided are in between, for example, "worry," "trepidation," "dread," "anxiety," "alarm," and "fear." From the point of view of choosing personnel for space flight it is clearly important to select individuals who are likely to employ their intellect consistently and coolly in an emergency, since extreme emotional reactions may produce either tremor, restlessness, inappropriate movement, and even convulsions on the one hand, or a state of "frozen fear," paralysis, or catatonia on the other.

No one knows all the determining factors for the eventual breakdown of strong men who are subjected to continuous severe emotional stress. Experience in the Second World War demonstrated that, though there are wide variations from individual to individual, every man has his breaking point (7). Physical fatigue, sleeplessness, hunger, thirst, discomfort, and illness were found to play important roles (8). Psychologically, the unremitting nature of the danger, lack of strong leadership, solitude or poor morale in the group, monotony and boredom, and uncertainty of the time of relief were shown to be highly significant (9). Psychoanalytically, it may be said that the ego succumbs whenever the combined forces attacking it, be they physical, psychological, or both, are more than it can bear. The concept of the ego can be of value here because it is known that the ego has large areas that are wholly unconscious, and these may be critical in determining the point of breakdown.

In the unconscious, threats to the ego may be divided into those that endanger it with (1) suffering, and (2) dissolution. In the former category are the familiar castration or mutilation threats; in the latter are desertion, abandonment, and death. Adequate attention is always given to the prevention of the former in the astronaut, within the limits of scientific knowledge, but interest in certain aspects of the latter is a relatively recent development.

Research in sensory deprivation has shown that the integrity of the human ego is critically dependent upon a continuous meaningful contact with the outside environment (10). Deprived of sensory input, the mind is cut adrift and regresses inexorably into that

Sargasso Sea of the primary process, where time disappears, where there is no order, quantity, direction, or rationality, where vivid, multicolored hallucinations swirl and befuddle the senses. Individuals differ enormously in their tolerance for the stress that is produced, but some "normal" subjects have been known to become frenzied and quite uncontrollable in their reactions. In our most recent work at Boston City Hospital we have been able to demonstrate that social isolation and immobilization, the usual concomitants of sensory deprivation experiments, are not necessary for the appearance of the characteristic results, though they tend to intensify them(11). The presence of a stranger in a "twin" experiment causes less serious mental aberrations; the presence of a wife, still less (12).

What does this mean with respect to our pioneering space astronaut? It has been recognized by a number of observers (13, 14) that aviators in high-level flight are subject to a "break-off phenomenon," characterized by dazed feelings, confusion, faulty perception, and judgment, and either anxiety or a peculiar exhilaration. Conducive to the appearance of this phenomenon are such conditions as monotony, inactivity, and lack of visual contact with the ground, in short, similar conditions to those which prevail in a sensory deprivation experiment.

It is our conviction that in assessing an individual's ability to withstand the stress of sensory deprivation, it is not sufficient to examine only his *conscious* reactions. Let me give you an actual case example of one of our subjects. This was a young man who was engaged in research in the problems of infection in dairy animals. He had taken both a bachelor's and a master's degree in dairy agriculture. Though he volunteered to participate in the experiment for thirty-six hours, he asked to be let out shortly after the end of the third hour. He moaned, "Please help me!" After the tank-type respirator, in which the subject was enclosed, had been opened, he lay motionless for about five minutes. He perspired freely, his face was immobile, and his limbs seemed to have lost their muscle tone. He had to be helped to remove his arm cuffs.

It developed that shortly after this subject had entered the respirator at the start of the experiment, he had taken a drink of eggnog from the automatic feeding device that was provided for the subject. He thought it tasted warm. Actually it was well refrigerated.

He imagined that bacteria were growing in the milk and would poison him. Anxiously, he then tried to imagine that he would produce an antidote in his own body which would counteract the effects of the poison.

During the last half-hour that this subject was in the experiment, he arched his back and looked toward the back inside wall. He thought he saw a grey curtain descend over the upper half of his field of vision, obscuring the feeding tube and the microphone. He looked forward toward the respirator and the film disappeared. He then thought he saw rays of light coming toward him from the microphone fixed on the tank.

In the interview that directly followed the experiment, the subject appeared guarded and controlled. In the twenty-four hours following the experiment, he suffered a severe anxiety attack with motor restlessness, profuse sweating, and preoccupation with the type of thinking he had experienced during the experiment. In contacts with members of the research group he was obviously anxious and needed frequent reassurance. He then recovered quickly and completely.

In psychiatric study it could be seen that this subject had severe deep-seated problems related to his parents and to authority figures generally. He was able to mask his dependence and resentment behind a well-poised, assertive façade—a defense which became brittle under stress. In the experiment it broke through in the form of claustrophobia, immobilization, and panic. His choice of profession, dairy agriculture, and the nature of his symptoms in his psychotic-like break, "poisoned" milk, both were intimately associated with his unconscious psychodynamic conflicts. It is reasonable to suppose that this subject, who might have passed many ordinary screening tests, would have fared badly as a space astronaut.

A candidate for space travel should have, along with all the other screening procedures that are applied to him, a thorough psychiatric appraisal which should include a psychoanalytically oriented survey of his *unconscious* emotional make-up. He should also be exposed to some standard sensory deprivation situation and be eliminated from consideration if he fails to withstand this kind of stress in reasonably satisfactory manner.

Prophylactically, during the course of space travel, every effort should be made to keep the voyager not only in constant communication with his scientific monitors on earth, but with close members of his family and friends. He should be given plenty of work to do, as variegated as possible. He should have a companion on the trip, and every precaution should be taken to avoid the insidious dangers of inactivity, monotony, and boredom. Let me reemphasize the desirability of a companion: most of our troubles on earth are caused by people; most of our troubles off earth may be caused by the lack of them.

REFERENCES

1. Solomon, P., P. H. Leiderman, J. Mendelson, and D. Wexler, Sensory deprivation: a review, Am. J. Psychiat., 114:357, 1957.
2. Mendelson, J., P. Solomon, and E. Lindemann, Hallucinations of poliomyelitis patients during treatment in a respirator, J. Nerv. Ment. Dis., 126:421, 1958.
3. Wexler, D., J. Mendelson, P. H. Leiderman, and P. Solomon, Sensory deprivation: a technique for studying psychiatric aspects of stress, Arch. Neurol. Psychiat., 79:225, 1958.
4. Mendelson, J., P. Kubzansky, P. H. Leiderman, D. Wexler, C. DuToit, and P. Solomon, Catechol amine excretion and behavior during sensory deprivation, Arch. Gen. Psychiat., 2:147, 1960.
5. Leiderman, P. H., J. Mendelson, D. Wexler, and P. Solomon, Sensory deprivation: clinical aspects, Arch. Intern. Med., 101:389, 1958.
6. Kubzansky, P. E., P. H. Leiderman, J. Mendelson, D. Wexler, and P. Solomon, A comparison of two conditions of sensory deprivation. Paper read at Amer. Psychol. Ass., Washington, D.C., Sept., 1958.
7. Grinker, R. R., and J. P. Spiegel, Men under Stress. New York, Blakiston, 1945.
8. Solomon, P., The use of plasma in the treatment of combat fatigue, Nav. Med. Bull., March, 1948, pp. 226–228.
9. Solomon, P., Incidence of combat fatigue, Arch. Neurol. and Psychiat., 57:332–341, 1947.
10. Hebb, D. O., The motivating effects of exteroceptive stimulation, Am. Psychol., 13:109, 1958.
11. Davis, J. M., W. F. McCourt, and P. Solomon, Sensory deprivation: (1) Effects of social contact, (2) Effect of random visual stimulation. Paper read at Amer. Psychiat. Ass., Philadelphia, April, 1959.
12. Davis, J. M., W. F. McCourt, J. Courtney, and P. Solomon, Sensory deprivation: the role of emotional support. (Unpublished manuscript.) Psychiatric Research Lab., Boston City Hospital.
13. Clark, B., and A. Graybiel, The break-off phenomenon: a feeling of separation from the earth experienced by pilots at high altitudes, J. Avn. Med., 28:121, 1957.
14. Bennett, A. M. H., Sensory deprivation in aviation, in P. Solomon *et al.*, eds., *Sensory Deprivation.* Cambridge, Harvard University Press (in press).

Time and Load Factors in Astronaut Proficiency

BRYCE O. HARTMAN

Once again, man stands at the threshold of a new era of exploration. Facing him is the most hostile environment he has ever invaded. Vast technological, biological, and human resources are being thrown into the battle. The accumulated skills and techniques of engineers, physicists, biophysicists, and specialists in the life sciences are being brought to bear on the unique problems of space flight. However, these problems are unique only in the sense of being unusual versions of problems which are already with us. Sustained research over the past two decades has found immediate application to space medicine. The psychophysiology of space flight does not represent a new field—rather, it is the application of psychophysiology to a set of special problems arising in the environment of space and in the missions our astronauts will fly.

THE ASTRONAUT'S JOB

Before evaluating the effects of time and load factors on the proficiency of man in space, it is important to consider the nature of the astronaut's job. Except for the special problems of controlling subsystems for maintaining the microenvironment necessary to sustain life, his task will not be greatly different from those of his earthbound brothers. Systems require certain kinds of operator skills and involve specific kinds of tasks, whether they are ground-based, airborne, or in space. Operator functions have evolved in a systematic fashion which warrants review.

Space flight is an extension of military aviation. If one views the development of military aviation from its infancy through current operational aircraft (or, more appropriately, current airborne

Dr. Hartman is Chief, Medical Psychology Section, Neuropsychiatry Branch, School of Aviation Medicine, USAF Aerospace Medical Center (ATC), Brooks Air Force Base, Texas.

weapons systems), we see a markedly accelerated development of automation. Hand in hand with this change has been a shift in the nature of the job performed by the man in this assembly of a man and a machine. There are a number of important differences which are obvious even in current systems. For example, pilots are no longer being taught airmanship in the sense of flying "by the seat of the pants." What we are teaching today is really more like "machinesmanship." Pilot proficiency today is highly dependent, probably by a factor of a hundred in comparison to the First World War, upon training and skill in *procedure*. The number of subsystems which the pilot controls has increased tremendously in just the last decade. The number of cockpit displays and other informational inputs in the modern cockpit is so much greater than in military aircraft of the early years of the Second World War that comparison is hardly useful. Consider also the huge increase in the communications load on the pilot in the past forty years.

What does this mean in terms of the functions of the man in the weapons systems with us today or under development? First, these changes are the natural result of the technical achievements being incorporated into systems. It is clear that increasing automation is ahead; the shift in the pilot's job of the future will be an extension of the changes we have already seen. Second, to an ever increasing degree, pilots are no longer flyers, but are operators of complex systems. The pilot of today has a job more like that of the flight engineer of the Second World War than any other job in the history of military aviation. It appears, in fact, that the creation of the position of flight engineer represents a historical turning point in the evolution of the pilot's job. As this trend continues, the role of the man in the air is becoming more like the task performed by ground-based operators in advanced weapons systems. This is probably fortunate for the researcher in human factors. Problems of the proficiency of operators of future systems hold promise of being quite complex, but at least we can look forward to a reduction in the number of job families with which we will have to be concerned.

What is the new systems operator's job like? Our best estimate of what the pilot's job is going to be comes from an analysis of what systems operators are doing in the most advanced systems of today. At first glance the situation is confusing. There are many different kinds of operators in today's systems. Which operator is most like the pilot of the future? It turns out that the sum total of the functions of the several operators in a system gives an excellent description of the job of the airborne operator pilot.

Parenthetically, it might be pointed out that many current systems utilize several operators, each with a different function and, in general, each working well below capacity. This is a luxury which is disappearing, so that ground-based operators are becoming more like airborne operators at the same time that airborne operators are becoming more like ground-based operators. Specifically, the functions of these two kinds of operators are coming together, but in different ways. For the operator-pilot, the job is changing. For the ground-based crews, the over-all requirements are remaining the same, but the division of functions is disappearing and the size of the crews is being reduced.

The keys to these new systems operators jobs are increasing automation and the assignment of an increasing variety of different functions to progressively smaller crews—to one or two men in the case of manned space systems. The most obvious results of these two trends can be seen in the complex array of displays, controls, and functions confronting systems operators. Detailed listings of individual tasks and functions performed by men for just a single system are an overwhelming job. A catalogue of human functions in all systems is a task of a magnitude which probably outweighs its value. What is needed is a summary of the operator's job to provide guidance in developing research on the human factors problems of the future. The tasks performed by the operators of these new systems have these general characteristics:

1. They are multivariate. The operator is required to perform a large number of different functions.

2. They involve a complex combination of skillful responses requiring precision and simple discrete responses such as throwing a switch.

3. There is an increasing requirement for the detection of signals, the interpretation of the information contained in these signals, and the making of decisions about alternate modes of system operation.

4. The rate of performance is variable, and involves intermittent responding and controlling interspersed with periods of monitoring.

5. The sequences of responses are highly variable. The requirements placed upon the operator are based upon minor deviations and major failures of automatic and semiautomatic machine processes which are basically unpredictable.

This summary of systems operator's tasks provides a framework within which to analyze the astronaut's job. Developing a more specific task description has proved to be difficult. We cannot, of course, talk in terms of specific task elements or known display-control configurations but there have been a few predictions. Bamford, Hanes, and Wilson (4) discuss the spaceman's functions in general terms. They see him carrying out four activities: sensing, interpreting, planning, and manipulating. They feel sensing will be limited primarily to the visual mode and will require vigilance and acuity. Interpreting, which involves an assessment of both the state of the system and the state of the system's environment, requires both long-term storage (through training) and short-term storage of ongoing events. The objective in interpreting is to analyze the difference between the actual and required output of the system. Planning is seen as the mirror image of interpreting, projected forward into time. Manipulating refers to overt operations, mostly in relation to specific controls or functions. They emphasize the importance of mission profiles in evaluating man's functions and efficiency in space.

Williams and Hopkins (47), in a stimulating analysis of the role of the pilot ten years hence, predict that future weapons systems will be primarily controlled by automatic equipment. They see man providing a flexibility in systems not economical by engineering approaches. In these highly automated systems, man's role will be that of a monitor and a mode-of-operation or flight-program selector. Central to this role of programmer will be the function of decision-making. They redefine decision-making in these systems. Rather than selecting from alternatives, which is the conventional concept, it will consist of detecting and identifying the state of the system. For most system states decision-making is completed at this point; each state has its own built-in mode of operation. This is an important breakthrough in understanding the system operator as a decision-maker. It emphasizes the unity of information-processing and decision-making, which are all too often regarded as separate functions. It is likely that research on trouble-shooting in maintenance tasks, which has been supported almost exclusively by the armed forces, may provide the basic information for future research on decision-making.

Procedural skills are another area of applied military research which provides basic information for analyzing factors influencing operator proficiency. The growth of procedural requirements in military aviation has already been mentioned. Procedural skills involve a series of discrete acts, largely operating simple controls such as switches or levers, carried out on a predetermined schedule with an invariant sequence. The chain of activities in locking on to a target, arming a weapon system, or fighting an engine fire in an aircraft are examples. The importance of this kind of an operator function is demonstrated by the large research and field evaluation program which was conducted by the Air Force Personnel and Training Research Center, now deactivated. This program should have provided us with some base line information on performance at procedural tasks, but unfortunately there seems to be no good summary and integration of the findings. All we can say for sure is that training is very important and the part-task trainers of simple design are exceedingly useful.

It is clear that procedural tasks will be part of the astronaut's job. It is part of any systems operator's job, but the applied researcher is not yet able to describe the primary characteristics of procedural skills.

There have been a few suggestions of specific tasks an astronaut might perform. Williams and Hopkins (47) point out that man will perform many switching operations, primarily because he is there and is a proficient "switcher." Ritchie (42) states that control systems will involve a kind of motor behavior which has received little study: the display will present information continuously, but the controls will be operated discontinuously, or with discrete movements to produce "bursts" of power. This kind of motor activity is, in effect, a discontinuous tracking task.

Sketchy though it may be, a picture of the astronaut's job emerges. He will be a monitor. While monitoring, he will be required to continuously diagnose the state of the system. When this state deviates from the desired one, he will be required to respond. If a new mode of operation is indicated, he will give the appropriate command to the system. If a malfunction or deviation from a specified mode occurs, he will give corrective commands. His display system will be multichannel, with some elements presenting information continuously and others only occasionally. His control system will also be multichannel, but will be composed only of discontinuous elements (switches) or short-term continuous elements (potentiometers, etc.). His work pattern will be variable, and execution phases will be intermittent. In general, he will perform a large array of discrete, discontinuous functions against a continuous background of monitoring and information-processing. In order to perform some of the more complex kinds of information-processing, he may need the assistance of an airborne computer. Such a computer would have both a short-term and a long-term storage function. It would integrate multiple bits of information and provide some interlocks (locking out some inappropriate decisions) in order to reduce the long-term storage load on the astronaut. In this case he would also be a computer operator.

Fortunately, performance at these kinds of tasks have been under study. Contributing factors to proficiency at any specific moment have been studied under the heading of speed stress and load stress. Changes over time in these sorts of tasks have been studied less intensively, but there is sufficient information available to make a first evaluation of the problems. The problem of proficiency at any given moment will be discussed next.

EFFECTS OF LOAD

Operator proficiency at any given moment is a function of the past history of the operator's performance, any residual effects from this past history, the sum of environmental stressors (both immediate and residual), and the load on the operator. Load, which is the primary concern of this section, refers to the sum of all requirements imposed on the operator at any instant by the system. It has both immediate and cumulative aspects. Task load is a continuum, probably best described by signal rate, which can vary from quite low levels to rates in excess of what the operator can handle. This continuum encompasses operator functions ranging from vigilance tasks (such as watch-keeping at sea) at the low end of the continuum, through monitoring multielement displays (which are a major part of all systems operators functions) in the mid-range, to high-load phases occurring in all complex systems.

A decade ago the concept of a continuum of task load would be unambiguous. Today it is not. Research since 1950 has identified speed and load as separate elements of task-load. The effects of speed stress and load stress on operator proficiency have received intensive study. The metric of the continuum is still valid. Signal rate, which is a direct measure of speed stress, is still the primary factor in operator proficiency (11, 37). Load, which is defined as the number of channels of information (frequently the number of displays), appears to be basically independent of the speed variable (10, 11, 12, 37, 45). Load is a stressor secondary to speed stress in most tasks. One way to conceptualize these two variables is to think of load as a task characteristic orthogonal to speed. In this schema, each operator's job can be described on a two dimensional surface, with signal rate on the base line and load (number of channels) on an axis at a 90° angle. Comparisons between several operator's jobs, or between phases of one operator's task, can be made quickly with this graphic presentation.

In view of new specificity of the term "load," the load continuum should be redefined as a continuum of "task-induced stress," using the definition by Garvey (16). Most research on operator proficiency in systems task has been concerned with high levels of task stress (40), but it is apparent that even jobs rated low in task-induced stress can be ordered on the task stress continuum. However, not all performance changes can be predicted from the position of an operator's job on the continuum, for most tasks at the low end require vigilance and monitoring functions, which will be discussed later.

Many studies of speed and load stress have used a task where the subject scans a continuous display, such as dials with revolving pointers which are continuously visible, and makes discrete responses, such as pressing a telegraph key. The speed and load variables are usually incorporated into a factorial design, with several steps on both the speed and load dimensions. Analyses of speed stress effects and load stress effects are made separately and then the interaction is evaluated. Both self-paced and externally paced studies have been conducted. Results have been presented in terms of over-all changes in error measures, reaction time, and more detailed analysis of performance in small segments of the task. Summaries of speed stress, load stress, and interaction effects will be presented separately.

Speed Stress Effects. An early study by Conrad (9), sparked by his previous work and that of Mackworth, used a four-dial display with moving pointers and a knob-turning, discontinuous response. While emphasizing the primacy of load in this study, Conrad reported that errors of omission were a logarithmic function of speed, but that the size of errors of commission were not affected by speed. He also found that the number of attempts were related to speed, although this measure did not increase as fast as speed. Errors of timing were not influenced by speed.

In a subsequent study (10), concentrated on display factors underlying omissions, Conrad found lapses of attention at low speeds, blocks and narrowed span of attention at high speeds. He noted that omissions occurred when other responses, both preceding and following, were close, and suggested that there is a period of diminished effector activity related to responses. This effect increased as signal speed increased, although it was independent of detailed changes in prevailing temporal conditions and only indirectly related to signal density at any specific point in the task. When this analysis was extended (11) to a more intensive study of these effects at only the favorable speed, similar effects could be seen. The analysis showed that the temporal structure of events (signals) is a primary determinant of the accuracy of any single response and that mean accuracy is a function of the frequency with which certain sequences of events occur. Conrad emphasized that mean speed was not appropriate for analyzing speed and load effects. Rather, it was the temporal characteristics of segments of the run and the frequency with which certain high density sequences occurred that determined the level of performance.

Conrad's studies to this point had used externally paced tasks. The temporal layout of series of responses was beyond the control of the subjects. In an attempt to determine whether subjects would modify these sequences to produce more favorable temporal characteristics, he ran two studies involving self-pacing. In the first (13), he compared performance in the self-paced and externally paced tasks. He obtained a smaller standard deviation for the self-paced condition, indicating that subjects were modifying driving speed to produce more favorable temporal characteristics. In the second (14), he added variations in load level in the self-paced task, to see whether the subjects would adjust differently for each load level. He found that subjects maintained the motor speed at an average rate for all load levels, despite the fact that effective adjustment requires a different speed for each load level. He was unable to account for this failure to adjust differentially.

By this time, the importance of overlapping signals has been established. In 1956, Mackworth and Mackworth published a study in which overlap was manipulated (37). Using a visual matching task with variations in the load and speed, they found increased errors and misses with increased speed. Drawing on Mackworth's earlier concepts of "crisis" (several signals in a short period of time) and "disorder" (confusion about the order in which to deal with signals), they reported that omissions increased more rapidly than the overlap index suggested, and felt that signal overlap accounts for most effects in these kinds of tasks. They noted that signals early in a crisis tended to be dealt with more effectively and that "lulls" were misleading because they tended to obscure the overload effects. Their results indicated that rate of *work* is the simplest index of speed and load stress and that periods of signal overlap are critical for assessing speed stress effects, rather than speed itself. They stated that speed stress can be defined as a combination of the number of signals per minute and the bunching of signals exceeding the maximum rate for decisions.

Systems-oriented researchers in this country became concerned with the problem. In 1954 Wagner, Fitts, and Noble (45) reported three studies in which subjects performed a moving-tape multichannel task, pressing a key when a spot and cross-line were in coincidence. Three speeds and three loads were used. Their results showed that performance deteriorated as speed increased. Using an information theory analysis, they obtained a decrease in the number of hits for a fixed number of signals as the rate of information increased. They emphasized the trade-off between signal speed and number of channels necessary to maximize information transmission.

In a recent paper, Jeantheau (33) required subjects to report symbol pairs in "messages" flashed on a screen. Both load and speed were varied. With increased speed, there was an increase in errors.

Load Stress Effects. In general, the load effects to be described comes from the same set of studies previously cited. Conrad's paper in 1951 (9) is a useful starting point. Using the multidial task characteristic of many of the British studies, he found that omissions increased with load and that the percentage of omissions was a function of load level. Number of attempts, on the other hand, was independent of load level. Errors of timing increased with increases in load, so that doubling the load doubled the timing errors. In his analysis of display factors underlying errors of omission (10), error increased with load, although speed had a greater influence. A more detailed analysis of missed signals (11), emphasizing the role of adjacent responses, added no further information to the effects of load. Conrad's study in 1955 (12) was directed specifically to load stress. Subjects performed the multidial task previously described. He obtained increased error with increased load, but the results showed that it was the temporal characteristics of the task produced by load which were important. There was no systematic concentration on any subset of the display elements. Conrad concluded that load should be specifically evaluated in terms of the perceptual content of the display, and that load stress analogous to speed stress was a useful concept in analyzing changes in performance. The findings in the experiment on the effects of load level on self-pacing (14), previously described, were unexpected and unexplainable. Despite variations in load level, the subject maintained the driving speed of the motor controlling display at an average constant rate.

In their visual matching task, Mackworth and Mackworth (37) varied load by having subjects attend to from two to twelve windows. They found that errors and misses increased with load, but that this effect was supplemental to changes produced by speed stress, which was primary. In a similar task, Jeantheau (33) also found that errors increased as load increased. The study by Wagner, Fitts, and Noble (45) used a multichannel display conceptually similar to the Conrad studies. Again the results showed that performance deteriorated as load increased.

The Interaction of Speed and Load. Varying results have been obtained on the interaction of speed and load. Conrad's basic study (9) did not demonstrate an interaction. He states, however, that speed needs to be qualified by load in evaluating multichannel performance, which leaves open the question of an interaction. Wagner, Fitts, and Noble (45) state that the interaction was not significant, but the same laboratory reported a study by Jeantheau (33) using a different kind of task. He found that the interaction was highly significant. Somewhat relevant was another paper from that laboratory (1) in which a significant interaction was obtained between speed and stimulus complexity.

Information analyses which produce a single curve describing performance across all cells of a factorial design leave the question up in the air. Such curves may account for an interaction not specifically discussed. Alluisi, Muller, and Fitts (1), in a visual comparison task requiring either key-pressing or verbal identification, studied the relationship between disjunctive reaction time and the average amount of information transmitted. They manipulated both speed and load, and obtained an increase in information transmission with an increase in alternative stimuli and corresponding decrease in stimulus presentation rate. Jeantheau (33), while obtaining a curve based on an information theory to fit all conditions, did not feel that this analytic technique added anything to the explanation of change in performance. Essentially, the question of an interaction is still a moot point, possibly biased by the emphasis the British researchers put upon the primacy of speed. The kinds of anticipation the task permits and the type of pacing employed, which will be discussed later, may be important factors in studying interaction effects.

Other Factors. Multichannel displays involve multiple elements of information, each of which varies in its relevancy in a number of ways. First of all, the relevancy of a signal varied according to how soon a response must be made to it. This is particularly true in displays providing a continuous flow of information. Those signals calling for a response in the future are temporarily irrelevant. This temporary irrelevancy is enhanced during periods of high signal rate, but has received no study. Secondly, where stimuli vary in complexity, the percentage of irrelevant information varies. Irrelevancy and stimulus complexity become additional load factors under such circumstances. They must be coped with, and so they add to the task load and contribute to further decrement in operator proficiency.

There have been a few studies on this aspect of task stress. In Conrad's study on load stress (12) it was found that irrelevant information play no part in performance changes. Gregg (23) required subjects to detect, discriminate, and respond to four levels of stimulus complexity in an array of stimulus-complexity conditions. He found that both reaction time and errors increased with increasing stimulus complexity (ordered according to a scaling technique based on the physical properties of the stimuli).

Archer (2) felt that these results were related more to the effects of irrelevant information, since subjects in Gregg's study had to abstract elements from the complex displays in order to make their responses. He gave subjects a similar task and controlled both the amount of irrelevant and relevant information. His results showed that response time increased as the amount of relevant information increased, but was not influenced by the amount of irrelevant information. Increasing the amount of relevant information is equivalent to making the display more complex. Archer, Bourne, and Brown (3) then studied the effect of task complexity on concept formation and problem solving. They developed visual stimuli with stimulus-complexity characteristics independent of specific stimulus dimensions and required subjects to classify them. The relevancy of a dimension changed on successive sessions. In contrast to their previous study, performance at concept identification degraded as an exponential function of irrelevant information. The study of Alluisi, Muller, and Fitts (1), previously described, also fits with the above results. They found that increasing the number of alternative stimuli required a corresponding decrease in presentation rate in order to improve information transmission. This area of task stress needs further study, but the results available so far suggest it is an important factor, probably having effects similar to those of load stress. We need to resolve the conflicting results obtained in the studies cited above. Many displays in real systems are more complex than those we use in the laboratory. Concept formation, in the form required by Archer, Bourne, and Brown, is too abstract for studying this aspect of the performance of the system operator. What is needed is a systematic exploration of the problem, using tasks which are meaningful variants of systems tasks. Of some importance is the analysis of the interaction between relevant and irrelevant information at increasing levels of task complexity.

Another factor present when displays provide a continuous flow of information is anticipation. The effects of anticipation on operator performance have been analyzed. Wagner, Fitts, and Noble (45) reported that anticipation does not affect performance on multiple channel situations, but that performance with anticipation sharply deteriorates in the one channel situation. They state that there was no evidence that anticipation has a negative influence on the magnitude of the interaction of speed and load. The two studies specifically reporting no interaction (9, 45) permitted anticipation, but the one study reporting a significant interaction (33) did not. Perhaps anticipation is the controlling factor for evaluating the interaction effects.

Pacing is also a factor that influences operator proficiency. Its effect is primarily on speed stress. Conrad (13) showed that subjects adjust signal rate to create more favorable temporal conditions for responding, but that they do so at an average rate across several load levels (14). Most systems do not permit the operator to control the time characteristics of signal onset or his rate of work, although Conrad points out that even in the externally paced situation operators can modify the rate of change by altering his rate of responding. This adaptation by the operator can be minimized by forcing the operator to respond as rapidly as possible. Alluisi, Muller, and Fitts (1) point out that this causes major alterations in performance, producing a ceiling in information transmission based on both the speed of responding and the range of stimulation.

In the above studies the subject responded discontinuously, i.e., by turning knobs or pressing keys. The emphasis was on the display, or input side of the task. Two studies have been primarily concerned with the motor or output side of performance.

Fitts (15) required subjects to perform several simple, overlearned motor tasks at varying speeds and loads. By an information analysis of the data he found an approximately constant rate of performance across tasks and over a wide range of movements and error tolerances. Outside this range, performance deteriorated. Garvey (16) required subjects to track under a variety of stress-inducing conditions. He found that performance deteriorated under stress, and that differences were accentuated under "good" and "stressful" configurations.

The studies reviewed to this point have been concerned with load and speed levels which did not vary within sessions. One of our current research programs has been directed toward a somewhat different operational problem. We are working on proficiency during sudden, short emergencies ("crises" in terms of the Conrad and Mackworth studies) as a function of base work rate. Using the Complex Behavior Simulator (Figure 1), a systems simulator designed to produce a task like that described earlier, we have varied base work rate. Base rates of 2,000, 1,000, 400, 200, and 100 signals per hour have been used. The load level has been maintained at a constant level of 29 subtasks. Sudden bursts of signals at a rate of 4,000 signals per hour occur on a schedule unknown to the subject. These bursts last for 30 seconds, after which the signal rate returns to the base level. Periods between bursts range from 5 minutes to 25 minutes.

Analyses to date have shown that differences within subjects across days and between subjects as a function of base work rate account for a large part of the variance. In tasks where speed and load levels are low most of the time, individual differences (both between and within operators) plays a major role. In a recent study of vigilance performance (where signal rate was low), Buckner, Harabedian, and McGrath (7) found that individual differences accounted for more than 90 percent of the nonresidual variance.

In a different kind of task, using a test called AUDIT, we have been working on the load variable. Subjects are required to listen to code signals occurring at a constant rate of one every 5 seconds. Three, four, or five different signals are used to vary load. The subject must keep a continuous count of each different signal, holding each count separate from the other, and press the appropriate key when he has counted four of a signal (i.e., four N's). Then he must start counting that signal again without losing his count on the others. The task must be performed for periods of 10, 20, or 30 minutes. This task has high requirements for detection, information-processing, and short-term storage in a complex kind of performance. Analyses to date show decrements due to load, as well as decrements due to duration. There also appears to be a "novelty"

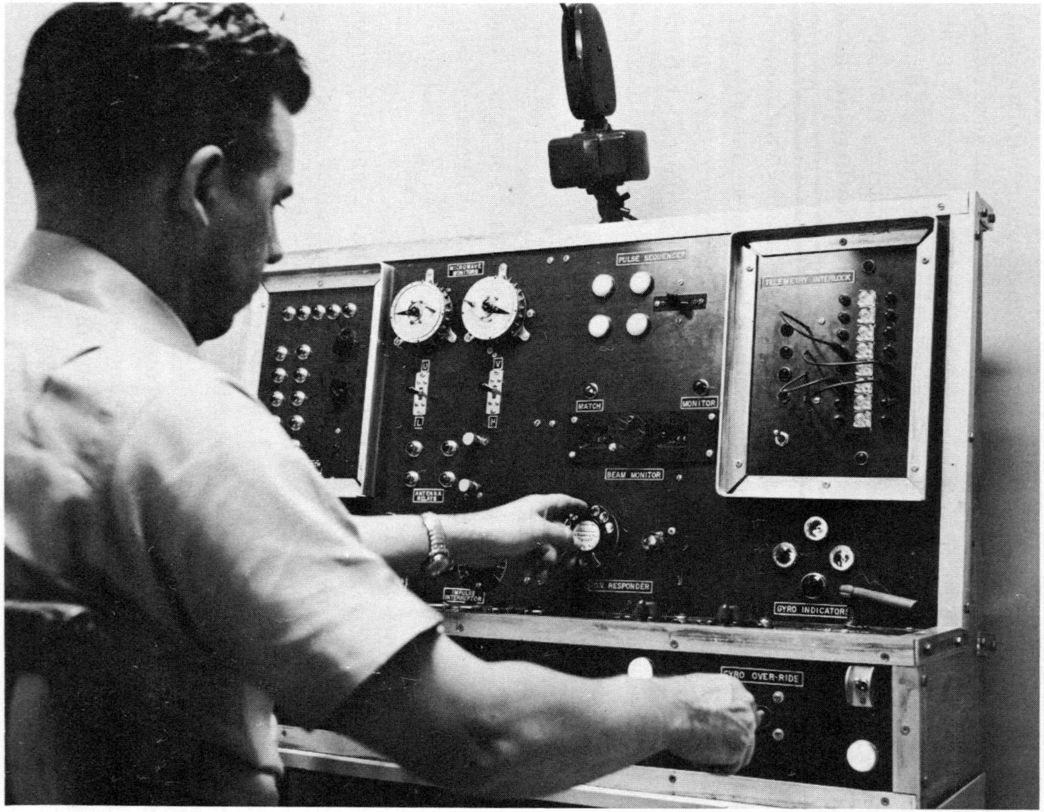

Figure 1. The Subject's Station in the Complex Behavior Simulator

factor related to relatively improved performance on a signal when it appears for the first time.

It is apparent that speed and load are primary factors in systems operator proficiency. Most effects can be accounted for in terms of the speed variable, which plays the major role in determining the temporal characteristics of sequence of signals. Load effects appear to increase the changes related to speed. The interaction of speed and load needs further study, but it may well be a function of task characteristics other than these two variables. Information analyses effectively demonstrate the trade-off necessary to maintain or improve performance at high levels of speed and load. In every case, systematic decrement has been repeatedly demonstrated for the high end of the task stress continuum.

Two kinds of methodological problems have been identified. The first deals with the analysis of performance changes. It is clear that one must analyze single responses in terms of the signal set from which it comes (10, 11, 12, 13, 37), rather than in terms of mean accuracy. The second concerns task characteristics in general. Anticipation, pacing, stimulus complexity, and amount of relevant and irrelevant information have received far less consideration than they deserve. Another important variable is multivariateness of the elements of these complex tasks. Studies to date have used multichannel tasks in which the channels are homogeneous. Tasks using multichannel, multivariate subtasks need to be studied. The Complex Behavior Simulator which we have developed is such a task.

Several writers (10, 15, 37) have hypothesized that there are central mechanisms involved in this kind of performance which have a fixed capacity. Studies contrasting simple reaction and choice reaction time suggest the same thing. Klemmer found that the subject could not respond to signals in a simple reaction time task at a rate faster than one second (34), but that with choice reaction time, they could perform at a faster rate (35). Broadbent (6) studied the effects of spatial separation on a multichannel auditory task. He states that spatial separation is desirable where the operator must attend to two or more channels, but that with rapid alternation, separation of signal sources may cease to have an advantage. He found that with alternation rates of 2 per second proficiency declined. This value is similar to that in the Klemmer studies and suggests the primacy of time in such a central mechanism. Assuming that the temporal characteristics of a sequency of events are the basic determinants of this fixed capacity of a central mechanism for organizing a behavior appears to be a useful way for accounting for load effects. Schaffer (43) suggests another kind of mechanism might be operating. After reviewing the literature on behavior under stress, he presents a neurophysiological hypothesis to account for changes. He cites two kinds of changes under stress: an increased rate of activity and disorganization, and a decreased range of activity or stereotyping of behavior. He suggests that disorganization (the main stress effect) is due to a "relative functional decortication" in which subcortical emotional centers become dominant over the cortex.

In our work with the Complex Behavior Simulator, we have seen changes during high signal rates like those described by Schaffer. In addition to observable breakdowns in previously systematic scanning behavior, we see "blocks" of several seconds duration, incorrect operation of controls despite a high level of overlearning, and a breakdown in the pairing of displays and controls, which is also highly overlearned.

One further point needs to be considered before terminating this section. Payne and Hauty (41) reported a study on a complex psychomotor task in which load was manipulated over longer blocks of time. They found that performance changes related to load could be described in terms of Hull's reactive inhibition (I_R) formulation. They stated that events such as crisis, disorder, and the pressure of irrelevant information can be regarded as periods of extraordinary expenditure of energy and the production of high levels of I_R. They point out that, in the final analysis, all experimenters on load are up against a lack of suitable scaling techniques for various loads in terms of energy expenditure. This point emphasizes the response side of performance. If the energy expenditure approach to speed and load effects turns out to be appropriate, the findings on speed stress will require reevaluation.

In any event, this much is obvious about the short-term effects of task stress on the reliability of the operator in a complex system. Operator proficiency at any point in time is determined largely by the machine. If it overloads him by imposing requirements high in load stress or speed stress, his performance will deteriorate. This decrement, which will be a loss from whatever level of proficiency the long-term effects permit, will occur almost instantaneously and will be a function of the temporal characteristics of the events (signals) imposed upon him during this "crisis."

It should be apparent that the engineer will have a more direct influence on this aspect of operator reliability than the human factors specialist. When designing a system, engineers parcel out the functions which the operator will perform. Designers of the several subsystems make these allocations in accordance with the functional requirements of the system, sometimes without regard for competing requirements from other subsystems. There is a natural tendency to exploit the operator's talents as a "switcher" and a decision-maker. Multiple demands at any point in system function can easily exceed the operator's capabilities—there is a maximum task load beyond which operator reliability will drop. Degraded system reliability is the inevitable result. The unique contribution of the human factors specialist will be to isolate these overload points through a segment-by-segment analysis of the operator's task, so that these overloads can be reduced to manageable levels.

LONG-TERM EFFECTS

Space flight will require periods of duty for operators which are well beyond those with which we have been concerned to date. In the previous section, we assessed factors which will alter operator proficiency during any specific period in time. At least two long-term factors will be equally important in changing the efficiency of man in space flight. These are fatigue and diurnal variation. Both problems have been with us for a long time, but few studies have been concerned with the effects of requirements of long-term performance interacting with the task of the systems operator. These problems are further complicated by the fact that we will be dealing with very small crews, one or two men, for the foreseeable future at any rate.

Fatigue Effects. Fatigue in complex tasks involves problems different from those in which gross energy expenditure is the primary characteristic. One summary of these changes (26) lists five kinds of decrement: loss of fine motor control, variability in performance, equivalence of stimuli, stereotyping of movements and responses,

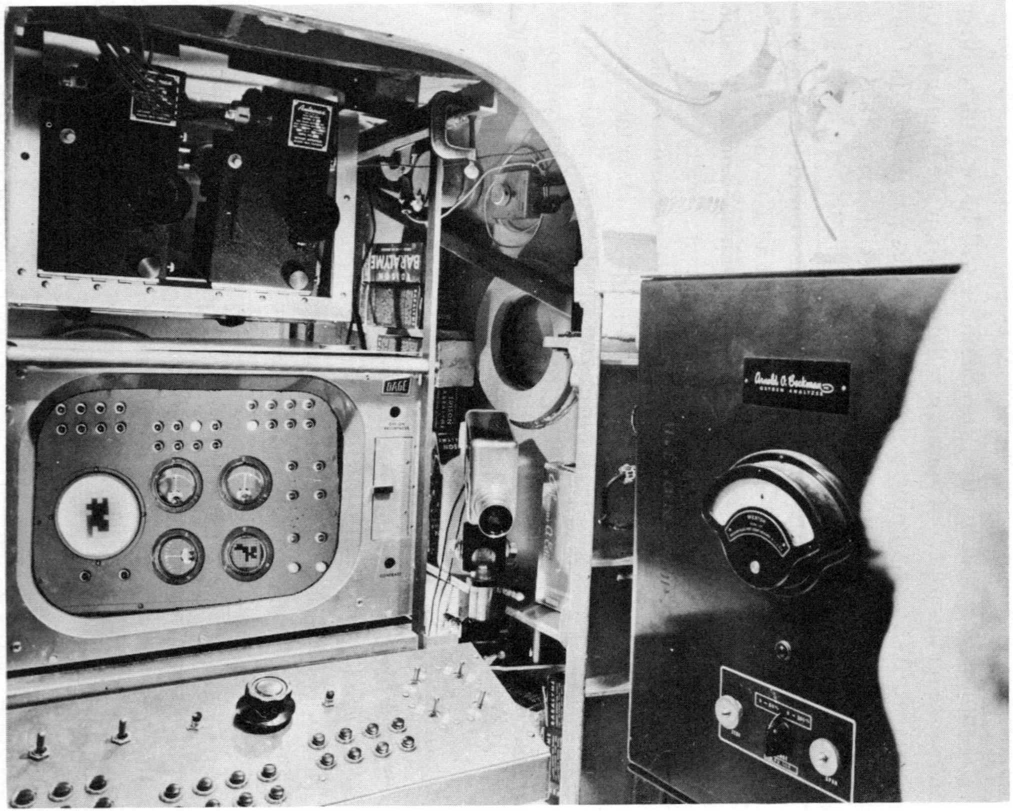

Figure 8. The Oximeter System Used in the One-Man Space Cabin Simulator

dysjunction of discriminations and responses. This study, concerned with changes in alertness overtime when performing complex tasks, suggested some more general mechanisms: loss in flexibility of set, change in controlling set, and an increase in subjective conflicts. It was pointed out, however, that man is able to bring all his capacities to bear on the completion of a task, and that this ability (termed "mobilization of resources") may offset potential decrements when the task can be brought to completion in a short time. This effect probably applies equally to some short periods of high task stress like that described previously. Welford, Brown, and Gabb (46), state that the compensatory and adaptive mechanisms of man are complex and surprising. They suggest that laboratory tasks for studying fatigue in complex performance need to be at least as complex as the task the operator normally deals with.

Hauty (28) emphasizes that the fatigue problem in space flight is complicated by the prolonged commitment of the astronaut to a set of complex functions and by the deleterious effects of loss of sleep. He points out that performance deteriorates rapidly in simple tasks requiring detection of single signals. Such simple tasks will obviously be a part of the astronaut's job. He also emphasizes the importance of individual differences in susceptibility to fatigue. Additional problems are the cumulative effects, deleterious subjective changes, and inadequate perception by the operator of the decrement in skills which have occurred.

In a subsequent paper, Hauty (30) further emphasizes the differential fatigue effects in different classes of tasks. The operator system in the SAM Cabin Simulator (Figure 2) required several different kinds of performance. Hauty concluded from his results that tasks based on gross, discrete cues are more resistant to fatigue than tasks based on *minute* cues, in which vigilance and alertness are important. He states that vigilance is the function most affected by fatigue. A recent investigation on signal detection in a vigilance task (25) showed that detection is better for high rates and short intersignal intervals. This is further support for the susceptibility of vigilance functions to fatigue.

In a report on seven-day flights in the SAM Space Cabin (44), Hauty presented data showing that four pilots maintained proficiency within days and across days when following a working schedule of four hours on and four off. In contrast, his data on a series of 30-hour runs requiring continuous work (29) on the same tasks showed progressive decrement. He concluded that human reliability cannot be extended much beyond 20 hours of continuous work, and that space flights should be programmed to maintain the most effective phase relationships between man's physiological cycle, the period of operation, and local time. He again emphasized that operator reliability could be improved by reducing the vigilance load.

In another paper based on prolonged runs in the SAM Space Cabin program, Gerathewohl (20) used Kraeplin's work performance test (addition of digits). Gerathewohl states that this test is particularly sensitive to changes in proficiency at a long monotonous task. In contrast to Hauty's results, Gerathewohl found that the volume of work done increased each day, and that errors and corrections also increased. It is apparent that, even in the systems environment, the kind of fatigue effect obtained is dependent on task characteristics.

The Problems in Vigilance and Monitoring. Vigilance seems to be a kind of performance susceptible to fatigue effects. We really do not know what happens to proficiency at vigilance tasks over long periods of time. Few vigilance experiments have gone beyond four hours of duty, and none have exceeded eight hours. Decrement in vigilance has received a considerable amount of study, however.

In their recent review of more than eighty experimental papers, McGrath, Harabedian, and Buckner (38) presented an excellent summary of the factors influencing vigilance behavior. There is general agreement that the major drops in proficiency occur within the first half-hour, and that after one hour performance stabilizes. Increases in response latency parallel errors of omission, but errors of commission (false reports) show no temporal changes within a session. Decrement is considerably less with multielement displays, but the over-all level of performance is considerably below that of single-element displays. Improving the detectability of signal increases the probability of detection. The percentage of signals detected is related to signal rate, though this effect may be contaminated by greater regularity of intersignal intervals at higher signal rates. Environmental stress degrades vigilance proficiency, but the introduction of artificial signals improves performance.

Bioelectrical measures show changes during a session, but not in a fashion directly related to signal occurrence and detection. Finally, individual differences play a large role, so it is important to select good "watch-keepers" where the vigilance requirements of a task are high. This is what we know about performance at vigilance tasks. What we do not know, except as suggested by Hauty's work, is what happens when the operator is committed to the task for extended periods of time.

Monitoring performance is another problem. Basically we do not know very much about monitoring behavior. Monitoring and vigilance functions tend to be lumped together. However, when we look at what operators are required to do in these two kinds of tasks, it is probable that there are important differences. In a vigilance task, the operator is required to detect single signals with low attention value and occurring only occasionally over long periods of time. Detection is a critical requirement. The discriminability of the signal is a major variable. In a monitoring task, on the other hand, the operator is usually dealing with multiple signals higher in attention value. Furthermore, many of the displays are presenting information continuously. Information processing is usually the critical requirement. If this is a valid distinction, changes over time should be different. Howland (32) used a task which has the characteristics of monitoring described above. His results showed a progressive increase in errors ("false reports") over a three-hour period. We do not know what happens to proficiency when the operator is committed to the task for extended periods.

Diurnal Effects. Diurnal variation is the other main factor involved in prolonged work. Shifts in proficiency as a function of this cycle are hardly acceptable for space flight. One way around the problem would be to develop techniques for adapting a man to a different cycle matched to the requirements of any specific space mission. But can man be adapted to other schedules? The seven-day runs in the SAM Space Cabin, previously described (44), examined this problem. Instead of the normal schedule of sixteen hours of activity and eight hours for sleep, subjects worked on a four-hours-on, four-hours-off schedule. Subjects quickly adapted to this schedule, sleeping part of every rest period both day and night. One subject showed only partial adaptation, sleeping little during the middle rest period, but this subject also had less total sleep than the others. The stability of performance across the three work periods each day is further evidence of effective adaptation. It appears that the diurnal cycle is easily altered.

In summary, there has been considerable concern in space medicine with fatigue effects as a major factor in reducing operator reliability. In contrast to the changes resulting from task load, long-term changes arise from internal factors in the operator. Under conditions of continuous performance, progressive decrement will occur. Data obtained in the normal 1g environment certainly suggest that it can be critical. Recent findings suggest that different kinds of functions will decline at different rates, so it will be important to engineer those functions most susceptible to fatigue out of the astronaut's job. Vigilance performance, in particular, needs to be eliminated from the operator's task. Displays for monitoring tasks need to be carefully human-engineered. With these kinds of adjustments in the operator's job, it is likely that performance can be maintained at a reasonable level, provided the operator is not required to perform complex tasks continuously. The diurnal cycle seems to be less of a problem. It appears that it can be easily altered with relatively simple procedures, at least in terms of proficiency effects and sleep schedule. As we shall see in the next section, these conclusions are subject to modification. Prolonged weightlessness may alter the long-term effects considerably.

THE SPECIAL PROBLEM OF WEIGHTLESSNESS

The effects on proficiency of weightlessness as an environmental stressor require special consideration here. Weightlessness represents a unique stressor in space flight. Engineering solutions to minimize this source of stress can at best be only partial solutions. There is every reason to believe that it will have systematic effects on operator efficiency. It is logical to assume that both the short-term and long-term effects, which are the concern of this paper, will be compounded by the stressors inherent in the weightless or nearly weightless state.

Weightlessness has proved to be an exceptionally difficult variable to study. No techniques for producing prolonged periods of true weightlessness have been developed. Centrifuges have been of some limited value. The use of elevators and parachute drops has also been suggested, but such techniques produced the weightless state for only a few seconds at a time. Flying an aircraft through a Keplerian trajectory has become a standard technique for producing longer periods of weightlessness. Weightless states of the order of a minute can be obtained by this technique, but it is apparent that this is far short of an effective procedure for analyzing prolonged periods of weightlessness.

Physiological, functional, and skills changes have been studied by this technique. Gerathewohl (18) has studied aiming precision during these short zero-gravity states and has observed systematic changes in the mean point of contact, average error, and the associated variances. Similar changes in eye-hand coordination have been reported by Von Beckh (5). It appears that these changes represent only a moderate disturbance in eye-hand coordination. In another paper (17), Gerathewohl analyzed changes in visual perception. He found an apparent displacement of perceived objects in a direction opposite to the changes in g-forces. He states that it is probable some minor impairment will occur, in the form of illusions and a hypersensibility of receptors.

These results have been concerned with entry into the weightless state. Reentry into the normal-gravity environment has also received some consideration. The data obtained by Von Beckh (5) suggested a reduced tolerance to g-stress upon reentry, but no performance data related specifically to the reentry problem was obtained. Henry *et al.* (31) reported that mice exposed to periods of two to three minutes of zero-gravity demonstrated normal dexterity and coordination upon return. Somewhat less relevant to the reentry problem, but still of interest, are two papers on tolerance to complex g-forces of the type for a vehicle reentering in an unstable state. Clarke and Headley (8) showed that monkeys could still make coordinated movements despite moderate disorientation after such centrifugation. Koehler (36) showed that subjects could continue to perform a motor task under these conditions.

None of these studies involved prolonged weightlessness. We might assume that weightlessness will pose no special performance problems for the astronauts. At the present time, this is only an assumption. We might maintain our concern with the effects associated with long periods in the weightless state. Gerathewohl

(19) in an excellent review of the physics of weightlessness and the history of research on the problem, emphasized that prolonged weightlessness will produce major changes in the astronaut. He suggested that man *will* be able to tolerate prolonged exposure, but that this is not the problem. The real difficulty will be readjustment to the 1g state upon return. He felt that the physiological effects (as in circulation, digestion, and muscular function) of returning to the normal gravity environment will involve major disturbances. He pointed out that the astronaut's job will be largely an "automatic, push-button affair" and that only on reentry will skill be required. It is precisely at this point, however, that major physiological disturbances (and concomitant performance disruptions) will occur.

In an earlier exploratory study we obtained exactly the kinds of effects predicted by Gerathewohl. A quasi-weightless state was produced by the water-immersion technique. The apparatus used in this study is shown in Figure 3. The subject was immersed for seven days. During immersion, systematic adaptive kinds of biological changes occurred (21). Accompanying this was a gradual decline in proficiency at a multielement systems task (27). In effect, the subject tolerated this quasi-weightless state well. However, dramatic decrements, primarily functional debilitation but reflected in performance, occurred upon return to the normal 1g state. To the observers, it was obvious that the subject would be markedly inefficient in performing complex tasks skillfully. If these results are valid, we have been dangerously complacent about the effectiveness of man in space flight.

Some concern has been expressed over the compounding of fatigue effects and lack of sleep in space flight. We analyzed sleep characteristics in the study just described, and found that the subject slept considerably less than normal without untoward effects (39). The subject averaged a little more than two hours of sleep each day over the seven-day period and appeared to be normally refreshed upon awakening. Furthermore, sleep states were characteristically drowsy or light sleep. This suggests that the astronaut will be easily aroused and reasonably effective in the event of an emergency during his sleep period. It also implies that fatigue in and of itself may be less of a problem during the weightless part of space flight. On the basis of our sleep results, we hypothesized that the major biological function of sleep is to permit recovery from a neuromuscular debt accumulated from the day-long task of counteracting gravity, and that the total amount of work performed in the weightless environment is considerably less than in a normal gravity environment.

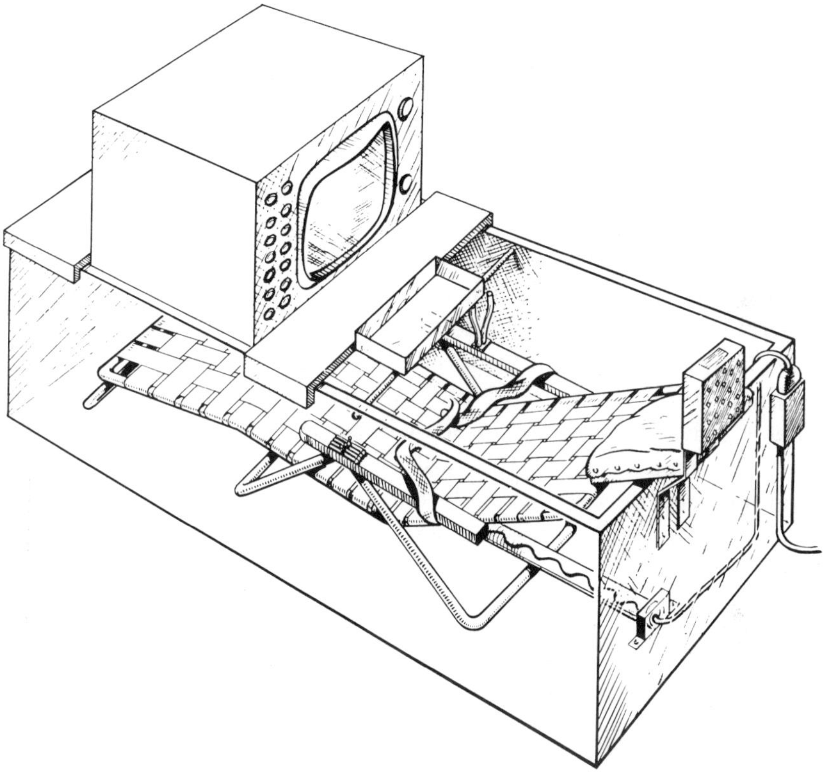

Figure 3. Apparatus for Studying Psychological and Biological Changes Resulting from Prolonged Exposure to Hypodynamic (Weightless) Environment

This hypothesis can be extended to fatigue. If correct, it means that an astronaut will be able to perform for considerably longer periods of steady work without deleterious effects.

In summary, it appears that weightlessness will be a problem primarily upon reentry. The magnitude of the problem has not yet been established, but reentry is a critical point in space flight and even minor decrements will be of considerable concern. Sleep will be less of a problem, if our results in the hypodynamic (water-immersion) environment are confirmed.

SUMMARY

This paper has been concerned with the effects of time and load factors on the reliability of man in space flight. The review of the literature has been restricted to studies in which men performed tasks like those of the operator of complex systems. The importance of conceiving the role of the astronaut as a systems operator cannot be underestimated—this concept is the key to evaluating the relevance of published and ongoing research.

The review has been broken down into two main aspects: short-term effects, which are a function of task load at any point in time; and long-term effects, which are a function of changes within the operator over time. Weightlessness, and its influence on long term effects, was given separate consideration.

Short-term effects are primary in determining operator reliability. These effects arise from the load imposed on the operator by the system. Signal rate is the basic variable. Signal density varies continuously during the operation of a system. When periods of high density occur, performance falls off almost immediately. When long periods of low density occur, performance drops off gradually, and the effects do not become apparent for some time. Although operator reliability is degraded in either case, different mechanisms are involved.

For the high task load situation, the operator is limited by a built-in, fixed ceiling in his ability to integrate, organize, and respond to a sequence of events. This limit is absolute, and its effects begin to occur automatically as soon as the operator's maximum capacity is reached. Acute disorganization can occur if exposure to this overload is extended. The mechanism is one involving higher cortical functions in the complex kinds of behavior which man performs so well.

Operator reliability can be achieved by redesigning the system to eliminate these periods of operator load. Only a segment-by-segment analysis of the operator's job can isolate those periods where the task has exceeded the operator's capabilities.

For the low task load situation, operator effectiveness is altered by a more primitive and biological mechanism. Though more obscure than man's fixed capacity, it appears to involve the concept of activation or arousal. The effect builds slowly over time, rather than appearing immediately. There is a gradual reduction in sensory efficiency, probably at cortical levels which are mediated by the ascending reticular activating system.

Detection, which is basic to vigilance tasks, is an example of a function which suffers in this situation. Basically, man is not a good "watch-keeper." Vigilance, which involves very low signal rates, is highly susceptible to fatigue effects and probably should be engineered out of the astronaut's job.

On the other hand, monitoring, which involves moderately low signal rates, is an inherent part of the job of a systems operator. When carried out against a background of related activities, monitoring can be maintained at an efficient level over extended periods. Such a background serves to prevent deactivation. Intensive human engineering to maximize the efficient presentation of information will be important.

A major problem in operator reliability will be proficiency during reentry. It is imperative that we study changes in the functional state of man immediately after a period of prolonged weightlessness. There is every reason to expect gross functional alterations in the operator as a result of biological adjustments to prolonged weightlessness. Reentry to the normal gravitational environment is sudden, and the astronaut is poorly prepared biologically to cope with g-stress. Gross functional disturbances will be reflected in critically degraded performance capabilities, which can be a major problem if the astronaut's functions are vital at this point in the mission. Admittedly, it will be difficult to study this problem. It may be necessary to make reentry largely automatic until space flight itself establishes the limits of man's capability at this point in the mission.

The long-term effects of fatigue and diurnal variation will probably be less critical than early workers in space medicine anticipated. It appears that diurnal variation will pose few performance problems. Fatigue may be somewhat more important, and consideration must be given to adjusting the work schedule of the astronaut to minimize fatigue effects. However, fatigue effects will certainly be secondary to short-term effects. It should be emphasized that the compound effects of sleep deprivation and fatigue are likely to be considerably less severe than we might anticipate from our 1g point of view. Exploratory research suggests that considerably less sleep will be required in the weightless environment.

Man is remarkably adaptive—he will function in space better than we have any right to expect. But reliability is not accidentally achieved. We must structure his job to insure that proficiency is maintained at a high level. The astronaut's contributions to the exploration of space can be fully realized only if we make our contributions with maximum effectiveness.

REFERENCES

1. Alluisi, E. A., P. F. Muller, Jr., and P. M. Fitts, An information analysis of verbal and motor responses in a forced-paced serial task, J. Exper. Psychol., 53:153–158, 1957.
2. Archer, E. J., Identification of visual patterns as a function of information load J. Exper. Psychol., 48:313–317, 1954.
3. Archer, E. J., L. E. Bourne, and F. G. Brown, Concept identification as a function of irrelevant information and instructions, J. Exper. Psychol., 49:153–164, 1955.
4. Bamford, H. E., L. F. Hanes, and S. E. Wilson, Missions for manned military spacecraft, Human Factors, 1:16–29, 1954.
5. Beckh, H. J. von, Human reactions during flight to acceleration preceded by or followed by weightlessness, J. Avn. Med., 23, 1952.
6. Broadbent, D. E., The role of auditory localization in attention and memory span, J. Exper. Psychol., 47:191–196, 1954.
7. Buckner, D. H., A. Harabedian, and J. J. McGrath, A Study of Individual Differences in Vigilance Performance. Tech. Rep. No. 2., Human Factors Research, Inc., Los Angeles, Calif., Jan., 1960.
8. Clarke, N. P., and R. N. Headly, Studies of primate tolerance to complex accelerations, Aerospace Med., 30:825–831, 1959.
9. Conrad, R., Speed and load stress in a sensory-motor skill, Brit. J. Indust. Med., 8:1–7, 1951.
10. Conrad, R., Missed signals in a sensory-motor skill, J. Exper. Psychol., 48:1–9, 1954.
11. Conrad, R., Adaptation to time in a sensory-motor skill, J. Exper. Psychol., 49: 115–121, 1955.
12. Conrad, R., Some effects on performance of changes in perceptual loads, J. Exper. Psychol., 49:313–322, 1955.
13. Conrad, R., The timing of signals in skill, J. Exper. Psychol., 51:365–370, 1956.
14. Conrad, R., and B. A. Hille, Self-pacing performance as a function of perceptual load, J. Exper. Psychol., 53:52–54, 1957.
15. Fitts, P. M., The information capacity of the human motor system in controlling the amplitude of movement, J. Exper. Psychol., 47:381–391, 1954.
16. Garvey, W. D., The Effects of Task-Induced Stress on Man-Machine System Performance. NRL Report 5015, Sept., 1957, Naval Research Lab., Washington, D.C.
17. Gerathewohl, S. J., Physics and psychophysics of weightlessness: visual perception, J. Avn. Med., 23:373–395, 1952.

18. Gerathewohl, S. J., Sensory-motor performance during weightlessness: eye-hand coordination, J. avn. Med., 28:7–12, 1957.
19. Gerathewohl, J. J., Weightlessness—the problem and the Air Force research program, Air Univ. Quart. Rev., X:No. 2:121–141, 1958.
20. Gerathewohl, S. J., Work proficiency in the space cabin simulator, Aerospace Med., 30:722–735, 1959.
21. Graveline, D. E., and B. Balke, Biological Hypodynamics: Implications in Prolonged Weightlessness. Sch. of Avn. Med., USAF, Rep. No. 60–88, Sept., 1960. Brooks AFB, Texas.
22. Graybiel, A., *et al.*, An account of experiments in which two monkeys were recovered unharmed after ballistic space flight, Aerospace Med., 30:871–931, 1959.
23. Gregg, L. W., The effects of stimulus complexity on discrimination processes, J. Exper. Psychol., 18:289–297, 1954.
24. Grissom, V., Wild 3-way tumbles in Mastif, Life, April 11, 1960.
25. Harabedian, A., J. J. McGrath, and D. N. Buckner, The Probability of Signal Detection in a Vigilance Task as a Function of Intersignal Interval. Tech. Rep. No. 3, Human Factors Research, Inc., Los Angeles, Calif., 1960.
26. Hartman, B., and P. M. Fitts, The Development of Techniques and Procedures for the Study of Alertness in Aviation Personnel. NRC Comm. on Aviation Psychology, Washington, D.C., 1950.
27. Hartman, B., R. E. McKenzie, and D. E. Graveline, An Exploratory Study of Changes in Performance in the Hypodynamic Environment. Sch. of Avn. Med., USAF, Rep. No. 60–72, July, 1960. Brooks AFB, Texas.
28. Hauty, G. T., Human performance in the space travel environment, Air Univ. Quart. Rev., 10:No. 2, 1958.
29. Hauty, G. T., Maximum Effort–Minimum Support Simulated Space Flights. Paper presented at the annual meeting of the Institute of Aeronautical Sciences, New York, Jan., 1960.
30. Hauty, G. T., Psychological Problems in Space Flight. Unpublished paper presented at the School of Aviation Medicine.
31. Henry, J. P., R. T. Ballinger, R. T., P. J. Mahn, and D. G. Simons, Animal studies of the subgravity states during rocket flight, J. Avn. Med., 23:521–432, 1952.
32. Howland, D., An Investigation of the Performance of the Human Monitor. WADC Tech. Note No. 57-431, July, 1958. Wright Air Development Center, Wright-Patterson AFB, Ohio.
33. Jeantheau, G., The Differential Effects of Speed and Load Stress on Task Performances. WADC Tech. Rep. No. 59-7, July, 1959. Wright Air Development Center, Wright-Patterson AFB, Ohio.
34. Klemmer, E. T., Time uncertainty and simple reaction time, J. Exper. Psychol., 51:179–184, 1956.
35. Klemmer, E. T., Rhythmic disturbances in a simple visual-motor task. Am. J. Psychol., 70:56–63, 1957.
36. Koehler, R. C., Human pilot performance during boost and atmospheric re-entry. Aerospace Med., 30:481–486, 1959.
37. Mackworth, J. F., and N. H. Mackworth, The overlapping of signals for decisions, Am. J. Psychol., 69:26–47, 1956.
38. McGrath, J. J., A. Harabedian, and D. N. Buckner, Review and Critique of Literature on Vigilance Performance. Tech. Rep. No. 1, Human Factors Research, Inc., Los Angeles, Calif., Dec., 1959.
39. McKenzie, R. E., B. Hartman, and D. E. Graveline, An Exploratory Study of Sleep Characteristics in the Hypodynamic Environment. Sch. of Avn. Med., USAF, Rep. No. 60–68, Oct., 1960. Brooks AFB, Texas.
40. Melton, A. W., and G. E. Briggs, Engineering psychology, Ann. Rev. Psychol., 11:71–98, 1960.

41. Payne, R. B., and G. T. Hauty, Reactive Inhibition as a Function of Task Load and Its Temporal Distribution. Unpublished study.
42. Ritchie, M. L., Man-machine dynamics in orbital vehicles, in *Human Control Dynamics in Air and Spacecraft*, B. J. Smith, ed., New York, Flight Safety Foundations, Inc., 1958.
43. Schaffer, H. R., Behavior under stress: A neurophysiological hypothesis, Psychol. Rev., 61:323–333, 1954.
44. Steinkamp, G. R., W. R. Hawkins, G. T. Hauty, R. B. Burwell, and J. E. Ward, Human experimentation in the space cabin simulator, Sch. of Avn. Med., USAF, Rep. No. 59–101, 1959.
45. Wagner, R. C., P. M. Fitts, and M. E. Noble, Preliminary Investigations of Speed and Load as Dimensions of Psychomotor Tasks. AFPTRC Res. Rep. No. 54-45, AF Pers. & Tng Res. Cen., Lackland AFB, Texas, 1954.
46. Welford, A. T., R. A. Brown, and J. E. Gabb, Two Experiments on Fatigue as Affecting Skilled Performance in Civilian Aircrew. Flying Personnel Research Committee 725, NRUPA Rep. No. 6, 1949.
47. Williams, A. C., Jr., and C. O. Hopkin, Aspects of Pilot Decision Making. Wright Air Development Center, Rep. No. 58-522, Dec., 1958.

Skill Maintenance under Adverse Conditions

PAUL M. FITTS

This paper will present a review of procedures than can be expected to lessen the effects of adverse environments on skilled performance. First, however, let us enumerate these adverse conditions and review briefly several theories regarding the nature of stress and its effects on skilled performance.

TYPES OF ADVERSE TASK ENVIRONMENTS

At least eight factors can be listed which usually have an adverse effect on skilled performance. These include (1) information overload (as already discussed by Miller and by Hartman); (2) danger or other conditions which result in fear, anxiety, or other emotional responses; (3) extreme environmental conditions such as cold, heat, vibration, intense noise, and glare; (4) noxious substances, including radiation effects; (5) restriction of movement and lack of sufficient variation in sensory inputs; (6) physical deprivations arising from restriction of food, water, or air intake; (7) long periods of intense work without adequate rest cycles (fatigue, etc.); and finally (8) inability to practice a skill under the conditions necessary for maintaining adequate proficiency may also be classed as an adverse condition.

THEORIES OF HUMAN RELIABILITY

One way to go about solving the problem of maintaining skills at a satisfactory level under adverse conditions would be by taking the steps indicated by well established theory. Therefore let us review briefly several of the better known theories which attempt to predict human reliability and see what they suggest about skill maintenance.

Interest in the topic of human reliability has centered on the

Dr. Fitts is Professor of Psychology and Director of Graduate Studies, Department of Psychology, University of Michigan.

topic of stress. The effects of stress on skilled performance have recently been reviewed by James Deese in a paper given at a symposium on training sponsored by the University of Pittsburgh. In this paper Deese points out that there are two views of stress. First, stress may be conceived as a mediating variable, a state aroused in an individual by particular environmental stimuli and chronically present in some individuals. This internal state presumably interferes with performance and thus contributes to unreliability. An interest that has been typical of investigators who have viewed stress as an internal state has been the identification of "high anxious" individuals, by psychometric devices such as the Manifest Anxiety Scale (16) or other diagnostic tools, and the prediction of ways in which these individuals will differ from "low anxious" individuals with respect to learning and performance. As far as large-scale practical applications are concerned, however, this approach has not proven very successful, since the correlations between the tests of manifest anxiety and subsequent performance have been uniformly quite low when applied to large groups of individuals. It may permit the elimination of a certain portion of the population from assignment to extra-hazardous occupations in connection with space, of course, as several previous papers have indicated.

Second, stress has been viewed as a collection of external (stimulus) events rather than as an internal state of the individual. This is in general the view which is characteristic of the previous papers which have dealt with stressful environments. Proponents of this view hold that stressful environments may have a quite different effect on different individuals—i.e., they assume differential susceptibility to stress.

Deese (5), while preferring to consider stress as a stimulus condition, has proposed that the effects of any particular set of environmental conditions upon skilled performance are specific to particular components of performance. A given set of conditions is not necessarily detrimental to all skilled tasks. As an illustration, stress may improve the force or speed of movements while at the same time reducing the precision of movements.

A further illustration of the differential effects of stress is the view held by most coaches that stress usually improves the play of athletes, such as football linemen, who must make simple, gross body movements, but may disrupt performance that requires more complex and varied activity, such as the play of a quarterback.

The view of stress that predicts differential effects on different tasks makes the topic of maintaining skills in adverse environments a complex one, since the procedure that is to be recommended is highly dependent on what skills are involved and what types of environmental stresses are encountered.

A MULTIPLE APPROACH TO SKILL MAINTENANCE

The present writer prefers the view of stress which holds that specific environmental conditions that are generally regarded as adverse or stressful will affect different aspects of skills and different people in different ways, not always detrimentally. Consistent with this view I should now like to discuss six different avenues to the maintenance of skill under adverse conditions. These six avenues are: (1) task simplification, (2) reduction of temporary input overload conditions, (3) feedback augmentation in low-input tasks, (4) overtraining in subroutines of complex tasks, (5) training for specific emergency procedures, and (6) use of optimum work cycles. Each of these avenues for improving the reliability of human skills will now be reviewed.

TASK SIMPLIFICATION

It is possible that the tasks assigned to a man may be underdemanding as well as overdemanding. However, let us start with a consideration of those tasks and situations where there are too many things for a man to do and too short a time in which to do them—situations such as Miller and Hartman have already analyzed. Thus we shall consider first the possibilities and advantages of task simplification when there is input overload, speed and load stress, or undue task complexity.

Given a particular task, such as stabilizing a space vehicle or solving a navigation problem, it has been shown by numerous experiments that the displays, controls, procedures, etc., which result in best performance under idealized conditions nearly always are the best for use under stressful conditions. Several lines of evidence for this conclusion will be reviewed.

Roger Loucks (10), conducting research at the Air Force School of Aviation Medicine during the Second World War, was the first to propose, as a fundamental concept of engineering psychology, that stress increases the importance of good task design. Loucks argued that under conditions of stress pilots and other operators of complex equipment would be likely to revert to "natural" modes of response. He wrote:

> The indicator which the novice can interpret most easily provides the minimal possibility of error when used by the more experienced pilot who has been trained on that same instrument. In contrast, the indicator which is difficult to master usually causes confusion because it tends to elicit perceptual-motor responses which conflict with those required for correct interpretation. The ambiguous instrument requires the subject to inhibit or block his immediate or direct response tendency and forces him to substitute an "unnatural" or sophisticated reaction. Inasmuch as an individual's perceptual habits are usually built up over a period of years and, in many instances, are based upon inborn reaction tendencies, an instrument which requires a subject to break up such well-established response systems is to be avoided whenever possible. Not only is a needlessly long period of training required, but the possibility can never be completely eliminated that under conditions of stress or fatigue the pilot may revert to his original and more "natural" way of interpreting the instrument. (p. 112)

Thus Loucks argued that stress does not result in variability or unreliability per se, but may elicit older, longer established habits.

In the years since Louck's article was published, a variety of studies have shown him to be correct in his basic assumption. Fitts and Jones (6), in critical-incident interviews with pilots, uncovered many instances of reversal errors made by highly experienced pilots in interpreting aircraft instruments, errors clearly due to the use of display designs that were contrary to long established perceptual habits which pilots possessed prior to training. Charles Simon (13) found evidence for an increase in reversal errors when stress was introduced into a laboratory task. Garvey and Taylor (9), in three separate experiments, found that initial differences between systems (displays, controls, etc.) became greater when the operator was stressed. They produced stress in a variety of ways, such as by prolonged work and by the addition of secondary tasks or other complications of the job to be performed. Recent work by Lt. Col. R. E. Murphy (12) also gave similar results.

In summary, it appears that one of the best ways of increasing the likelihood of reliable performance under unfavorable environmental conditions is to insure that the responses that will be required of a man are compatible with his long established habits, i.e., are "natural" ones.

REDUCTION OF INFORMATION OVERLOAD DURING PEAK PERIODS OF WORK

Dr. James Miller and Dr. Bryce Hartman at this symposium, and Mackworth (11) and Conrad (3) in earlier publications, have emphasized the limited nature of man's capacity for dealing with information when it is received at too great a rate, or from too many sources at once.

It hardly needs to be pointed out that one important way to improve human reliability is to minimize the effects of these temporary periods of overloading. This can be done in several ways.

At the U.S. Naval Electronics Laboratory a short-term storage device has been tried out with men who had to work at a task, such as that of an airport control tower operator, where several messages may come in simultaneously. The device stored one or more of the voice communications, permitting the operator to listen to the message he wanted to hear at the moment. Thus the operator could avoid the stress of having to cope with several simultaneous auditory inputs.

A promising technique for reducing information overload effects has been perfected recently by Lindquist at Minneapolis Honeywell in connection with work on Project Mercury. He performed a microanalysis of the information to be handled from second to second during potential critical periods of orbiting flight and reentry, and then adjusted the operator's task so that there was no chance that the total information rate during these critical periods would exceed the capacity of the operator. This type of analysis involves the estimation of the net information rate for the varied aspects of the task, as this changes from time to time, plus the estimation of the operator's peak capacity.

Still other avenues to the reduction of peak overload effects have been studied by psychologists at Rand and at the System Development Corporation (2). This group has been especially interested in analyzing the means used by a team of operators in adapting to increased work loads. One such procedure is the balancing of loads among operators who learn to assist each other when a temporarily heavy load falls on a particular person or work station. Capacity for load-balancing depends on several factors, including training and the ability of operators to share information.

In all of this discussion it has been assumed that there is no control over the input itself, only control over the ways in which the input is displayed, stored, distributed, etc. If the input load itself can be controlled, then the problem is considerably simplified. A forced-paced task can be changed into a self-paced task, or the operator can be given control over the rate of input information.

It is often possible to reduce the peak information loads on a system by redesign of system components. Consider an example from Project Mercury. One of the most critical aspects of this flight is the maintenance of proper vehicle attitude during retrorocket firing. Attitude maintenance is important because the direction of the thrust exerted by the rockets relative to the flight path is critical if proper reentry is to be achieved. The present design of the rocket system produces a very high information rate for a period of about thirty seconds, a rate which may come close to exceeding human tracking ability. This high information rate results from the fact that the three retrorockets fire in rapid succession with periods of overlap. If it were possible to effect the application of reverse thrust over three separate periods of time, a three-dimensional tracking task would be reduced to a considerably simpler one- or at most two-dimensional task, and the information load on the operator might be reduced and the reliability of his performance increased correspondingly.

FEEDBACK AUGMENTATION

The importance of feedback as a factor in the regulation of skilled performance has long been recognized. However, the role of achievement feedback as a means of heightening motivation and of maintaining alertness has only recently been demonstrated experimentally. Two series of experiments deserve special mention.

Smode (14) studied the effects of achievement feedback on learning and performance in a tracking task. In such a task the subject already uses two sources of feedback: (a) internal or proprioceptive feedback arising from his own movements, and (b) external visual feedback which is available from the tracking display. Smode added a third information source, in the form of a decade counter which accumulated a score based on the subject's performance in the task. The latter is called achievement feedback, as distinct from the previously mentioned sources, which are called intrinsic and action feedback respectively.

From one point of view, achievement information feedback might be expected to act as a distraction and thus to interfere with tracking performance. Note that the accumulated score displayed on Smode's decade counter was of no help to the subject in indicating what he should do next; it only told him how well he had been doing in the past. Thus, if he looked away from the tracking display in order to check his accumulated score he risked getting off target. Nevertheless, in Smode's experiment the group of subjects which was given achievement information feedback was markedly (and statistically significantly) superior to the subjects in the control group which used the same tracking display but were only told their score at the end of each 1-minute trial (see Figure 1). In interviews at the end of the experiment, subjects said that the achievement information made the task much more interesting.

The effects of achievement information feedback are not specific to a tracking task. In fact, Smode's experiment was an extension of some earlier work done in collaboration with the present writer and Alfred Leonard (7), in which similar results were obtained in a pattern recognition task.

From a theoretical standpoint, these results are important in suggesting that both learning and performance are dependent on moment-to-moment availability of information regarding the level of success being achieved in a task. It is precisely this kind of information that is so often lacking in military and industrial tasks. The worker sees and feels his own responses as he works, but often has little opportunity to evaluate his over-all achievement against an objective standard. By way of contrast, most preferred leisure-time activities do provide good achievement feedback. Every golfer, for example, carries a score card and knows at all times exactly where he stands with respect to par for the number of holes he has played.

Many industrial, military, and space-flight tasks can be designed to incorporate scoring equipment which the operator can use in performing quality control checks on his own work.

Now I would like to turn to a different use of feedback in maintaining performance. This use was dramatically demonstrated by the work of the late F. V. Taylor and his associates, who used

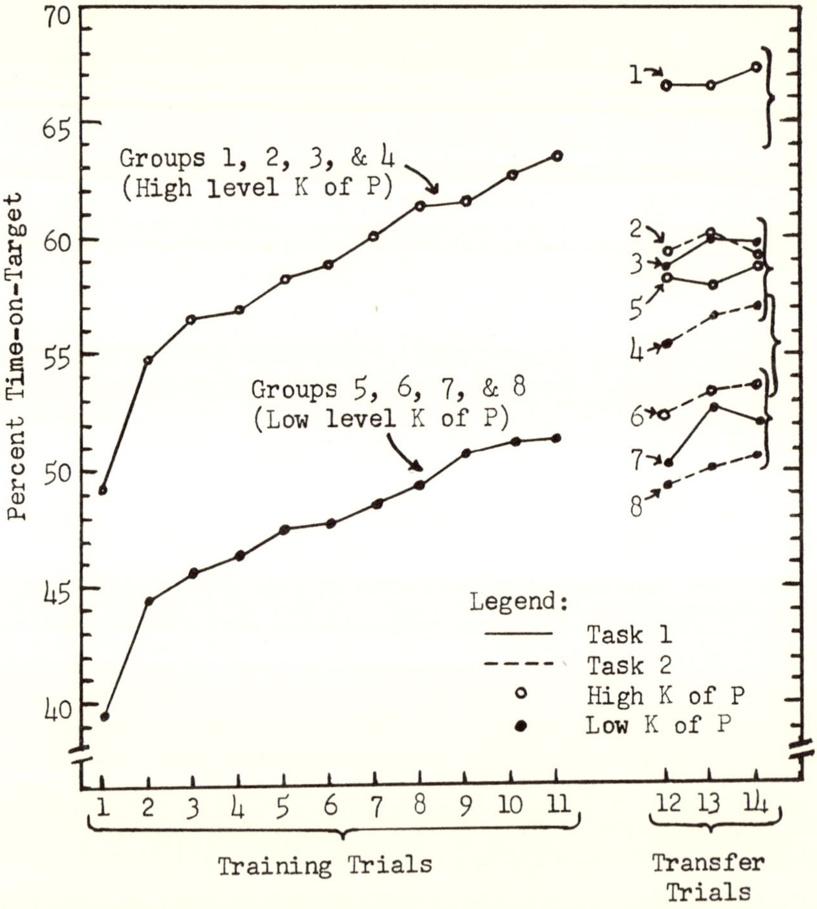

Figure 1. Percentage Time-on-Target Scores

Scores are for high-level and low-level knowledge of achievement (K of P) groups over training and transfer trials (20 Ss per group). Brackets indicate groups that did not differ significantly on the three transfer trials (Duncan's Multiple Range Test). From Smode, 1958.

artificial signals, plus immediate achievement feedback, to maintain the level of alertness in monitoring tasks. In space flight there are likely to be long periods during which very little is happening. It is important to maintain the level of performance under these low information input conditions.

Garvey and Taylor (8) reported a series of studies investigating several of the variables which would be involved if artificial signals were to be employed to enhance monitoring performance in an operational man-machine system. The operators in their experiments searched a bank of dials for two-hour periods, watching for infrequently occurring deviations from normal readings. Seven experiments in all were conducted. The results showed that the addition of "artificial" signals consistently increased speed and accuracy in reporting infrequently appearing "real" signals. These effects apparently were the result of achievement feedback which was given following the appearance of the artificial signals, and perhaps also to the somewhat higher over-all level of resulting activity in the task.

In summary, it appears that achievement feedback, either with respect to a real task or in connection with artificial signals or test problems, can be used (a) to increase motivation, (b) to increase alertness, and (c) to warn operators or their supervisors of any drop in their level of performance during long and monotonous duty assignments. A ground station, for example, could use the feedback to monitor the performance of a monitor in a space vehicle, and the astronaut could monitor himself. With proper attention to feedback in the design of space vehicles, it appears that there should be no occasion where sensory deprivation would interfere with performance.

OVERTRAINING

In most training programs it is customary to specify some level of performance or skill, called the criterion level, which is considered satisfactory for the particular task. This is also known as a training standard. Ordinarily training is terminated as soon as this standard is reached. Overtraining refers to training that is continued after the criterion level is reached. Evidence will now be presented as to the importance of overtraining as a means of improving performance under stress. It will be necessary here to connect two different experimental findings.

The first point to be emphasized is that skill learning, as evidenced by continued improvement in many difficult tasks, appears to go on for many years although at a progressively decreasing rate. Snoddy (15) was one of the first investigators to point this out. Plotting log scores in a mirror drawing task against the log of the number of

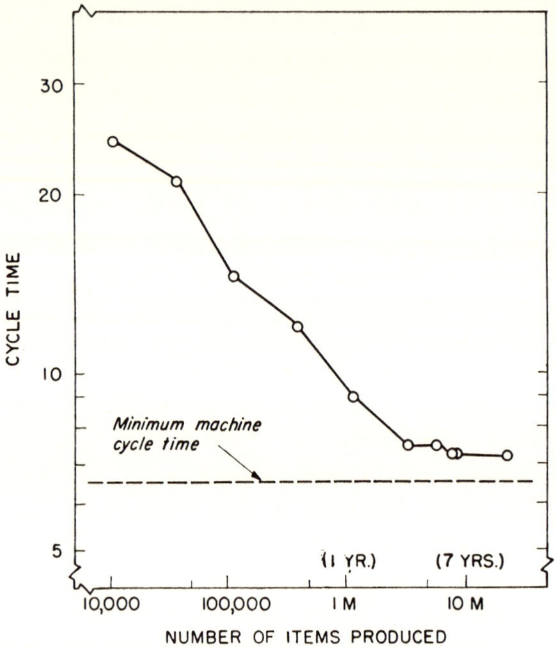

Figure 2. Increase in Speed with Continued Practice in an Industrial Task (Cigar Making)

The ordinate is the total production by the operator since beginning work, a period of over seven years. From Crossman, 1959.

trials, he found that after the first few days learning continued as a straight line with positive slope. Recently Crossman (4) has reviewed the literature on speed skills. He concludes that the important factor that limits improvement over periods of several years of daily practice on the job often is the cycle time of the machine which a worker is using. An example is shown in Figure 2.

The extent of the improvement in skills that is possible from several hours of daily practice is also indicated by another source of evidence. This is the age at which peak or championship performance is achieved. In many skilled activities, such as the production of music, professional sports, and the practice of surgery, individuals reach their peak performance only after ten years or more of work at their specialty.

What does this long-continued improvement in skill mean for the maintenance of performance under stress? Coupled with another experimental finding it has profound significance. This other finding is that overtraining increases the resistance of a skill to interference or disruption from information overload effects or other forms of stress.

Bahrick, Noble, and Fitts (1) showed, for example, that overpractice in an information-transmission task, involving responses to visual stimuli by the right hand, increased resistance to interference from a second task that required the use of the left hand in responding to auditory stimuli. The point to emphasize is that overpractice apparently benefits performance under stress, long after the operator has reached the criterion or standard which was established for the first task.

These results appear to warrant a specific conclusion. Men who are being prepared for an especially difficult and critical task will profit from as much as an hour or more a day of training for periods of a year or more, even if the task itself may last for only a short period of time. In the case of operators who are being prepared for space-flight duties, such training would have to be given in a simulator, of course.

TRAINING FOR THE UNEXPECTED

Another point with regard to training needs to be emphasized. This has to do with practice in emergency procedures. It is a widely accepted design practice today to automate most functions that are repetitious or that can be programmed in advance, reserving for the human operator those functions which must be performed infrequently, under unspecified conditions, and if unforeseen contingencies should arise. It is true that man is capable of solving novel problems, of improvising, and of using ingenuity. However, it is equally true that his capacity for performing novel tasks is greatly enhanced by training. The conclusion is obvious. A great deal of emphasis, in training, should be given to practice in procedures that may never have to be used. In this way performance under the stress of an emergency may to a considerable extent be converted to a routine performance in which the operator relies on well established habits.

An earlier conclusion, regarding the importance of designing the displays and controls so that they are compatible with old habits (population stereotypes) should be reemphasized in connection with this discussion of emergency procedures.

USE OF OPTIMUM WORK-REST CYCLES

Another important source of stress is that arising from long periods of work without adequate rest.

Data reported in preceding papers have shown that tasks which require continuous alertness and a high level of activity usually are performed at peak efficiency for only relatively short periods of time. It is true that man can, if sufficiently motivated, perform feats of remarkable endurance. Fighter escort missions during the Second World War and the Indianapolis Memorial Day automobile races provide examples. Nevertheless, scientific data indicate that relatively short work-rest cycles are to be preferred. Studies of radar observer performance on antisubmarine patrol during the Second World War indicated that peak performance (as evidenced by the number of sightings) was maintained only for an hour or less at a time. The same was true of submarine lookouts who were watching for the patrol planes.

Previous speakers have emphasized the importance of man's diurnal cycles. Perhaps the most significant work during the past decade on the problem of duty cycle has not yet been published. These studies are now underway at Lockheed Aircraft in Marietta, Georgia, under the direction of Oscar Adams and Jack Kraft, and are being supported by the Behavioral Sciences Laboratory, Wright Air Development Division. Recent tests on Strategic Air Command Crews have shown that highly motivated and well trained crews are able to work at a series of exacting tasks for a period of 15 days following a 4-hour-on, 2-hour-off cycle (16 hours of work a day for 15 days without a break). This finding lends encouragement to the belief that a three-man crew might be able to maintain a continuous duty cycle in which one man would rest while the other two would work, provided the duty cycle was sufficiently short. However, it is too early to draw any firm conclusions regarding optimum duty cycles for missions in which a crew of minimum size must continuously perform monitoring and other perceptual and motor tasks in space flight.

SUMMARY

In summary I would like to reemphasize the conclusion that there is no single or simple way to increase the reliability of skilled human performance under environmental and task stress. I have reviewed six avenues to the improvement of reliability. Three have to do with design of equipment and the man-machine system (task simplification, reduction of input information overload, and use of augmented feedback), two have to do with training (overtraining, and training for emergency procedures) and one has to do with the work-rest cycle. There are still other avenues to increased human reliability; for example, I have not touched on the possible use of drugs.

I would like to close on an optimistic note. I believe that man, under reasonable circumstances, is capable of highly reliable performance. Instances from everyday life provide perhaps the best examples. Consider the symphony orchestra as an illustration. This assemblage of highly skilled men is capable, on any given evening, of performing for two hours with a good probability that not one of the notes struck by approximately one hundred musicians will be rendered improperly or occur at the wrong time. Another example of a highly reliable skill is the proper identification of the signature pattern on a check by a clerk in a bank. Millions of times a day people trust their funds to this procedure for transferring money, secure in the knowledge that the chances of an error in signature identification is negligible. A further example of a reliable skill is that involved in passing an automobile on the open highway, the closing speed often being 120 miles an hour or more and the lateral clearance as little as 5 or 6 feet. Unfortunately head-on collisions do occur; the wonder is that they do not occur more often! I estimate that many drivers may pass about one million cars a year, with less than 0.1 percent chance of colliding head-on with any one of them. This gives a probability of less than 1^{-10} of a gross error by either driver in what is actually a complex sequence of perceptual-motor behaviors.

Automata may eventually replace man in performing each of the activities I have cited here as examples, if they become cheaper or more reliable than man. However, the fact remains that man is capable of quite reliable performance in situations where he realizes that reliability is important.

REFERENCES

1. Bahrick, H. P., M. E. Noble, and P. M. Fitts, Extra-task performance as a measure of learning a primary task, J. Exper. Psychol., 48:298–302, 1954.
2. Chapman, R. L., and J. L. Kennedy, The background and implications of the Systems Research Laboratory studies, in G. Finch, and F. Cameron, eds., *Air Force Human Engineering: Personnel and Training Research*, pp. 65–73. ARDC TR 56-8, 1956.
3. Conrad, R., Speed and load stress in a sensorimotor skill, Brit. J. Indus. Med., 8:1–7, 1951.
4. Crossman, E. R. F. W., A theory of the acquisition of speed-skill, Ergonomics, 2:153–166, 1959.
5. Deese, James, Skilled Performance and Conditions of Stress. Paper read at a symposium on training, University of Pittsburgh, Feb., 1960.
6. Fitts, P. M., and R. E. Jones, Psychological Aspects of Instrument Display: I. Analysis of 270 "Pilot Error" Experiences in Reading and Interpreting Instruments. Dayton, Ohio, USAF Air Material Command, Report TSEAA-694-12A, Oct., 1947.
7. Fitts, P. M., and J. A. Leonard, Stimulus Correlates of Visual Pattern Recognition. Final report on Contract Nonr-495 (02), Ohio State Univ. Research Foundation, Columbus, Ohio, Oct., 1957.
8. Garvey, W. D., and F. V. Taylor, The use of "artificial signals" to enhance monitoring performance, in P. M. Fitts, ed., *Human Engineering Concepts and Theory*, pp. 16.1.1–16.1.14. Ann Arbor, Univ. of Michigan Publication Distribution Service, 1959.
9. Garvey, W. D., and F. V. Taylor, Interaction among operator variables, system dynamics, and task-induced stress, J. Appl. Psychol., 43:79–85, 1959.
10. Loucks, R. B., An experimental evaluation of the interpretability of various types of aircraft attitude indicators, in P. M. Fitts, ed., *Psychological Research in Equipment Design*. Washington, D.C., U.S. Govt. Printing Office, 1947.
11. Mackworth, N. H., and J. F. Mackworth, The overlapping of signals for decisions, Am. J. Psychol., 69:26–47, 1956.
12. Murphy, R. E., Effects of threat of shock, distraction, and task design on performance, J. Exper. Psychol., 58:134–141, 1959.
13. Simon, C. W., The Effects of Stress on Performance in a Dominant and Non-dominant Task. Unpublished Ph.D. thesis, Ohio State University, 1952.
14. Smode, A. F., Learning and performance in a tracking task under two levels of achievement information feedback, J. Exper. Psychol., 56:297–304, 1958.
15. Snoddy, G. S., Learning and stability, J. Appl. Psychol., 10:1–36, 1926.
16. Taylor, J. A., The relationship of anxiety to the conditioned eyelid response, J. Exper. Psychol., 41:81–92, 1951.

Measurement of Cognitive Process

SATOSI WATANABE

Investigation of human cognitive process under stress is of importance for two reasons. One obvious reason is that the success of a space flight, partially or totally under human control, depends critically on the adequacy of the cognitive process of the navigating personnel under unusual conditions which prevail in such a flight. A second and less obvious reason is that the study of any property of an object is, as history of science shows, considerably enhanced when the object under investigation is placed under various extreme conditions. An extremely high or low temperature, or a high pressure has proved to be instrumental for the understanding of a physical property of matter under a normal condition. Thus, space flight may become a useful testing laboratory for human cognitive processes in general.

Human cognitive processes may be broadly divided into deductive and inductive process. An example of the deductive process is an effort to answer a question of the following type: Given the speed V of the vehicle, what is the time required for it to reach the destination D miles away? This type of cognitive process can be mechanized relatively easily by the use of a simple computer. More subtle and less easily mechanizable is the process of induction. For instance, two meters on the pilot's control-board suddenly show some irregularities. There are hundreds of possible causes which can give rise to these irregularities. The pilot has to decide his action quickly, basing his decision on his evaluation of the probabilities of various possible causes. This is a typical inductive process, for there is no logically unique solution to the problem except in a special case, and the decision depends on the evaluation of probabilities of various possible causes.

Dr. Watanabe is a Senior Physicist with International Business Machines, and Adjunct Professor of Electrical Engineering, Columbia Univesity.

I do not want here to enter into the old question as to whether inductive process can be entirely performed by a machine or not. My personal view is that in so far as the body of experience is finite, which is always the case with human experience, the machine can be a help but does not give an unambiguous answer to an inductive problem. Whether or not this view is ultimately tenable, there is no doubt about the fact that the human element in a space flight becomes particularly important when an inductive process is involved.

If this thesis is true, it will then be very desirable to measure numerically the amount of inductive reasoning done by a human subject in a given situation. If such a measure can be well defined, it may become possible to compare the inductive ability of a human under normal and adverse conditions. What I want to present in this paper is a method to define such a numerical measure of inductive process. The details of the work on this subject have been published (1), therefore I shall refer here to only a few of the results.

In deductive as well as inductive processes there are usually two sets of propositions, $\mathscr{H} = \{H_1, H_2, H_3, \ldots\}$ and $\mathscr{D} = \{D_1, D_2, D_3, \ldots\}$, and we are interested in two kinds of probabilities, $p(D_i/H_j)$ and $q(H_j/D_i)$. Characteristic of this problem is that one of the two probabilities, say p, is determined by the nature of $\mathscr{H}$ and $\mathscr{D}$ only, while the other, q, is not determined by $\mathscr{H}$ and $\mathscr{D}$ only. If p and q are thus defined, then $\mathscr{H}$ becomes a family of hypotheses and $\mathscr{D}$ becomes a set of possible observed data. The quantity $p(D_i/H_j)$ is the probability of obtaining an observed datum D_i on the assumption that H_j is true. Therefore, p is a deductive probability. The quantity $q(H_j/D_i)$ is the probability of the hypothesis H_j being true on the basis of the observed datum D_i. Thus q is an inductive probability.

In most cases, we can repeat the same experiment which may yield various results contained in $\mathscr{D}$. Suppose we repeat the experiment ν times and let $q^{(\nu)}(H_j)$ be the inductive probability we attach to hypothesis H_j on the basis of ν observed data. Then introduce the entropy function $U^{(\nu)}$ by

$$U^{(\nu)} = -\sum_j q^{(\nu)}(H_j) \log q^{(\nu)}(H_j). \tag{1}$$

This inductive entropy has to decrease with time at least on the average, for our inductive probabilities attached to various hypotheses must become more and more concentrated on fewer and fewer hypotheses. This is a tendency opposite to the usual H-Theorem. Thus we can expect an "*inverse H-Theorem*":

$$\frac{dU^{(\nu)}}{d\nu} \leqslant 0 \tag{2}$$

on the average. When $U^{(\nu)} = 0$, induction is completed, for all but one hypothesis are discredited. For this reason $-dU^{(\nu)}/d\nu$ may be called the *rate (speed) of induction.*

If the observed data are distributed according to the law of independent events and if we use Bayes' Theorem for the evaluation of $q^{(\nu)}(H_j)$, we can indeed mathematically prove (2) as the expected behavior of the inductive inference. In the case where only one hypothesis finally survives ($U^{(\infty)} = 0$), we have usually $U^{(\nu)} \propto \nu e^{-a\nu}$ for large ν. (a = a positive constant.)

It will be an interesting experiment to find out the $U^{(\nu)}$ curve as a function of ν in a human subject. Of course, this presupposes a possibility of experimentally determining $q^{(\nu)}(H_j)$ of a human subject.

We may here adduce an extremely simple example just in order to clarify the meaning of various symbols. $\mathscr{H}$ may consist of two hypotheses, H_1 which says that a particular coin is a regular coin, and H_2 which says that the coin is a double-headed one. D_1 may be that a toss of the coin gives head and D_2 may be a toss of the coin gives tail. Then $p(D_1/H_1) = p(D_2/H_1) = 1/2$ and $p(D_1/H_2) = 1$, $p(D_2/H_2) = 0$.

Suppose we repeat the coin toss and we obtain only heads all the time. If this continues indefinitely, it is obvious that $q^{(\nu)}(H_2)$ and $q^{(\nu)}(H_1)$ become respectively 1 and 0, for $\nu \rightarrow \infty$, no matter what values they may have at finite ν. By a simple calculation using Bayes' Theorem, one can show that for large ν, $U^{(\nu)}$ behaves as $\nu(1/2)^\nu$. How would a human subject react under normal and adverse conditions?

It is granted that decision on an action based on a hypothesis has to be made by a human before the credibility of the hypothesis, say, $q^{(\nu)}(H_k)$, becomes unity (which would usually require an infinite time). It seems natural to assume that an action based on a hypothesis H_k is taken as soon as the relation

$$q^{(\nu)}(H_k)/[1 - q^{(\nu)}(H_k)] \geqslant \theta_1 \tag{3}$$

or the relation

$$q^{(\nu)}(H_k)/q^{(\nu)}(H_i) \geqslant \theta_2 \quad \text{for all } i \text{ such that } i \neq k \tag{4}$$

is satisfied. This threshold, θ_1 or θ_2, measures obviously the degree of prudence in taking an action, hence it may be called "prudence threshold." It can of course depend on the magnitude of the reward and possible disaster risked by this decision. In the normal life, θ_1 or θ_2 may have a fairly constant value characteristic of a person. However, under abnormal circumstances or in an emergency, a person will be forced to lower this threshold in order "not to be too late." The threshold in (3), θ_1, however, must be larger than 1/2. Here, estimation by the human of the allowed time for decision-making may become another estimation problem. In any event, it may be an interesting psychological problem to try to determine θ_1 or θ_2 experimentally in a person.

Finally, as regards the reliability of cognitive process (here, I mean mainly a deductive inference), it may be emphasized that it is very important to establish the functional relationship between the probability P of error in a cognitive process, and the time T allowed to complete this process. From experience in the reliability problems in electric networks, I conjecture that P, as a function of T, will be approximately expressed as a function lying between

$$P \propto \exp(-\alpha T) \tag{5}$$

and

$$P \propto \exp(\exp - \alpha T) \tag{6}$$

where α is some positive constant. If the actual function is close to (5), the performance (of temporal improvement) may be said to be mediocre, while if it is close to (6), it may be said to be good. If, for instance, a person repeats the same calculation twice, each time with a probability of error p then the probability of both calculations being erroneous is of course p^2. This corresponds to (5). The formula (6) is a temporalistic analogue of the Moore-Shannon model of reliability. See Moore-Shannon (2), and also Kochen (3). It will be an extremely interesting project to determine the experimental function $P = f(T)$, since in a space flight the time factor is very important. It may even turn out that this function $f(T)$ is not a monotonous function of T as (5) or (6) suggests.

REFERENCES

1. Watanabe, S., Information theoretical aspects of inductive and deductive inference, IBM J. Res. and Devel., 4:No. 2:208, 1960.
2. Moore, E. F., and C. E. Shannon, Reliable circuits using less reliable relays, J. Franklin Inst., 262:Nos. 3, 4:191, 281, 1956.
3. Kochen, M., Extension of Moore-Shannon model for relay circuits, IBM J. Res. and Devel., 3:No. 2:169, 1959.

PART 4

Special Techniques of Control

Prolonged Hypothermia

F. JOHN LEWIS, PETER J. CONNAUGHTON, *and*
GORDON HOLT

Hypothermia would appear to be suitable for the passengers of a space vehicle. To match the shortage of oxygen, the shortage of food, the monotony, and the small cabins the greatly reduced metabolic activity and the deep narcosis produced by hypothermia should be ideal. Attractive, indeed, for the space traveler would be the choice of hibernating during long periods when there was nothing that he had to do. Mammals capable of hibernating achieve winter sleep easily when food is scarce and there is little need for activity; then, with their body temperature only a few degrees above the environmental temperature, they rest safely for many days. Unfortunately, this desirable state can not be attained yet in homeothermic animals.

Short, intense cooling to near-freezing temperature is quite well tolerated by warm-blooded animals, even though prolonged cooling is not. Our earlier studies (9, 10) as well as those of Andjus (1) and Smith (14) have shown that homeothermic animals may be cooled to near-freezing temperatures by simple means for short periods with complete recovery. Monkeys withstand these low temperatures well (11), and we were able to show that man, too, could be cooled to a low temperature (9° C.) with complete recovery using only a respirator and surface cooling (12).

Going down the thermometer scale, cooling has been carried an important step further with single mammalian cells (spermatazoa) which will withstand solid freezing at −70° C. for long periods with complete functional recovery (13); this intense cooling should be possible for the whole animal. At the present time, however,

Dr. Lewis, Dr. Connaughton, and Dr. Holt are on the staff of the Department of Surgery, Northwestern University Medical School. The research described in this paper was supported in part by United States Air Force Research Contract 29(600)-1729 and U.S. Public Health Service Grant H-2879.

subfreezing temperatures of the intact homeothermic animal are not tolerable, near-freezing temperatures are only tolerable for short periods of time, and even moderate cooling (20–23° C.) of long duration is dangerous. This last type of cooling—a type which might be suitable for passengers of a space vehicle—is the subject of this report.

We have studied hypothermia prolonged for twenty hours or more at body temperatures below 25° C. in dogs. Though a great number of articles have been written about hypothermia, these articles are almost all about hypothermia of short duration. Fisher and his associates have been an exception (3, 4, 5, 6). Our work confirms some of their studies of prolonged hypothermia and adds tests of agents which we hoped would make prolonged hypothermia safe. In some of our test groups we have achieved a higher survival rate than has hitherto been reported.

Though in some of our preliminary studies using these techniques, animals were cooled for only 4 to 12 hours, we will describe only the experiments in which dogs were kept at a temperature below 25° C. for more than twenty hours.

METHODS

Mongrel dogs weighing from 8 to 18 kg. were anesthetized with pentobarbital sodium and cooled by surface cooling. Thermistor thermometer probes were placed in the esophagus in all dogs, and additional probes were placed in other parts of the body in a few of the animals. A femoral artery and vein were cannulated in order to measure venous and arterial blood pressure and obtain blood samples. Before cooling, and at intervals thereafter, blood samples were analyzed for hematocrit, CO_2 content, oxygen saturation, pH, and plasma hemoglobin. Blood volume studies were done on some of the animals. During the entire process the animal was attached to an automatic respirator (8) and given either air or a mixture of 5 percent CO_2 in 95 percent oxygen.

Cooling and body temperature regulation were achieved with a special apparatus[1] (Figures 1 and 2) which has reservoirs of cold and warm refrigerating fluid, either of which may be pumped through a conventional refrigerating blanket which is wrapped around the dog.

[1] Autotherm Corp., P.O. Box 25122, West Los Angeles 25, California.

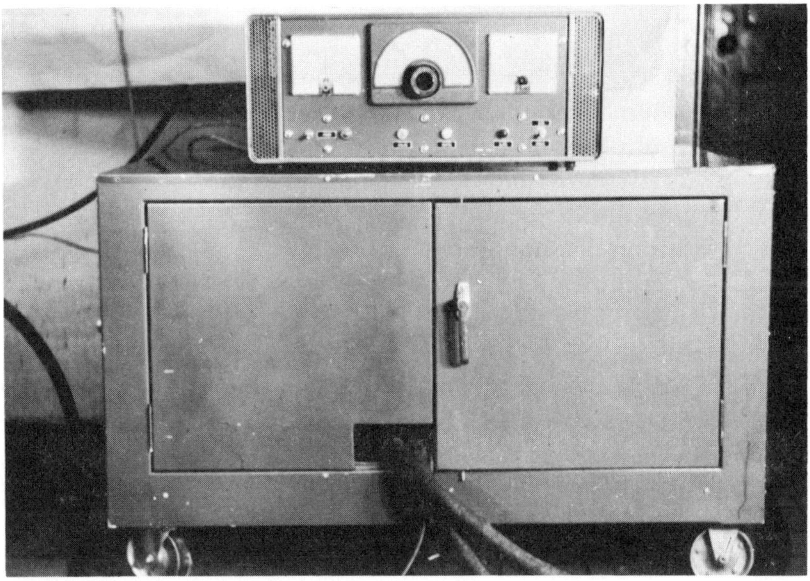

Figure 1. Automatic Cooling Apparatus

The control unit with its registering dials and the knob with which to set the desired temperature is on top. The refrigerating unit, heating unit, pump and valves are in the lower cabinet.

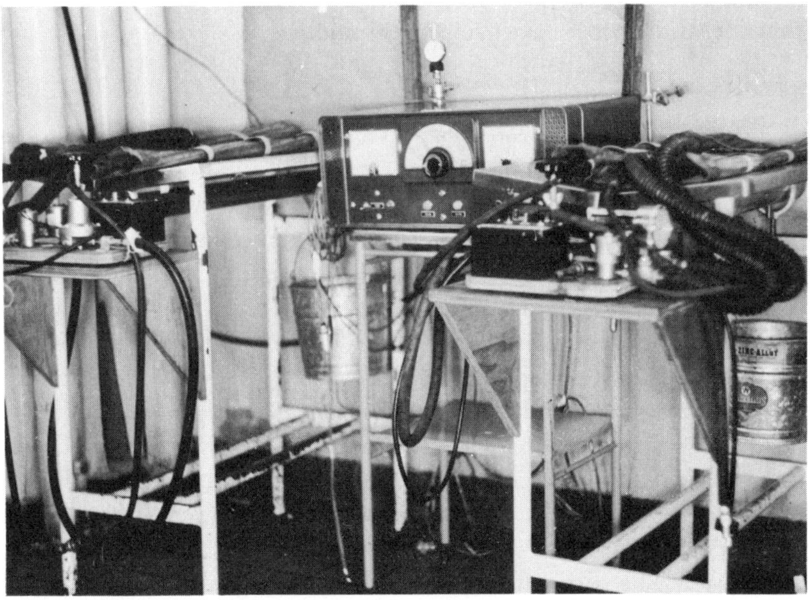

Figure 2. Automatic Cooling Apparatus Ready for Use

There are tables for two dogs but only one dog can be attached to the automatic control unit at a time.

The electronic control unit monitors both the dog's temperature and the temperature of the blankets, and it operates valves that regulate the temperature of the fluid which is pumped through the blanket. A knob on the control unit allows the operator to choose a temperature, the animal will then be cooled to this temperature and kept at that temperature automatically.

In many of the animals the technique was varied or medications were added in order to try to improve the survival rate. When Dibenzyline was given, it was given in doses from .05–.10 mgm:/kg. one hour before cooling. Chlorpromazine was given in a total dose of 150–300 mgm. in saline intravenously. It was started as a slow drip at the beginning of cooling and continued while the animal was cold. Vasoxyl was given in a dose of 40–80 mgm. in 300 cc. of normal saline during the cooling period. Cortisone was given in doses of 15 mg./kg. four times a day for four days prior to cooling. Reserpine was given in doses of .05–2.4 mg./kg. before cooling was commenced. Heparin was given in doses of 1–10 mg./kg. prior to and during cooling. When saline was given, it was given in a volume of approximately 700 cc. during the cooling. The dogs in the exsanguination group had 200–400 cc. of blood removed one week before cooling. The dogs which had splenectomies underwent this operation two weeks prior to cooling.

RESULTS

Anesthetic Effects of Hypothermia. We found that each dog had to be cooled below a certain critical temperature in order to eliminate anesthetics during prolonged cooling. This point was sharp. A rise of as little as one-half of one degree Centrigrade above the critical level resulted in movement, and this movement stopped when the temperature was again lowered. The critical level was a little above 23° C. in most dogs, and thus, after a few preliminary experiments, all the animals were kept at or slightly below 23° C. Temperatures this low are not usually employed when surface cooling of short duration is used during cardiac surgery or neurosurgery in man, but if the complications of additional anesthesia are to be avoided during prolonged hypothermia a temperature this low is required, at least in the dog.

Survival. The survival rate among the 98 dogs in which an effort was made to keep the body temperature below 25° C. for more than 20 hours was 32 percent (31 dogs). Dogs designated as survivors lived through the prolonged cooling period and rewarming to a normal temperature. Some died during the next day or so. The total number of dogs cooled is broken down into groups in Table 1.

Table 1. Survival Rates

Group	*Number of Dogs*	SURVIVORS *Number*	*Percent*
Early controls	9	2	22
5 percent CO_2	12	6	50
Dibenzyline	7	3	43
Chlorpromazine	7	1	14
Vasoxyl	5	0	0
Cortisone	7	0	0
I.V. saline	11	2	18
Heparin	18	4	22
Exsanguination	6	2	33
Splenectomy	4	1	25
Reserpine	5	5	100
Reserpine controls	7	5	71
Total	98	31	32

In some of these groups the survival rate was about the same as in the early control group. The addition of heparin, intravenous saline, or chlorpromazine, partial exsanguination, or splenectomy did not seem to improve the survival rate. All of these treatments may not have had adequate trial, but the results achieved were not encouraging.

Two drugs which tended to keep the blood pressure up (Figure 4), cortisone and Vasoxyl, appeared to affect the animals adversely, for no dogs in either of these groups survived.

In four groups the rate of survival seemed to be higher than it was in the earlier control group. On statistical analysis with a Chi-square test, however, survival in the group respired with 5 percent CO_2 and in the group prepared with Dibenzyline was not significantly greater than in the controls. A significantly greater survival rate was found in the reserpine group and in the group labeled reserpine controls. This later group, the reserpine control group of animals, was studied after success in the reserpine group.

A number of small changes in technique had been made in the reserpine group, and we felt that these changes, even without the reserpine, may have led to an increase in the survival rate. This may be the case, for there is no clear-cut difference in survival rate between the reserpine group and the reserpine controls. Both of these groups have a higher survival rate than any of the other groups. The small changes in technique which may have been effective were as follows: Prone position of the animal was used in contrast to the earlier supine or lateral position. A shorter inspiratory phase was used with the respirator, and intratracheal pressure was not allowed to exceed 12–14 mm. Hg. Deeper anesthesia was probably used during induction of cooling than was employed for most of the earlier dogs. Thorough and frequent tracheal aspiration was carried out during the rewarming phase to prevent atelectasis which may have complicated the earlier experiments. Intravenous sodium bicarbonate in a dose of 25–30 milliequivalents was given just before rewarming to counteract metabolic acidosis which is a regular feature of prolonged hypothermia.

Physiological Changes. The trend during prolonged hypothermia of several physiological measurements is graphed in Figures 3 through 8. In most of the figures the average measurements are graphed separately for animals that survived, those that died during hypothermia, and those that died during rewarming. In some of the graphs a difference is noted between animals that died and those that survived, but more striking is the profound change that occurred during prolonged hypothermia in all dogs.

Both the heart rate and blood pressure fell and remained down at a relatively constant level during hypothermia, as is illustrated in Figures 3 and 4. The heart rate was the same in the survivors and nonsurvivors, but the blood pressure was significantly higher at 20 hours among the survivors. Efforts to keep the blood pressure up failed to increase the survival rate, however. The graph shows the high blood pressure which was maintained in animals given cortisone or Vasoxyl, but none of these animals survived; in fact, none in the Vasoxyl group lived for even 20 hours.

The hematocrit rose (Figure 5) in confirmation of most previous studies of hypothermia, and it seemed to continue rising for as long as the animals were cooled. It did not level off, and in some animals

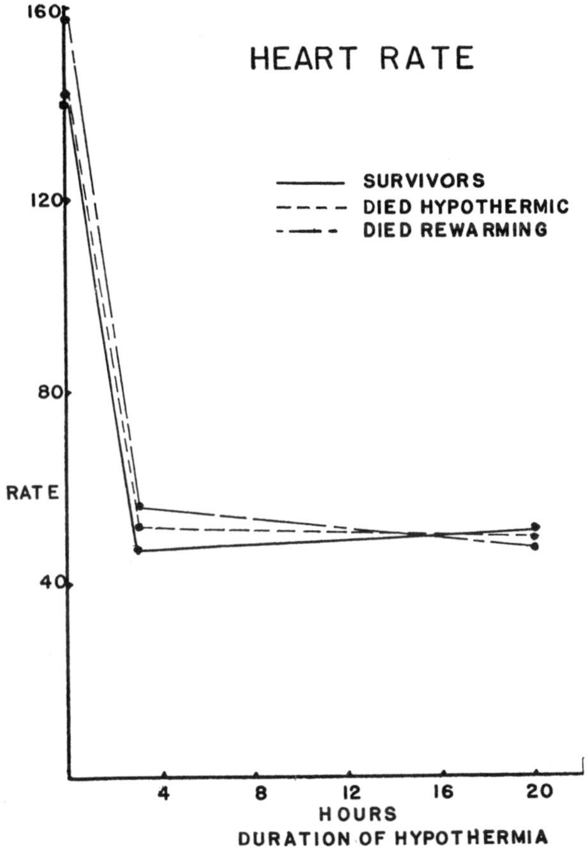

Figure 3. Average Heart Rate

This shows a slowing of the heart rate with cooling which then remained unchanged for 20 hours.

it reached strikingly high values—67 percent in one dog that survived. The difference in hematocrit between survivors and dogs that died during rewarming was statistically significant at 4, 12, and 20 hours. Hematocrits in dogs that died during cooling were not significantly different from either of the other groups. The rising hematocrit went along with the falling plasma volume in the 13 animals in which this was studied.

Oxygen saturation of the venous and arterial blood followed a pattern illustrated in Figure 6. Though arterial saturation remained

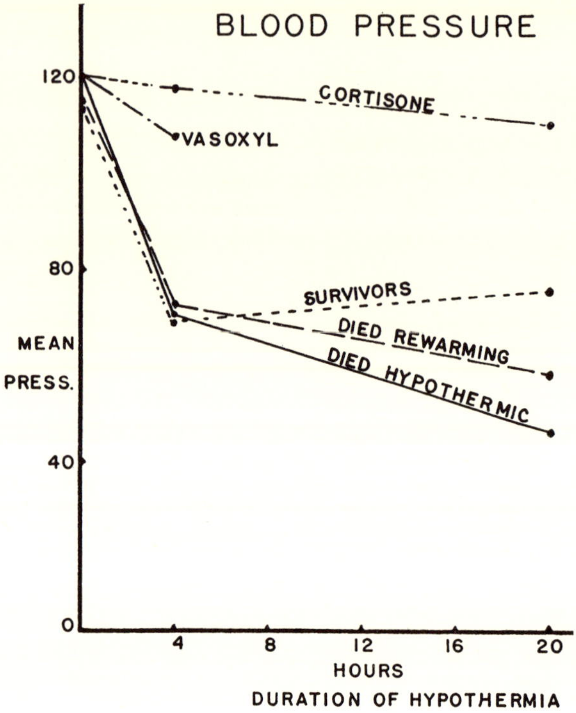

Figure 4. Average Mean Arterial Blood Pressure

Unless maintained with cortisone or Vasoxyl blood pressure dropped. At 20 hours it was higher in the animals destined to survive than in the dying animals.

high throughout, there was a striking drop in venous saturation as time passed beyond 4 hours of cooling. The drop was statistically significant, and none of the medications used altered this pattern. Venous saturation was higher at 4 hours than at normothermia, indicating adequate tissue perfusion then; but, as hypothermia progressed, tissue perfusion apparently failed to keep up, even though metabolic needs had been reduced. The oxygen content of the arterial blood remained normal, but an unusually large amount of this oxygen was extracted by the tissues, even though the shift in the oxyhemoglobin curve caused by the lower temperature would not favor this extraction. Tissue oxygen tension must have reached a low level.

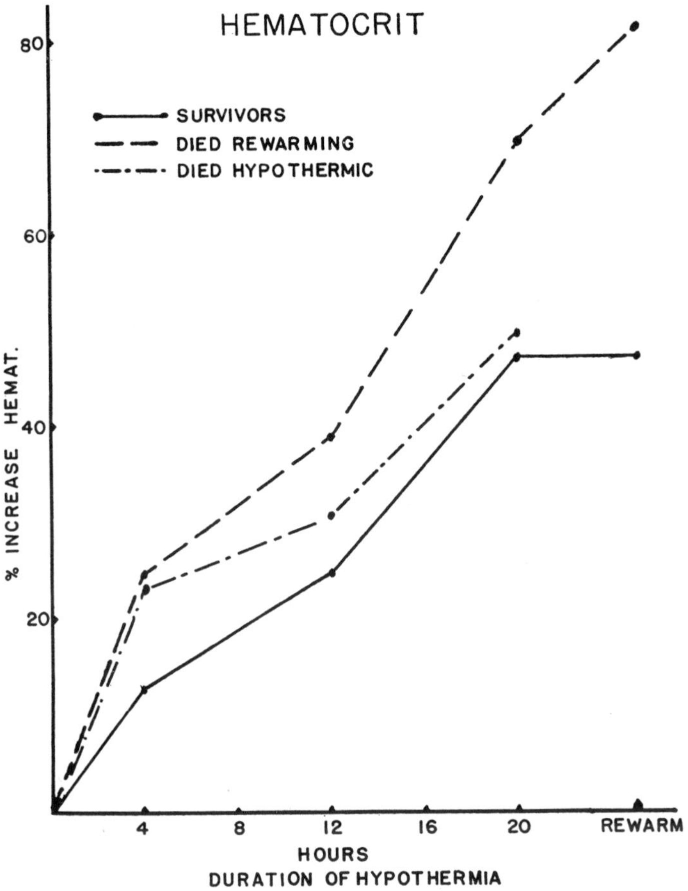

Figure 5. Average Hematocrit Determinations

The hematocrit kept going up as long as the animal was hypothermic.

The relatively poor perfusion indicated by low venous oxygen saturation is also reflected in the falling pH shown in Figure 7. It takes some time for this fall to occur. At 4 hours in the dogs breathing room air the pH is actually up. This rise, which occurs regularly in hypothermia of short duration, when an efficient respirator is used, can be prevented by using CO_2 (10) as is shown in the lower line of the graph. Beyond 4 hours, however, in either the dogs respired on room air or on CO_2, the pH drops. Apparently the metabolic

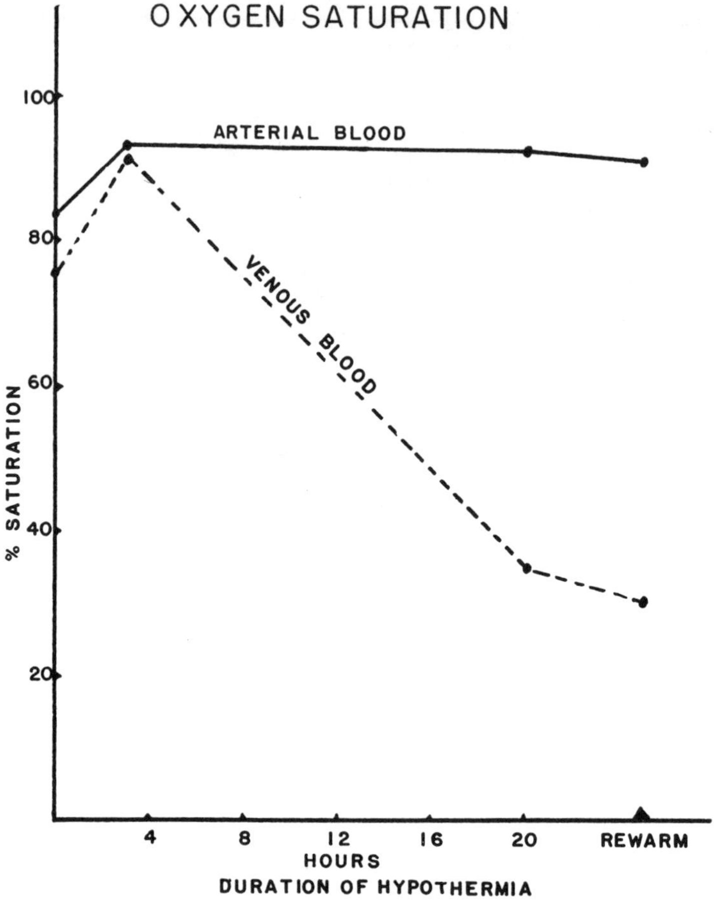

Figure 6. Venous Oxygen Saturation

This had fallen significantly at 20 hours of hypothermia.

acidosis which developed during hypothermia (2) and which is probably due to inadequate perfusion, can no longer be compensated for by hyperventilation. There is no significant difference between the survivors and the animals that died in respect to pH changes, and the data did not prove that 5 percent CO_2 in 95 percent O_2 had any advantage over room air in prolonged hypothermia, though the survival rate was higher in the animals receiving 5 percent CO_2.

Plasma hemoglobin rose on the average (Figure 8), though it did not reach levels usually considered lethal.

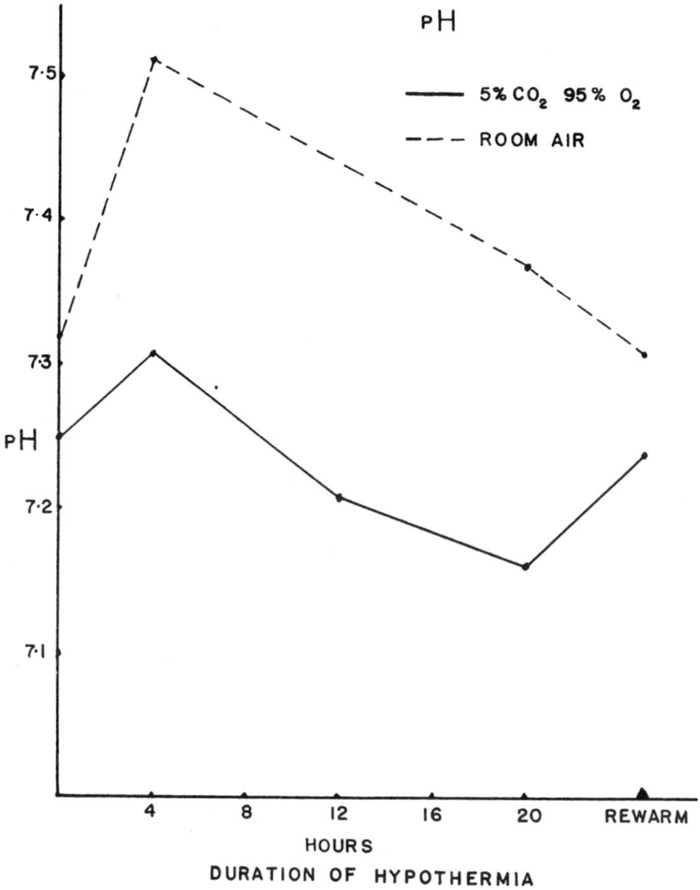

Figure 7. Average Arterial pH Determinations

The pH tended to continue falling as long as the animal was hypothermic.

Electrocardiography. With progressive cooling the ECG showed sinus bradycardia with prolongation of the P-R interval, the QRS complex, and the QT segment. Often a diphasic T-wave appeared which might become deeply inverted as cooling progressed. A "current of injury" sometimes appeared, but this or other changes did not help us in prognosis.

We do not know how often ventricular fibrillation may have been the cause of death. Since temperature regulation was controlled automatically, the animals were not under constant observation

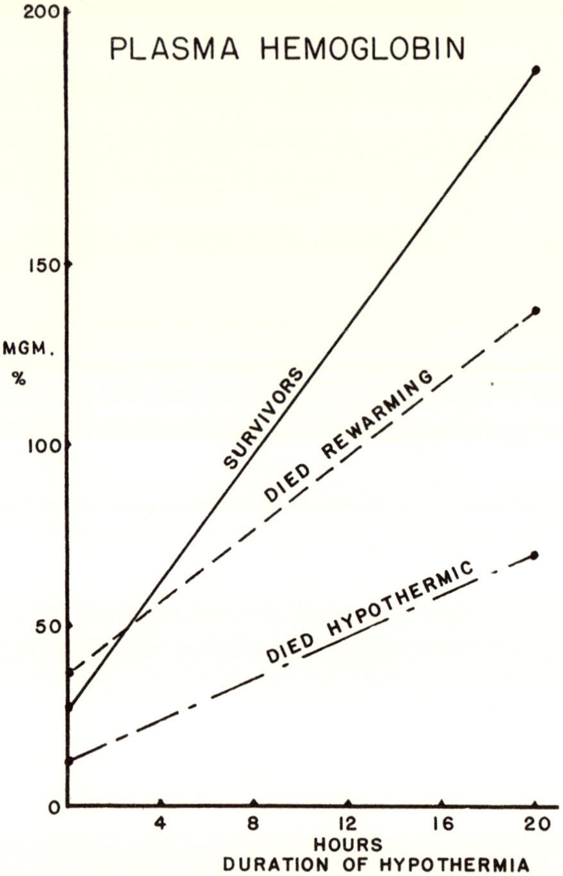

Figure 8. Average Plasma hemoglobin

while cold. Forty-four deaths occurred during hypothermia, and it is possible that ventricular fibrillation was the final mechanism of death in many of these animals. By the time a zero blood pressure was noted it was too late to tell.

DISCUSSION

Hypothermia maintained for many hours by the techniques we use is not safe for the dog. A picture of shock occurs with a low blood pressure, reduced blood volume, and metabolic acidosis. These changes all become more severe as time passes. The longer hypothermia lasts the more dangerous it is. Perhaps due to unsuitable small blood vessel reactivity (7), or due to a cardiac output that is too low, or due to a combination of factors, tissues are not perfused adequately at low temperatures. If the inadequate perfusion continues long enough the shock is irreversible, and the animal will not recover.

In the most recent experiments, the reserpine group and the reserpine control group, the survival rate has been significantly higher than in previous groups, but even these animals still show the ominous signs of a progressive increase in hematocrit and a fall in pH. The high survival rate we now achieve may be attributable to the attention we now pay to a number of small features of the technique which we have come to believe are important on the basis of experience. We have not been able to alter basically the response of the animal to prolonged hypothermia.

Reserpine has been employed with the idea that it would do away with the adverse effects of epinephrine and norepinephrine (15). Its use has been followed by the highest survival rate we have achieved, but it will have to be studied further and animals receiving reserpine will need to be cooled for longer periods of time before we can be certain that it helps.

The automatic control system for maintaining body temperature accurately at the desired level works reliably.

SUMMARY

1. An automatic control system has been used to maintain the body temperature of dogs below 25° C. for 20 hours. Once this low temperature has been reached no anesthesia other than hypothermia was required.

2. Blood pressure and pulse rate remained low throughout the cooling periods and as time passed the hematocrit rose, plasma volume fell, pH fell, and venous oxygen saturation fell.

3. Of the 98 dogs cooled in this fashion 31 survived rewarming.

4. A number of agents and medications have been used in order to try and increase the survival rate. Best results were achieved with the most recent technique which features a number of small changes such as deeper anesthesia during induction of hypothermia. Reserpine may also have led to a higher survival rate.

REFERENCES

1. Andjus, R. K., Sur la possibilité de ranimer le rat adulte refroidi jusqu'à proximité du point de congélation, Compt. rend. Acad. d.sc., 232:1591, 1951.
2. Deterling, R. A., Jr., E. Nelson, S. Bhonslay, and W. Howland. Study of basic physiologic changes associated with hypothermia, Arch. Surg., 70:87, 1955.
3. Fedor, E. J., B. Fisher, and S. H. Lee, Rewarming following hypothermia of two to twelve hours, Ann. Surg., 147:515, 1958.
4. Fisher, B., C. Russ, E. Fedor, R. Wilde, R. Engstrom, J. Happel, and P. Prendergast, Experimental evaluation of prolonged hypothermia, Arch. Surg., 71:413, 1955.
5. Fisher, E. R., E. J. Fedor, and B. Fisher, Pathologic and histochemical observations in experimental hypothermia, Arch. Surg., 75:5, 1957.
6. Fisher, B., E. J. Fedor, and S. H. Lee, Rewarming following hypothermia of two to twelve hours: II. Some metabolic effects, Ann. Surg., 148:1, 1958.
7. Haddy, F. J., M. Fleishman, and J. B. Scott, Jr., Effect of change in air temperature upon systemic small and large vessel resistance, Circulation Res., 5:58, 1957.
8. Lewis, F. J., An electronically controlled respirator for the experimental laboratory, J. Thoracic and Cardiovasc. Surg., 38:408, 1959.
9. Niazi, S. A., and F. J. Lewis, Tolerance of adult rats to profound hypothermia and simultaneous standstill, Surgery. 36:25, 1954.
10. Niazi, S. A., and F. J. Lewis, Profound hypothermia in the dog, Surg., Gynec. & Obst., 102:98, 1956.
11. Niazi, S. A., and F. J. Lewis, Profound hypothermia in the monkey with recovery after cardiac standstill, J. Appl. Physiol., 10:137, 1957.
12. Niazi, S. A., and F. J. Lewis, Profound hypothermia in man, Ann. Surg., 147:264, 1958.
13. Polge, C., A. U. Smith, and A. S. Parkes, Revival of spermatozoa after vitrification and dehydration at low temperature, Nature, 164:666, 1949.
14. Smith, A. U., Frost-bite in golden hamsters revived from body temperatures below below 0° C., 11:1255, 1954.
15. Woodson, R. E., H. W. Younghen, E. Schlittler, and J. A. Schneider, Rauwolfia: Its Botany, Pharmacognosy, Chemistry and Pharmacology. Boston, Little, Brown and Co., 1957.

Drugs, Space, and Cybernetics: Evolution to Cyborgs

NATHAN S. KLINE *and* MANFRED CLYNES

A wanderer is man from his birth.
He was born in a ship
On the breast of the river of Time;
Brimming with wonder and joy
He spreads out his arms to the light
Rivets his gaze on the banks of the stream.

As what he sees is, so have his thoughts been.

"The Future" by Matthew Arnold

Man must first conceive that which he would create. Viewed from a cosmic time scale, today we fumble and crawl, having barely crossed the threshold of existence; because a rattle responds when we shake it, we are swollen with instant pride and label ourselves "masters of the universe." We have not yet even learned to conquer disease, we are ignorant as to the basic nature of electric, magnetic, and nuclear forces—of the very nature of force itself. We can only communicate with each other in the most inarticulate fashions, and we do not know how to create life. Our presumption is even greater than our ignorance: when we cannot understand something we call it UNKNOWABLE MYSTERY OF ULTIMATE. The Epimetheans among us then cry "sacrilege" when the problem is even approached. As if God's infinity were but a finger's grasp beyond our own limitations!

Participant Evolution. The challenge of space travel to mankind is not only to his technological prowess, it is also a spiritual challenge to take an active part in his own biological evolution. The great scientific advances in the years to come may be utilized to permit existence under environments radically different from those provided by natural circumstances today. This task of adapting his body to whatever milieu he chooses will be made easier by increased knowledge of homeostatic functioning, the cybernetic aspects of which are just beginning to be investigated and understood. It is also likely that through a study of his psychological and physical needs in unusual environments a clearer understanding of man's needs in his home environment will be found.

In the past, the altering of bodily functions to suit different environments was accomplished through evolution. From now on, at least in some degree, this can be achieved without alteration of heredity by suitable biochemical, physiological, and electronic modification of man's existing modus vivendi.

Homeostatic mechanisms found in organisms are designed to afford a stable operation in the particular environment of the organism. Three examples of some successful alternate solutions provided by biological mechanisms to the body-environment problem, with regard to operating temperature, are man, hibernating animals, and poikilothermic fish (organisms with blood that takes on the temperature of the environment).

Various biological solutions have also been developed for another regulatory problem: respiration. Mammals, fish, insects, and plants have each a different biological solution with its inherent limitations but eminently suitable for its field of operation. Should there be a desire for an organism to live outside its field, an "insurmountable" problem exists. The problem, however, is only apparently insurmountable. If a fish wanted to live on land it could not readily do so. If, however, a particularly intelligent, dissatisfied fish could be found who had studied a great deal of biochemistry and physiology, and who was a master engineer and cybernetician and had excellent laboratories, this fish would be able to design an instrument that would allow him to go on land and breathe air quite readily. To what degree this instrument would resemble lungs is an interesting question which we clearly cannot answer today because we are not as intelligent as this fish would have to be. However, it is apparent that we will have sufficient knowledge in the future to design our own instruments to make it possible for our bodies to do feats no less difficult than breathing on land would be for a fish.

The environment wished for by man at this present stage of development is that of empty space. Biologically, what are the changes that would be necessary for man to live adequately in such surroundings? The solution of artificial atmospheres encapsulated in smaller or larger enclosures is only temporizing. It is also a dangerous temporizing, much as it would be dangerous for the fish to take a small quantity of water with him to live on land. The bubble all too easily bursts.

The Problems. In the following pages some of the biological difficulties which others feel exist in respect to space travel are reviewed, as well as some new problems. Two sets of possible answers are furnished. One provides solutions which probably could be devised with presently available knowledge and techniques. The others are projections into the future which, by their very nature, must resemble science fiction. To illustrate, there are possibly much more efficient ways of carrying out the functions of the respiratory system than by breathing, which in space is cumbersome. One proposed solution for the not too distant future is relatively simple—don't breathe!

Even though they offend terrestrial common sense, eventualities predicted of space travel, such as time distortion, will be hard realities, and resultant physiological and psychological conditions must be considered. We must consider not only flights of days, months, or years, but also journeys of several thousand years' duration.

The New Frontier. If man attempts a partial adaptation to the conditions of space instead of being insistent that he carry his entire environment with him, a number of new possibilities appear. One is led to ask what are then the biologic changes that would have to be made in his homeostatic mechanisms for man to be able to live in space *qua natura?*

Cybernetic Aids for Space Life. The autonomic nervous system and the endocrine glands cooperate in man to maintain the multiple balances required for his continued existence. They do this without conscious control, although they are amenable to its influence. The necessary readjustments of these automatic responses and levels under extraterrestrial conditions require the aid of control theory as well as extensive physiological knowledge.

What are some of the devices necessary for creating self-regulating man-machine systems? This self-regulation needs to function without the benefit of consciousness, in order to cooperate with the body's own autonomous homeostatic controls. For the artificially extended homeostatic control system functioning unconsciously, one of us (Manfred Clynes) has coined the term Cyborg. The Cyborg deliberately incorporates exogeneous components extending the self-regulatory control function of the organism in order to adapt it to new environments. If it were necessary for us to continuously check to maintain our heart at the appropriate rate, keep our respiratory rate at approximately 16 per minute, and see that digestion was proceeding with proper peristaltic waves, there would be little time left for other activities. If we also had to adjust these rates upward or downward depending on whether we were doing more or less activity, we would be a slave to keeping the human body functioning. Similarly, if a man in space, in addition to flying his ship must be taking continual checks and making continual adjustments in order to keep himself alive, he becomes a slave to the machine. The purpose of the Cyborg is to provide an organizational system in which these robot-like problems are taken care of automatically and unconsciously, thus freeing man to explore, to create, to think, and to feel. One device helpful toward the construction of Cyborgs, which is already available, is the ingenious osmotic pressure pump capsule developed by S. Rose (1) for the continuous slow injections of biochemically active substances at a biological rate. This Rose osmotic pressure pump capsule is incorporated into the organism and allows administration of a selected drug at a particular organ and at a continuous variable rate (as low as 0.01 ml a day or less), without any attention on the part of the organism.

The whole device can be buried in an animal, which can lead a reasonably normal life while the injection is going on. The mode of force of the injector depends on the osmotic pressure developed by a saturated aqueous solution of Congo red against water. This solution is contained in a partially collapsed rubber compartment and is separated from a second water compartment by a semipermeable cellophane membrane. Water moves by osmosis into the Congo red solution and expands the rubber compartment. It is this expansion which provides the mechanical force to eject the drug out of the apparatus. The pump need be only two and a half times the total volume that it is intended to deliver. The rate can be changed by altering the area and/or thickness of the cellophane which separates the water and the Congo red solution. If blocked, the injector is capable of developing two atmospheres of pressure. This means that any resistance which develops in the fine plastic tubing going to the site of injection is easily overcome and thus does not alter the rate of injection. The following description is abridged from Rose (1).

Figures 1 and 2 show component parts and assembled apparatus. It consists of three compartments: a drug compartment, a water compartment and a Congo red compartment with a clamp to hold the semipermeable cellophane membrane. When 16.5 square mm. of membrane are exposed the injector delivers fluid at 0.12 ml per diem. However, any desired rate can be achieved by using a suitable cellophane and an appropriate sized hole in the clamp. The Congo red compartment consists of a latex bag of 3.0 ml capacity. Distilled water in the quantity of 0.5 ml and Congo red (.06 gm) are placed in the bag. This makes a saturated solution with 0.52 gm of excess Congo red out of solution. The bag is partially collapsed to remove all the air and is then tied over the clamp. The clamp and latex bag are fixed in the glass ampoule by means of ties which utilize the splayed edge as fixation points. The drug compartment (H) consists of the space between the Congo red bag and the glass ampoule. When the bag expands, fluid is forced out through the nipple of the glass ampoule and is then carried by means of plastic connecting tubing to the desired organ. The water compartment consists of a second latex bag (I) which is tied over the splayed edge of the glass ampoule. This compartment is filled with distilled water either at the time the apparatus is assembled, or later, by means of a syringe and needle when the injector is buried in the animal. The water can now move under a constant osmotic gradient through the cellophane membrane into the Congo red compartment. More dye dissolves and a saturated solution is maintained. The Congo red bag expands and forces fluid containing the drug through the nipple. The whole arrangement is such that at least 2 ml of water can diffuse into the bag. Thus 2 ml of drug will have been slowly and constantly forced through the nipple down the plastic tube to the desired organ. Apparatus is already available which will deliver 0.01 ml per day for 200 days, and there exists no reason why this time could not be considerably extended. The apparatus has been used on rabbits, dogs, large rats, and for continuous heparin injection in man. It should be noted that polythene tubing is superior to stainless steel for needles as well as connecting tubes. No untoward general effect

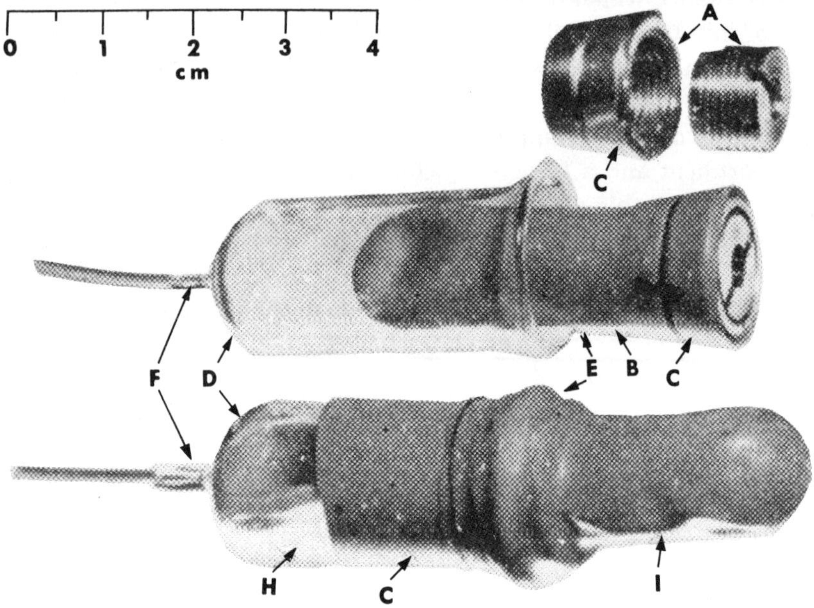

Figure 1. Rose Osmotic Pressure Pump

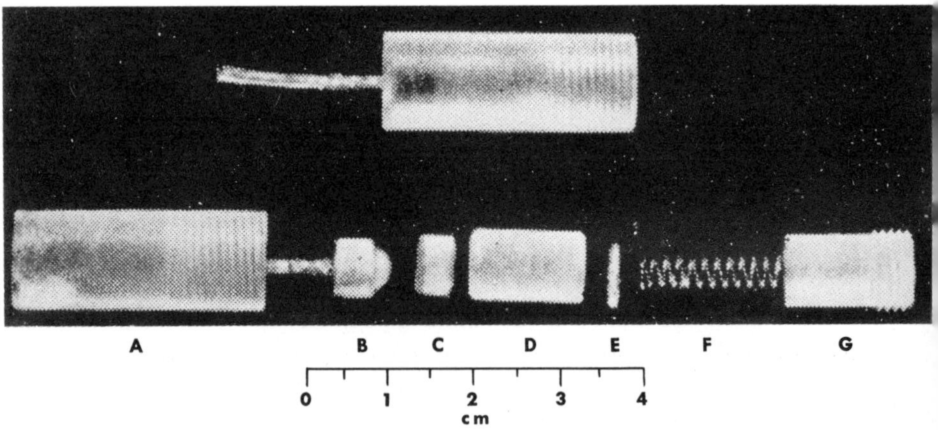

Figure 2. Component Parts of Rose Osmotic Pressure Pump

on the animal's health was noted when the small injector was buried in a large animal. Even five years ago an injector 7 centimeters long and 1.4 centimeters in diameter weighing 15 gms was successfully buried in rats weighing 150–250 gm. Figure 3 shows a rat weighing 220 gm. with an injector in situ (1).

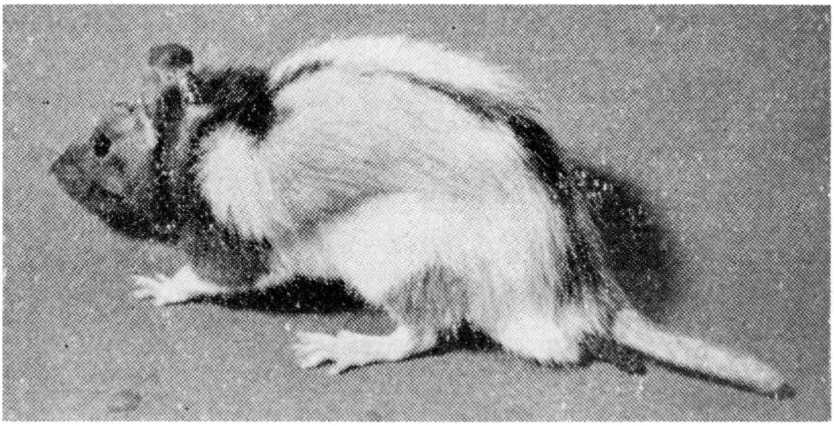

Figure 3. Rose Osmotic Pressure Pump In Situ

The combination of the osmotic pressure pump capsule with sensing and controlling mechanisms can form a continuous machine-man controlled loop which will operate as an adjunct to the body's own autonomous controls. In this way these controls can be changed to the desired performance characteristics under various environmental conditions. Such a system is possible today, with the selection of appropriate drugs. For example, systolic blood pressure may be sensed, compared to a reference value dependent on space conditions encountered, and regulated by letting the difference between the sensed pressure and reference value control the administration of an adrenergic or a vasodilator drug. Of course, it presupposes that we should be cognizant of what the optimum blood pressure under various space conditions should be.

The "Natural" Biological Boundary. How are we to set the upper limits of "natural" human physiological and psychological performance? We can take as minimal the capabilities demonstrable under control conditions such as yoga or hypnosis.

At such institutions as the yoga colleges in India, the human imagination is stretched by the muscular control of which even the average undergraduate is capable. Hypnosis per se may prove to have a definite place in space travel, but there is prior need for much more information about the phenomena of dissociation, generalization of instructions, and abdication of executive control.

We are presently working with a new preparation which may greatly enhance hypnotizability, so that pharmacological and hypnotic approaches may be symbiotically combined.

The Physical Parameters. At the time of this writing a cluster of eight rockets is sufficient to place a 25,000-pound pay load in orbit. As to the ultimate future, we cannot assume a set limit on either pay load or power. It is entirely conceivable that there might exist a space station more than a mile in diameter and capable of creating its own gravitational field. Once established it would be difficult to change the orbit of such a space station, but if properly placed it would be able to traverse a considerable part of the solar system. Under these circumstances it might even be possible for the object to create its own atmosphere. It is rumored that the Russians among others are already operating on such a space station—known as Earth.

SPECIAL PROBLEMS

Wakefulness. On August 2, 1958, Marion "Pat" Boling completed a solo nonstop flight of approximately 7,000 miles from Manila, in the Philippines, to Pendleton, Oregon, in a single-engine Beachcraft Bonanza. Almost the entire flight was made over water, and it was without radio communication for sizable periods of time. Except for a very brief period the pilot was awake for the 24 hours preceding the flight and almost all of the 48 hours during which he was airborne. Upon arrival he was feted and it was almost 48 hours longer before he obtained any substantial amount of sleep. Certainly the conditions of the trip required the highest degree of alertness, involving both clear judgment and full executive control. As a veteran airline pilot Captain Boling was quite familiar with many of the difficulties he would face, and highest on the list of physiological problems was the questions of how to remain awake and alert. It was decided to try one of the group of drugs known as psychic energizers, which were capable of reducing fatigue and increasing the ability to concentrate.

Preliminary testing was done because of variations in individual sensitivity, latency, and side effects, and since there was no information available as to the effects of altitude with its concomitant change of physiological conditions. Medication was started on May 13 at 3:00 P.M., and total sleep that night occurred between 0400 and 0600. The next night, however, with the same dosage, there was a full night of nine hours' sleep; but, on May 15 there were a total of only two hours sleep again, and on May 16 only one hour. Medication was continued for approximately one more week on half the former dosage without side reactions. It was then discontinued because it appeared to potentiate the Pyribenzamine which had been started for hay fever on May 19. A letter describing the experience states: "During the time I was trying the medication, I never felt any nausea or any of the possible effects you mentioned except possibly a slight headache for a few minutes . . . . I sent the cabin of the plane up to 10,000 feet for several hours and felt, if anything, slightly better than I had in the past."

A preparation containing 5 mg. of amphetamine was provided for emergency use. It should be noted that this dosage of a stimulant is usually quite temporary, and certainly one tablet is an impossibly low dose to counteract marked fatigue for any extensive period when used alone. The pilot continues: "I felt real fine on generally about 3–4 hours of sleep a night and the (amphetamine) worked very well in conjunction with it. There was a very slight drowsiness immediately after taking it, changing to an alert exhilaration within 20 minutes." Essentially the same regime was followed during the actual flight.

For flights up to a few weeks or even a few months it would thus appear desirable pari passu to utilize one of the psychic energizers. If reduced temperatures are used to lower metabolic rate (to be discussed later), the energizers should be tested to determine if they are capable of enabling the individual to retain alertness. It should be pointed out that another possible advantage of a psychic energizer is resultant reduction in physiological and psychological "stress." In a paper which has been submitted for publication (2) there was reported a highly significant decrease in eosinophile count following cortisone injections after patients were placed on psychic energizers as contrasted with their reaction without such medication. Certainly, the energizers should also be tested for their effect on sensory deprivation, sensory invariance, action limitation, and sensory overload. Because of the increase in nitrogen retention resulting, the energizers, which are also monamine oxidase inhibitors, may also make for more efficient food utilization.

Radiation Effects. There are experts far better informed in respect to chemical protection against radiation than the present authors. We will consider the Cyborg to handle chemical radiation protection. Dr. Walter H. Whitcomb of the Radiobiology Branch of the School of Aviation Medicine at Brooks Air Force Base reported on increase of radiation resistance resulting from combined administration of aminoethylisothioronium and cysteine to monkeys. This is not a complete feedback loop, because there is no sensor to measure radiation protection, but for practical purposes an open loop is adequate.

For the present we must assume that radiation is unavoidable and work toward the development of improved drugs for protection against radiation damage. It would appear most sensible to administer such drugs only during the periods when they are indicated rather than continuously. Here a servomechanism responsive to background count with proper anticipation would be ideal, since a self-regulating mechanism could be retained without the pilot's direct attention and he would be free to carry out some of the other functions which cannot be automatically regulated in this manner.

Metabolic Problems and Hypothermic Control. In view of the estimated consumption of ten pounds a day of human fuel (two pounds of oxygen, four pounds of fluid, and four pounds of food) the supply problem becomes immense even with reutilization of extractory products. Except for hop-skip orbiting the question must be asked as to whether all this consumption is necessary. The purpose of flight is to make certain observations and to carry out certain control functions. In the short flight periods, up to a month or two, through the use of physic energizers and adjunctive medication no more than a few hours a day of sleep would be required in the normal environment. This regime has been tried for periods ranging from a few days to a number of months, and in addition to sleep reduction there is evidence that efficiency increases rather than decreases.

Patients have been on this regime for as long as three years, so that extended usage appears entirely feasible.

For *prolonged* space flight, however, it would appear highly desirable to follow exactly the opposite approach. During a flight of months or years, assuming that the space ship itself was performing satisfactorily, there would be little or no reason for the passenger to be awake unless he were passing close to some interesting object or through some field which required observation. It should not be too difficult to create a system which would arouse the passenger to become a pilot if any of the flight conditions being followed passed outside the safety threshold. Similar arrangements could be made in respect to observational data, so that the passenger could be aroused to become an observer if detection apparatus indicated phenomena worth observing. The psychological advantages of this will be discussed subsequently, but the present relevance is to the possibility of radically reducing the metabolic needs of the organism. Antithyroid preparations which are presently available commercially are not entirely satisfactory. Their use tends to disturb the balance of other endocrine organs, and a number of them appear to possibly be carcinogenic. Ablation of the thyroid would also tend to throw other endocrine organs out of function in addition to producing some of the unwanted effects of hypothyroidism.

At present the most practical solution would appear to be a reduction of body temperature, somewhat in the nature of that used in certain types of heart surgery.[1] Much work needs to be done in respect to determining the nature of metabolism under these circumstance. It is probable that quite different enzyme systems will be dominant. Eventually enzymes and drugs might be used to establish body temperature through a change affecting the brain center controlling temperature rather than through external refrigeration.

The recent brilliant investigations of C. H. Li demonstrate that the pituitary growth hormone acts differently on the brain than on other parts of the body. Mice hypophysectomized shortly after birth died at the end of one month. Although the skull and other organs stopped growing the brain did not, with the result that death was

[1] It would be interesting for experimental purposes to lower body temperature via a vascular shunt in which the blood passes through a miniature thermoelectric cooling device and is returned to the vascular system. C. William Hargens of the Franklin Institute is working with this type of instrument adaptable to small animals.

caused by cerebral compression. The differential action between the brain and the rest of the body suggests some intriguing possibilities. It may be feasible with hormone action to lower metabolism in the rest of the body but to maintain it in the brain so that, although there are over-all reduced food and oxygen requirements, mental activity will tend to be unimpaired. Alternatively, the entire body may be cooled homeostatically, but the brain heated electronically.

The extensive and original work of Dr. William Sacks of our staff utilizing radio-tagged glucose has provided a technique of measuring cerebral metabolism in vivo. He has demonstrated in humans that glucose was not the sole brain metabolite as was at one time widely believed. (There is also a difference between schizophrenics and nonschizophrenics which may open the way to a clearer understanding of the nature of the disease.) It would be most interesting and appropriate to determine changes in glucose consumption and brain metabolism measured in this way under conditions of low temperature.

Presumably hibernation is also under pituitary control, and if the hormone controlling this can be identified and reproduced (or at least accumulated) it becomes possible to reduce metabolism without resorting to external cooling devices. In view of the differential hormone action on the brain relative to the growth hormone it suggests that it may not be impossible to reduce metabolism in the rest of the body by means of the hibernating hormone but to maintain the brain in an alert state.

Oxygenation and Carbon Dioxide Removal. Breathing is an excellent system for metabolism in an atmosphere with adequate oxygen supply and low carbon dioxide content. In space and on other planets atmospheric conditions are all wrong for this purpose. Carrying sufficient oxygen for any length of time is prohibitive in terms of weight (2 pounds a day), and even a closed ecological system is awkward and must allow for major losses due to low efficiency and possible disruption by meteorites.

Ideally, an artificial organ should be provided to replace the lung. Blood should be shunted from the pulmonary artery through a microsystem capable of reducing the CO_2 and adding appropriate quantities of O_2 after which it returned to the pulmonary vein. Theoretically, an inverse fuel cell process might convert the CO_2 to

C and O_2 with the latter remaining in the blood stream. Energy for such a system could be supplied either externally from solar energy or from atomic processes within the system.

Under these conditions breathing would be not only unnecessary but impossible. The mouth could be opened for food intake and speech articulation for limited periods of time. Alternatively, a digestive tract tube (entering through the rectum) or intravenous feedings might be preferable.

Because of the great acceleration at blast-off, it appears possible that if respiration is carried out in the usual manner there will likely be a period ranging from four to eight minutes during which no breathing can be accomplished. One possible solution is prior oxygen saturation, which was discussed some three years ago in a Russian journal (3).

The removal of carbon dioxide during this blast-off period presents a more critical problem but there has been little literature on this subject. The fuel-cell technique possibility would appear to take care of both of these problems.

The reduced (or absent) oxygen and pressure in the space ship also reduces the danger resulting from puncture by meteorites.

Fluid Intake-Output. Even with lowered temperature, the maintenance of fluid balance is a major problem. Following the same general approach as before, we believe that the development of an "adaptive" system should be attempted. It is theoretically possible to reshunt the urine after suitable processing directly into the bloodstream. The greatest problem in utilizing urine as a source of fluid is the occurrence of urea which amounts to 25 to 30 grams a day. If the urine could be fed directly from the ureter through a shunt containing urease, the urea would be converted into carbon dioxide and ammonia. The carbon dioxide could then either be handled by our postulated fuel pump or, if this were not available, serve as a source of substrate for conversion to oxygen by algae. The amount of carbon dioxide produced in this manner would incidentally form an excellent check on the adequacy of kidney function, since the quantity of urea produced is quite stable. Ammonia could be handled by the use of nitrifying bacteria with conversion to nitrates or nitric acid. At the present time this would be largely discard and could not be fed directly back to the bloodstream. On the other hand, the remaining filtrate could be treated with ion exchange resins and predetermined levels of blood sodium, potassium, chlorides, and phosphates released to maintain appropriate homeostasis. There are unquestionably alternate systems, but even the one proposed here would be portable so that it would not preclude long periods of travel away from a "space womb."

The 7 grams of feces produced daily in fasting man or the 10–12 grams if intravenous feeding is used would be measurably less under conditions of lowered metabolism. Through the use of a miniaturized septic tank, CO_2 would be produced and could be handled in the manner described above. The residual fluid could be again passed through columns and the filtrate containing the trace metals reinjected into the vascular system. By sterilizing the gastrointestinal tract even the 7 grams of feces might be largely eliminated. Appropriate pathogens could be reintroduced when needed as has been done in animals. This would also reduce the possibility of dangerous bacterial mutations which might be produced by radiation.

The absence of breathing will conserve the substantial amount of fluid which is normally lost in this manner so that replacement will be complete, except for a small quantity disappearing through surface evaporation, which would be minimized by a reduction in body temperature and appropriate insulation through clothing and/or plastic coatings suitably applied.

Enzyme Systems. Under conditions of lowered body temperature it is already known that certain enzyme systems would tend to remain more active than others. For instance, those enzymes acting on lipids and lipid derivatives continue to function even at 0° C. (in other words, butter will turn rancid at temperatures that would act to prevent spoilage of other foods). The extent to which pharmaceutical or chemical agents could influence this enzyme activity has not been systematically investigated but, beyond question, will play an important role.

Since the metabolism is subject to the control of the enzyme systems, there exist a number of intriguing possibilities. Following radiation it may be possible to convert certain organisms from aerobic to anaerobic states and by studying the changes in the enzyme systems possibly to adapt them to eventual human use. In the same manner selective atmospheres of other types could be investigated, as well as the possibility of developing enzymes which would convert CO_2 to O_2 in vivo (as in plants) which would eliminate the necessity for a fuel-cell conversion.

Since many enzymes when crystallized have a charge, there appears to be no reason why they could not eventually be accelerated electronically in a cyclotron, which would give us some idea of possible performance under special condition of space travel. In point of fact, there is no reason to expect the slightest change! If acceleration force exceeds cohesion force changes might be expected, but this bears no relation to speed; relative to distant galaxies we are already traveling better than 50,000 miles per second. Even if the enzymes (or a biological organism of any kind) were to race along at 180,000 miles per second, not only would there be no change, but the organism would be unaware of its speed. Enzymes would be excellent material for testing the biological properties under these circumstances, since it is relatively simple to determine whether they have retained catalytic activity. Speed should have no effect if acceleration is not excessive. Some biologists have questioned whether chronological age and biological age parallel each other. By rapid acceleration of a radio-tagged organism with a known half life it would be possible to compare biological aging and physical time.

Vestibular Function. A possible source of misinformation during space flights might be through vestibular function. At the present time either the astronaut will exist in a situation of weightlessness or the rotation of the space ship could be deliberately increased so that sufficient centripetal force is created to establish a "pseudo-gravity." Even under the latter condition the vestibular organs might provide disturbing misinformation, since any change in distance of the head from the outer shell could upset such adaptation as had occurred. The extremely "primary" nature of vestibular function makes it less adaptable to begin with. The conditions of pseudo-gravity require almost continuous readaptation, while under conditions of weightlessness any random movement of the head is likely to spread the endolymph in an unpredictable manner. The conflict of vestibular sensations with those derived from other sense organs could only contribute to disorientation and probably produce nausea and vomiting.

Rather than depend entirely on pharmaceutical means which reduce sensitivity of the vomiting center, there are a number of alternate solutions. The vestibular organs could be rendered temporarily nonfunctional in a reversible manner by temporarily draining off the endolymphatic fluid or, alternately, filling the cavities completely. This ought to be done well in advance of actual flight, in order to permit the individual to become adapted to a universe without vestibular cues. This problem of vestibular function has also been of concern to the Soviets, since they have reported on alteration of vestibular function both by drugs and surgery with substitution of touch and sight receptors under conditions of weightlessness and tumbling. Streptomycin and a number of its cogeners produce loss of vestibular function as an unwanted side effect in sensitive individuals. Most desirable, of course, would be a procedure whose effects were entirely reversible. The nearest approach to this available at the present time is the introduction into the endolymph of an anesthetizing substance of the cocaine series or paralyzing injections into the vestibular branch of the eighth nerve, but the duration of action tends to be rather limited. Using the Rose osmotic pressure pump administration technique it may be possible to greatly prolong such action.

Hypnosis must also be considered as a means of control of vestibular function, but it cannot be depended upon from present evidence. Some fifteen years ago one of us ran a series of experiments using a modification of the Barany chair (4, 5) in which, under hypnosis, it was possible to induce the nystagmoid reactions characteristic of acceleration and deceleration with the subject in a stationary position. Despite a trance extending to a depth of negative hallucinations, it was impossible to eliminate nystagmus while the patient was accelerating or decelerating. It therefore appears unlikely that hypnosis would eliminate the subjective clues produced by the vestibular organ.

It is also possible that vestibular function will not be a problem at all, but at present we cannot be sure and must be prepared to deal with the contingency.

Cardiovascular Control. At the present time a beginning is being made in the quantitative study of the multiple homeostatic functions of the cardiovascular system, from a control system point of view (6, 7, 8, 9). In this field the application of control system theory of biology (10) has already yielded some fruitful results. It can be expected that, eventually, enough will be known about the system dynamics involved to make it possible to alter the homeostatic functioning by the Cyborg technique.

By reason of different metabolic needs, as well as haemodynamic considerations, the biologically optimum heart rate and blood pressure under extraterrestrial conditions may be considerably different from that on earth. If a reduced body temperature is maintained, further adjustments of cardiovascular functioning would be necessary to regulate appropriate blood flow. Presently available drugs, which may be used in the Cyborg technique applied to the cardiovascular system, include epinephrine, nor-epineprine, reserpine, digitalis, quinidine, amphetamine, apresoline, ephedrine, and a host of others. Some of these act on specific portions of the system, while others have a more widespread effect. By a suitable rate of administration of these drugs and hormones through Rose osmotic injectors, cardiovascular functioning can be altered in the required directions through external commands. These commands can be made a dynamic function of the sensed cardiovascular functioning of the organism.

Cyborg technique also envisages the alteration of the specific homeostatic references within the brain. Through this approach, regulation of function might be obtained with a minimizing of expected strain, since in this method the regulated homeostatic level is changed without interfering with the organic control loop itself.

Electric stimulation may replace drug action in certain respects. It may eventually become desirable to regulate heart rate through electric stimulation. The possibility of affecting selected brain centers through appropriate electric stimulation, in order to control cardiovascular functioning, should also be considered.

It is thus clear that, eventually, man will have techniques available to radically change the cardiovascular functions so as to biologically optimize them for the particular environment chosen. Such a step, previously carried out by evolution through selective survival, would now eventuate through the purposeful construction of Cyborgs.

Muscular Maintenance. If prolonged sleep or limited activities are enforced for periods of months or years the maintenance of adequate musculature becomes a real problem. Quite possibly the reduction of body temperature and metabolism may defer this process but it cannot entirely avoid it. Although there are pharmaceuticals which help maintain muscular tonus, one must really understand the chemical reasons for atrophy to develop methods of pharmaceutical protection.

Perceptual Problems. The lack of atmosphere will create markedly different conditions of visual perception than those to which we are accustomed. In all probability it would be most desirable to make observations through a medium which would reintroduce some of the distortions to which we are accustomed, and to which the subject could be acclimated before the flight began. Part of the problem will result from searching for an adequate "frame of reference." In this regard it is possible that the factors which influence autokinesis may have an influence on space problems of perception (5). Whether pharmaceuticals would influence autokinesis has yet to be determined. There is nothing to stand in the way of such investigation at the present time. The effect of tonus-inducing stimuli on visual perception has been described (11).

There are a number of articles, such as that of Yarbus, in the Soviet literature indicating interest on their part in this same area (12).

Pressure. Under pressure lower than 60 millimeters of mercury man's blood begins to "boil" at his normal body temperature. Therefore, if he is to venture out of his space ship without a pressure suit he will have to reduce his normal operating temperature sufficiently so that the vapor pressure of his fluids is no greater than the internal tissue pressures. This is no problem as far as arterial blood pressure is concerned, but it may become problematical for venous blood pressure. This is another in the series of reasons why body temperature must be lowered if we are to avoid constrictive pressure suits. The device previously referred to for the selective cooling of blood might be useful here under special circumstances. The Russians, too, have described "decompression tissue emphysema" (due to vapor formation) in the brain and have found that this can be controlled by the lowering of temperature (13).

Not referred to in available literature on this subject is the presence of cold agglutins which appear to be much more prevalent in certain individuals than others. Since their presence can cause cardiovascular difficulties, the blood of potential candidates for space travel should be tested for this in advance.

Variations in External Temperature. At the real extremes of temperature man will require the protection of a space ship or space station. There are quite likely to be intermediate conditions, however, which are within, or close to, the limits of human tolerance. If pressure is not excessive, oxygen consumption–CO_2 disposal regulated by the mechanism previously described, and internal body temperature lowered it might then become possible for man to walk about relatively unencumbered, except that the absence of an atmosphere would produce almost unbearable contrast between sunlight and shadow. Even in such mundane places as Mexico City or Kabul, stepping from daylight to an enclosure is a surprising experience. With unsuitable enough conditions the part of the body turned away from the sun (or its equivalent) could be in deep freeze while the part turned toward the sun would be overdone.

The same approach to handling this problem could be used for the humans as is used on the space vehicle itself, i.e., the control of reflectance and absorption. This could be in the form of clothing, but, ideally at least, the hands and face should be protected directly so that they need not be encased. There are already in existence pharmaceuticals which produce changes in pigmentation, while substances like para-aminobenzoic acid provide quite effective protection against actinic rays as they reach us here on earth. Needed is a chemically regulated system responsive to incident light as a homeostatic process to adjust to its own reflectance in such a way as to maintain the desired body temperature.

If space travel for weekends on excursion flights ever becomes common, a super-sunburn heat-insulating preparation offers alluring promotional possibilities—"Try Solar-Polar on your next Space Flight"; "Use Planet-Aire, the All Purpose Celestial Cream"; or, "Star-light, the Space Resistant Face Lotion."

Gravitation. The effectiveness of the force available to a biological organism for its own locomotion and for its encounters with other objects or organisms is a function of the ratio of molecular (f) to gravitational ($\vec{g}$) and inertial forces ($\vec{m}$), i.e., $\frac{f}{\vec{g} + \vec{m}}$. The forces generated during contraction of a single muscle fiber are primarily molecular forces. These are independent of gravitational and inertia effects. The effective relative mobility which they produce is a function of the ratio of the total muscular forces developed to the total inertia and gravitational effects. If we consider organisms of different sizes, such as an ant, a man, and an elephant, it is clear that the available mobility ratio is largest for the ant. The average man can lift his own weight with some effort. The elephant cannot, while the ant, of course, can lift many times his own weight. This is not surprising, since the ant muscle cells are basically utilizing the same molecular forces as those in the elephant muscle cells. To explain this apparently strange phenomenon we may consider a similar behavior pattern displayed by a liquid. In a pail, water is unable to overcome the effects of gravitation and the level rises only at the very edges of the surface. Surface tension, which is a molecular force phenomenon, is effective against gravitation only to a minute degree. If we consider, however, a porous material, the water has no difficulty in climbing up such material to great heights, overcoming gravitational forces. This is merely because the small space of the pores of this material allows the molecular forces of the liquid a greater ascendancy over the much smaller gravitational forces, since the molecules are of fixed size. This illustrates that whenever the ratio of molecular to gravitational forces is changed a considerable change in behavior can result. It is clear that biological size is not an accident, but is in part dictated by an appropriate ratio of molecular to gravitational and inertia forces.

Until now there was no possibility of significantly changing this ratio under the normal living conditions of an organism. Space life alters this ratio by changing the gravitational component while the molecular and inertia effects remain the same. On earth the elephant can run faster than man. On the moon, could man beat the elephant in a race, or would he be left behind even more? The limit of running speed is given by the maximum speed of moving the legs in the opposite direction. With low gravity the legs are relieved of their supporting function and can consequently concentrate exclusively on their propelling function. The inertia forces the elephant has to contend with in moving his legs are considerably greater than man's even in proportion to his strong musculature, so that man would benefit more from an increase in rapidity of his leg motion. On the moon, or planet X, with reduced gravity, it is likely that man would be able to catch up with an elephant. On the other hand, because of his long and slender legs, the giraffe would be relatively many times swifter than he is on earth.

However, since the inertia forces remain the same, a change in direction would still require similar muscular effort at a given speed. Thus, the general mobility pattern is basically altered.

The molecular forces available are, however, influenced by temperature. It is, therefore, a possibility that for smaller gravitational fields than those found on earth a low body temperature would be desirable and for larger gravitational fields a higher than earth-normal temperature would be optimal. It is here that suitable drugs could be highly useful in establishing a different homeostatically controlled temperature. It may even be possible for a servomechanism to work in conjunction with homeostatic human controls so that the body temperature is automatically regulated by the prevailing gravitational field. In this way the reference inherent in the biological homeostatic temperature regulating mechanism would be adjusted according to the gravitational field prevalent so as to set the temperature of the body at a higher level in strong gravitational fields and at a lower temperature for weak fields. To the already existing biological control loop an additional control loop would be added, designed by man for his better homeostatic operation, i.e., Cyborg. Of course the drugs developed would have to be specific, so that side effects due to change of body temperature would be avoided or controlled. Note that abnormal temperature is not necessarily synonymous with disease.

The body temperature chosen by the evolution of an organism is optimal only in its own gravitational environment. It determines a ratio of molecular to gravitational and inertia forces as well as the speed of biochemical reactions. Thus, the speed of molecular concentration leading to muscle movement is also linked to the speed of molecular action leading to biochemical change. The biological rhythms inherent in a given organism are conditioned by the $\frac{f}{\vec{g} + \vec{m}}$ ratio as well as diurnal variations. Thus the optimal heart rate, for example, may be significantly altered (for a biological optimum) under conditions of existence different from those found on earth.

Magnetic Fields. In the past there has been relatively little reason for concern with the effects of strong or weak magnetic fields. The nature of magnetic forces and the possible effects they may have constitute two of the unknowns of space travel. We do know that in the Soviet there is a considerable amount of research in this area. In our own country Heller has demonstrated that strong magnetic forces could play a role, and perhaps a quite important one, in biological organisms. If magnetic forces do have an important influence it may be that chemicals and alteration of temperature might act to either retard or facilitate specific effects. At this juncture the most useful action is to identify the problem and indicate which areas are capable of investigation.

Sensory Invariance and Action Deprivation. It is a truism that asking the proper question constitutes a large portion of the answer. The search for phlogiston occupied several centuries because of an inappropriate conceptualization of the problem. It may well be that current research in "sensory deprivation" may lead to a good deal of fruitless research if caution is not exercised.

As is so ably stated in the introductory paragraph of a recent review of the subject,

Isolation phenomena have received wide attention since the first newspaper reports, some eight years ago, of experiments performed at McGill University on problems described by the term "Sensory deprivation." This work made a profound impression on both the medical and the lay press. A volume of magazine and newspaper stories resulted, generalizing from the technical reports and drawing conclusions that have given rise to some gross misconceptions. It was implied that a new psychologic technic had been demonstrated which (a) involved isolation and reduction of sensory stimulation, (b) had the power of reducing normal healthy people to mental incompetency, and (c) was probably involved in the "mysterious and diabolical technics of brainwashing and thought control" practiced by the Communists. Fact and fancy, intermingled in these second- and third-hand reports, were repeated indiscriminately by responsible men of several scientific disciplines. (14)

Original investigators such as Hebb and Lilly have been careful to define in operational terms what it is that they are doing. The general conceptualization, however, is less discriminating, and many investigators have started work along this line assuming as a proven fact that the crux of the problem is sensory deprivation. We would first like to point out that it is often not sensory deprivation but sensory invariance which has been evaluated in past studies. It makes comparatively little difference whether there is a continuous sound of the same pitch and volume or whether there is "silence." It is the *lack of change* in kinesthetic, proprioceptive, auditory, and visual fields rather than the *absence* of perceptions which has been the common denominator.

In a preliminary study now in progress we have hypothesized that it is not sensory invariance but action invariance (or action deprivation) which is the key point.[2] The conditions under which "sensory deprivation" have been capable of producing hallucinations, delusions and other psychotic behavior have also served to limit the activity of the subject. Some of the circumstances under which hallucinations, delusions, or psychotic reactions can be induced in normal subjects do *not* limit sensory intake in any common sense meaning of the word. In a recent experiment simulating space flight (reference withheld on request), two of the four subjects developed marked visual hallucinations despite the fact that they were allowed to move about the simulated space vehicle, were in radio contact with a transmitting station, and in visual communication via a television screen. Thus, although the senses were allowed to function in an unimpeded manner, hallucinations and delusions nevertheless developed. Rather than sensory deprivation the situation is better described as one in which action is severely circumscribed. It may be that either sensory invariance or limitation of activity (or a combination of the two) is capable of producing psychotic behavior. In view of the emphasis on the sensory aspects we believe it useful to stress the activity limitation.

There exists a constant feedback between activity and sensation,

[2] Shurley, in a paper given at the American Psychiatric Association in May, 1960, referred to the "desire for action" on the part of the individuals who were subjected to "sensory isolations." Dr. George E. Ruff in the discussion of this paper pointed out the desire of subjects he tested under similar circumstances "to make their actions or thoughts meaningful ones."

with the latter providing confirmation of the functioning of the former. In recent work it was shown that the occurrence of "meaningless" stimulation did not prevent hallucinations. Similarly, we would predict that meaningless or purposeless activity would not prevent psychotic symptoms. In contrast, if sensory invariance or action restriction were meaningful or purposeful, according to our thesis, they would *not* produce abnormal symptoms. Thus, the monotonous roar of a plane motor or confinement to a sick bed may be irritating but not psychotogenic because they are each "for a reason." This is not pure speculation but a theory capable of experimental confirmation or disproof. The shape of future research in this area will in large part be determined by the conceptualization of the problem, and with the adequacy of the concept rides the probability of success.

During prolonged flights of many months or years there will be very little to see, and that will be of negligible interest. To reduce both sensory invariance and action limitation the most practical way of dealing with the problem might well be to have the pilot sleep twenty-three of the twenty-four hours. This could be done either through the use of pharmaceuticals such as are used in Dauerschlaf, with the addition of an amphetamine-like compound to arouse the pilot rapidly or, perhaps more practically, by the use of an apparatus which could induce sleep by the passage of an electric current through the brain in the manner of the Soviet Electroson apparatus.[3] The control device of the machine governing sleep and wakefulness could be preset for regular periods but, in addition, geared in such a manner that the pilot will be aroused by any emergency condition. With the increase of speeds and the lowering of metabolism, consideration of flights running several hundred or even thousands of years cannot be off-handedly dismissed as mere fantasy.

For a number of reasons it would appear desirable to render the passenger unconscious during blast-off. The extreme physical and psychological discomfort which would result from wakefulness does not serve any useful purpose. Obviously anesthesia could be induced pharmacologically, but it would appear simpler to utilize an apparatus to induce sleep by the passage of an appropriate electric

[3] Interestingly, S. Rose whose osmotic pump we have described, wrote on electrical anesthesia over 15 years ago (15).

current through the brain. The waking time could be automatically preset and a safety precaution introduced by also providing control over this apparatus from an earth station.

During the period when he is awake, mere observation is probably not sufficient to ward off psychotic reactions, and the pilot should be involved in a series of actions which serve a measurable and known purpose. An individual of creative ability would be able to carry out much more satisfying activity in a circumscribed space than one who required "the thousand nothings of the hour" to benumb him. Writing is one obvious way of usefully occupying time, but of more pertinence would be the ability to play a musical instrument which would provide activity and direct pleasure. A violin would seem to be an ideal instrument for space travel. The opportunity to increase one's skill and musical understanding would be a welcome motivating factor, coupled with the ease with which the violin may be held in the absence of gravitation.

Erotic and Emotional Satisfaction. Recent work by Olds has demonstrated the existence of a so-called "pleasure center." The animal will choose stimulation of this brain center in preference to other activities. The existence of a subjective feeling of pleasure can, of course, only be inferred. Whether there exists an analogous center in humans and whether it will provide a substitute for erotic satisfaction is not known. Since emotions involve considerably more than sensations it remains to be seen whether stimulation of the brain area will produce complex reactions of this type. In any case, a careful evaluation is needed to make certain that other judgments and reactions are not negatively influenced or distorted by stimulation of this type.

Psychoses. Despite all the care exercised there remains a possibility, if not a probability, that somewhere in the course of events a psychotic episode might occur. This is one condition for which no servomechanism can be completely designed at the present time. An emergency osmotic pump containing one of the high potency per milligram phenothiazines together with reserpine would be included in the complete picture of the well-armed space man. Not infrequently the individual undergoing an acute psychotic episode denies that his mentation, emotions, or behavior are abnormal. Under these circumstances he would obviously refuse to voluntarily accept medication. For this reason, assuming that monitoring is adequate, there should also be a release device capable of being activated from the earth station or by a companion if there is a crew.

It is important to point out that knowledge as to the effect of pharmaceuticals in alleviating hallucinations induced by sensory invariance or action limitation may provide valuable information as to the nature of hallucinations in mental disease and also serve as a screening technique for new treatments. We could learn a great deal about the use of pharmaceuticals in mental disease as well as in space travel if facilities were available for studying the area of overlap.

Limbo. The contingency of possible extreme pain or suffering as a result of unforeseen conditions must also be considered. The pilot should therefore be able to elect a state of unconsciousness if he feels it necessary. Prolonged sleep introduced either pharmacologically or electronically seems most obvious.

Ad Nauseum. There exist quite a number of medical problems amenable to pharmacological influence which we have not dealt with in the present paper. This is because both too much and too little is known (the former by others and the latter by us). We merely wish to state our awareness of having neglected to include conditions such as nausea, vertigo, motion sickness, vibration tolerance, and the like, so that although our presentation may be exhausting, it is not equally exhaustive.

SUMMARY

It is proposed that man should use his creative intelligence to adapt himself to the space conditions he seeks rather than take as much of earth environment with him as possible. This is to be achieved through the Cyborg, an extension of organic homeostatic controls by means of cybernetic techniques. Both chemical and electronic means are to be used in the control systems to be built, which will cooperate with the body's own autonomic controls. The necessary change of these controls for space survival cannot be conveniently supplied for us by evolution; they have to be created by man himself, using his acquired knowledge of cybernetics and physiology. Thus, man's activity in this regard complements evolution, freeing him from the need of conscious attention to the regulation of his own internal environment.

Methods applicable to several control systems are suggested. Particular use is made of the Rose osmotic pump for the continuous injection of drugs at biological rates, simulating secretory activity. The object of these controls is to achieve a biological optimum, considerably different for various extra-terrestrial conditions from the earth-normal. Control of levels of cardiovascular operation, body temperature, metabolic systems and psychic energy are discussed.

It is suggested that such existence in space may provide a new, larger dimension for man's spirit as well.

REFERENCES

1. Rose, S., and J. F. Nelson, A continuous long-term injector, Austral. J. Exper. Biol., 33:415–420, 1955.
2. Kothari, N. J., J. C. Saunders, and N. S. Kline, Effect of phenothiazine and hydrazides on pituitary-adrenal response. In press.
3. Voyenno-Meditsinki Zhurnal No. 6, pages 65–72, June, 1957.
4. Shepperd, L. A., N. S. Kline, and J. W. Hopsopple, Vestibular function, in Fred A. Mettler, *Selective Partial Ablation of the Frontal Cortex: A Correlative Study of Its Effects on Human Psychotic Subjects*, pp. 117–137. New York, Hoeber, 1949.
5. Heath, R. G., M. B. Carpenter, F. A. Mettler, and N. S. Kline, Visual apparatus: visual fields and acuity, color vision, autokinesis, in Fred A. Mettler, ed., *Selective Partial Ablation of the Frontal Cortex: A Correlative Study of Its Effects on Human Psychotic Subjects*, pp. 138–147. New York, Hoeber, 1949.
6. Warner, H. R., The frequency-dependent nature of blood pressure regulation by the carotid sinus studied with an electronic analog, Circulation Res., 6:35–40, 1958.
7. Grodins, F. S., Integrative cardiovascular physiology: a mathematical synthesis of cardiac and blood vessel hemodynamics, Quart. Rev. Biol., 34:No. 2:93–116, 1959.
8. Clynes, M., Computer analysis of reflex control and organization: respiratory sinus arrhythmia, Science, 131:300–302, 1960.
9. Clynes, M., Respiratory control of heart rate: Laws derived from analog computer Simulation, I. R. E. Transactions, Medical Electronics, ME-7:2–14, 1960.
10. Clynes, M., Application of control system theory to biology, in O. Glasser, ed., *Medical Physics*, Vol. 3, pages 72–80. Chicago, The Year Book Publishers, 1960.
11. Kline, N. S., Effect of Tonus-Inducing Stimuli on the Perceived Movement of a Stationary and of a Moving Point of Light. Master's thesis, Clark University, Worcester, Massachusetts, 1951.
12. Yarbus, A. L., Research on the laws of eye movement in vision, Doklady Akad. Nyuk, 96:No. 4:733–735, 1954.
13. Annals of the Academy of Sciences U.S.S.R., No. 3, 1957; New Surgical Archives No. 4, Vol. 208, pages 51–55, Kiev, July–August, 1957.
14. Wheaton, Jerrold L., Fact and fancy in sensory deprivation studies, Aeromed. Rev., Review 5–59, August, 1959.
15. Rose, S., and D. Rabinov, Electrical anesthesia, Med. J. Austral., 1:657–659, 1945.

Hypnosis as a Tool for Investigating Some Problems of Space Flight

ROY M. DORCUS

Hypnosis has a long history, and a serious appraisal of the application of hypnotic techniques to problems related to space flight indicates that there are a number of areas in which it might be a valuable research tool. It might be utilized in these areas:

1. In the selection of individuals who may become candidates for manned space ships.
2. In the creation of "realism" in "models" constructed for simulation of space conditions.
3. In implanting ideas for reducing fear and anxiety involving unknown situations.
4. In reducing boredom by compressing unoccupied time and creating illusions of stimuli to fill time.
5. In directing attention to specific tasks to be performed under stress.
6. In lowering metabolic rate and reducing oxygen intake.
7. In maintaining uncomfortable positions in such a manner as to make them more tolerable.
8. In training individuals to induce self-hypnosis so that they may bring about sleep when desired and awaken at any time in an alert condition.

While these applications of hypnosis to problems of space flight have not been made, there is sufficient evidence of a related nature in the experimental literature on each of these points to indicate that we might expect some degree of success if hypnosis were utilized as a tool.

I should like to examine each of these areas in more detail and to

Dr. Dorcus is Professor of Psychology and Dean, Division of Life Sciences, University of California, Los Angeles.

indicate briefly some experimental data which may have relation to the specific problem under discussion.

The selection of individuals for space flight on physical as well as psychological bases is almost certain to be inadequate, since all the physical and mental stresses to which the individual will be subjected can at present only be surmised. Even though our surmises about the stresses to be encountered turn out to be correct in large measure, we cannot predict how the human organism will react to unknown and new stresses.

The conventional way of determining individual reaction to such situations is to construct or create models that duplicate or simulate the projected stresses as nearly as possible. The candidate is then placed in an operational "setting" in which his behavior is measured in a multitude of ways. Study of the records yields data that we hope will indicate whether individuals A, B, or C will be a suitable candidate for space flight. We usually assume in any selection procedure that we know or can determine the characteristics necessary for the "job." In this situation we do not know in any precise way what the desirable characteristics are. We can only infer from performance in models or model situations. There is one element that is quite imponderable in the models situation as applied to space flight. This element relates to whether or not we can create a situation that will convince the candidate that it is the real thing and not a "model." The long list of illusions and hallucinations which have been produced in subjects in a hypnotic trance covers practically all of the sense modalities as well as distortions of thinking and imagining. Pain, warmth, cold, pressure, and color sensations have been suggested to subjects in whom appropriate reactions are attained. Reactions of fear, anger, or hostility can readily be evoked, or the reverse is possible. Fear evoking stimuli can be so controlled that the individual may become aggressive in a situation which normally would involve fear and withdrawal.

Subjects have been induced to perform asocial and dangerous acts, such as placing their hand in a container of supposedly poisonous reptiles or attacking their superior officer, whom they were told was an enemy agent. If such illusions and hallucinations can be produced in hypnotic subjects, we might expect that it would be possible to persuade subjects that "model" situations were at least partially real.

Similarly, if we can reinstate under hypnosis tragic or fear-evoking situations which have been so painful that the situations have been repressed from consciousness, it would also seem probable that we could implant ideas which would reduce fear and anxiety. We know that such is the case, from studies on surgical patients who have subsequent to hypnosis undergone the most difficult and painful forms of surgery without evidence of anxiety or pain. Further evidence that anxiety is reduced in surgical patients can be found in the decrease in requests for anodynes during the postsurgical recovery.

Most of the hypnotic experiments dealing with time have been directed toward comparing subjective (or "psychological") time with clock time. In general, time estimates of performing a given task under hypnosis tend to agree with the times normally required to carry out the tasks. When subjects are requested to hallucinate an experience, the actual time elapsing will be only a few seconds or minutes, which corresponds roughly to the time elapsing in long complicated dreams. There would not seem to be any logical reason why this situation could not be reversed. If we suggest to the subject that one hour will seem to be the equivalent of only a few minutes, we might anticipate that this would occur. Subjective estimates of time are accelerated or decelerated in relation to sensory experience and would likely be controlled by the creation of hallucinations or amnesia.

The process of inducing hypnosis very often involves a narrowing of the field of attention, so that the subject tends to ignore distracting stimuli. We know that loud sounds, unwanted visual stimuli, and even the discomfort of pain can be removed from the attention of the subject. It is safe to argue, therefore, that the attention may be directed successfully to tasks to be performed to the exclusion of distracting stimuli and situations. Evidence on this point can be found in the initial attempts at learning new material under hypnosis. In general, it has been shown that more material is learned in the first few trials under hypnosis than occurs during a similar number of trials in the waking state. The usual explanation for this fact is given in terms of the greater degree of concentration which exists in the hypnotic state.

We may argue that if we can increase attention, reduce anxiety, and increase motivation in a favorable way, there would be little reason to question the fact that hypnotic subjects would be able to perform tasks involving great stress more successfully than normal subjects could perform them.

We have already referred to the selective nature of attention under hypnosis, which can be so concentrated that even the most demanding stimuli can be ignored. This facility in the hypnotic state seems to be much greater than in the normal state; hence we might anticipate that the individual could maintain attention to specific details for long periods of time without distracting stimuli intervening.

Maintaining efficient operational capacity with a minimum expenditure of energy would seem to be another desirable requisite for space flight. Studies indicate that respiration, cardiac activity, peristalsis, and basal metabolic rate can be altered by hypnotic suggestion. While the induction of hypnosis does not in itself alter these functions, suggestions of relaxation, drowsiness, and calmness will bring about a slowing down of these activities. How greatly these can be modified is open to conjecture at the present time.

While drugs may be used to modify these functions, they usually produce other reactions which may be undesirable and may require a time lapse before the subject will be completely alert and active. If drugs are used to produce sleep, the individual is incapable of awakening completely and responding alertly in an emergency. When hypnosis is used for such purposes, there is no time lag or wearing off period; hence the individual is completely alert instantly. The subject can be taught self-hypnosis to bring about sleep or relaxation and can awaken at any desired time or upon any designated signal.

Minimal movement as well as fixed positions for long periods of time pose problems of discomfort, muscle atrophy, and joint disintegration. If positions of the body are maintained by mechanical controls, the problems of movement and weight become quite significant. There is no question but that movement of large members of the body will have to be restricted in part by mechanical means, but from an operational point of view the least mechanical fixation possible is the most desirable. We can through hypnosis maintain fixed positions of members of the body for several months without complaint from the subjects. For example, in a plastic surgical procedure, we maintained the patient's arm in a position which normally would be very uncomfortable for about twelve weeks. There were some muscle and joint problems, although these might have been overcome by means of appropriate suggestions to the subject. Hypnotic subjects will submit to great physical stress with no apparent reaction.

I believe, therefore, that we are safe in maintaining that hypnosis may be a valuable tool in investigating a number of problems, such as those described above, related to space flight.

REFERENCES

Dorcus, Roy M., ed., Hypnosis and Its Therapeutic Applications. New York, McGraw-Hill Company, 1956.

Hull, C. L., Hypnosis and Suggestibility. New York, Appleton Century, 1933.

Weitzenhoffer, A. M., Hypnotism: An Objective Study in Suggestibility. New York, John Wiley and Sons, 1953.

Conclusion

BERNARD E. FLAHERTY

This symposium was concerned with man, his comfort, and his safety. Dr. Philip Solomon summed up this concern when he said: "An astronaut is not going to be a very large mouse, cat, dog, or monkey placed in an apparatus which carries him off Earth. He is a unique kind of creature who has emotional needs and reactions which play an important role in his general behavior and the way in which he will approach the tasks necessary on space flights."

These problems in preservation were examined over a wide range, from the viewpoint of the research scientist studying the parts of a single cell to that of the engineer concerned with the immediate deadlines necessary to get our Project Mercury astronauts into space. It is significant, though somewhat paradoxical, that the basic human theme of the symposium was introduced by Dr. Ernst Stuhlinger, an engineer, as he discussed technical objectives and requirements. It is inevitable, said Dr. Stuhlinger, that man "will be guided and driven into space by the same motives that drove him to the poles of the earth some sixty years ago." Although we cannot separate the individual strengths of man and machine in a man-machine system, the "human mind is still far superior to any electromechanical device" in terms of memory, logical associations, decision in the presence of multiple variables, and distinction between the usual and the unusual. These human advantages will be of utmost importance in early space flight, when it is imperative that man must supply information about himself in a strange and hostile environment, where he must not only analyze the adequacy of instrumentation, but also note its deficiencies.

The accounts of the personal experiences of pioneers like Colonel Simons and Captain Kittinger give us a realistic base from which to project the conditions to be encountered in space flight. They further intensify the already deep concern of scientists for the human beings who will extend the limits of the vertical frontier. The opinions and observations of Dr. Simons, who personally piloted a balloon to the threshold of space (101,000 feet), demand careful consideration. In addition to his balloon flight Dr. Simons has participated as subject in a simulated flight chamber experiment, and his listing of the differences and similarities between actual and chamber-run flights is of great potential value to workers in simulated space-flight experiments. Colonel George Steinkamp and Dr. George Hauty, who have had more experience with simulated space flight than any other workers in the field, concur in a demand for realistic simulation. They also indicate convincingly the great value of realistic simulated experience as a training tool.

The existence of a twenty-four-hour cycle rhythm was established at the symposium. Does this mean that the space traveler will be forced by an internal "clock" to observe the same periodicity of action which was determined by the Earth's revolution? Or can he learn a new rhythm which will permit increased efficiency in his tasks? Can we predetermine the natural adaptability for change in astronaut candidates? Only further research can answer these questions.

What will happen when man leaves the terrestrial environment which has determined his nature through evolutionary processes which began when life was first created on this planet? Before we can know what effects the alien environment of space will have on the human psychophysiological system we must know more about the intricate workings of this involved mechanism we call man. The papers on cybernetics represent efforts to understand some of the complex processes which are involved in normal behavior and learning as well as in reduction of sensory input and sensory overloading. More data are needed in this field.

From these considerations the symposium proceeded to problems of performance under stress; sensory alteration and sensory deprivation were matters of primary concern. The conditions of isolation, weightlessness, and boredom might cause an astronaut to lose control of his situation and abort the mission. However, as was pointed out, future astronauts will have a variety of tasks and the companionship of a fellow crew member. Further, the astronaut's sense of being will be fortified by communications with his family and friends on Earth, and his time will be occupied with important observations, reports, and instrument readings and adjustments. It is also possible that he can be encouraged through advance training to develop a resistance to these conditions. Individual resistance to the symptoms which mark sensory deprivation can be partially determined by tests in a space cabin simulator and through depth interviews of the astronaut candidates. Each of the methods is inadequate, however, since intense motivations of the men who are in the real situation may obviate some of the weaknesses which appear in the laboratory situation. Perhaps new methods will be developed which will more closely approximate the real situation.

Further basic physiological research is also necessary, as the papers presented by Dr. Horace Magoun and Dr. Mortimer Applezweig indicate. Dr. Clark T. Randt, of the National Aeronautics and Space Administration, pointed out: "Evidence presented here and elsewhere indicates that there is continuously operating tonic activity in the central nervous system which is modulated by the sensory input. Sensory deprivation involving decreased input in animals and in man has been shown to be associated with fluctuating states of consciousness and mental aberrations, as well as vasomotor instability associated with elaboration of epinephrine. Further, these effects can be traced to a relatively small epinephrine-sensitive area in the rostral portion of the brain stem reticular core, upon which collaterals of all sensory systems, including the special senses, impinge. Demonstration of continuous tonic activity in the brain and the resultant lack of modulation from restriction of the sensory input may reflect a fundamental aspect of brain function which has been brought to light by space-related research."

In this connection it is well to emphasize the broad importance of this symposium and the whole program of space medicine. What was discussed here is not only space oriented. It has implications throughout the field of mental health. Medicine and biology will benefit in their broad aspects from research into the problems of space flight.

Although some of those present felt that, through engineering, the space ship could reproduce terrestrial conditions, others saw the need for extending man's performance through drugs, hypothermia, hypnosis, or a series of electronic devices. The need for further research into the side effects of drugs was emphasized, and the question of the complete awareness of the hypnotized subject was raised. Although investigation of hypothermia for extending performance is in an early stage, the participants were nearly unanimous in urging an intensive research program in this area. While the possible use of special devices to further automate man be extending autonomic responses is still in the speculative stage, it offers interesting opportunities for research that will benefit not only space travel but general medicine as well.

There are many questions which have yet to be asked, many more which are as yet unanswered. Meetings such as these are designed not only for the scientists of today, but, through the colleges and universities, for the scientists of the future. The men and women who will extend the boundaries of the vertical frontier will, in so doing, broaden our understanding of the processes of life itself.

Index